HUMAN ANATOMY AND PHYSIOLOGY

BIOPHYSICS OF SYNOVIA

HUMAN ANATOMY AND PHYSIOLOGY

Additional books in this series can be found on Nova's website
under the Series tab.

Additional E-books in this series can be found on Nova's website
under the E-book tab.

HUMAN ANATOMY AND PHYSIOLOGY

BIOPHYSICS OF SYNOVIA

LEONID SEMENOVICH PINCHUK
AND
YULIYA MICHAILOVNA CHERNIAKOVA

Nova Science Publishers, Inc.
New York

For permission to use material from this book please contact us:
Telephone 631-231-7269; Fax 631-231-8175
Web Site: http://www.novapublishers.com

Library of Congress Cataloging-in-Publication Data

Biophysics of synovia / editors, Leonid Semenovich Pinchuk, Yuliya Michailovna Cherniakova.
p. ; cm.
Includes bibliographical references and index.
ISBN 978-1-61942-006-9 (hardcover)
I. Pinchuk, L. S. (Leonid Semenovich) II. Cherniakova, Yuliya Michailovna.
[DNLM: 1. Joint Diseases--therapy. 2. Synovial Fluid--physiology. WE 300]

616.7'2--dc23

2011042518

Published by Nova Science Publishers, Inc. ✝ New York

CONTENTS

PREFACE

Synovia is vital as a lubricant for joints, reducing friction and protecting bone contact surfaces against attrition. Nevertheless, its unique structure, properties, and functions tend to receive insufficient attention in the medical literature. This book aims to redress the balance. It fully describes the physical, biophysical, and physicochemical properties of synovia and explains the variety of methods used to assess the condition of synovia and its substitutes. Up-to-date information is provided on the most effective chondroprotectors, and a key part of the book is the presentation of a new minimally invasive method of joint treatment involving preparations based on the patient's own blood serum. First encouraging clinical results obtained with this new method are documented. *Biophysics of Synovia* will be of interest to traumatologists, orthopedists, physiologists, biophysicists, and specialists in material science and tribology.

INTRODUCTION

A joint is the conjugation of bones allowing them to move freely relative to each other. The limb joints enclosed in a joint capsule are termed synovial joints. They provide a record-low friction and compensate for the wear of the joint ends of articulating bones. Owing to synovial joints, human locomotor activity is maintained for many years. Such a long functioning of friction units implies optimal lubrication conditions to be ensured in them.

Synovial fluid contained in the joint in insignificant amounts serves as a lubricant for joints. It decreases friction efficiently and protects the contact surfaces of cartilage-covered bones from attrition. This indicates that the lubrication system of a healthy joint is close to perfect and synovial fluid is characterized by a very high lubricity. In addition to tribological function, synovial fluid transports wear products from joint cavity to lymphatic bloodstream, feeds joint tissues, and contains cellular elements, enzymes, and immune-competent agents that suppress the activity of foreign cells and substances penetrating into the joint.

That is why the structural parameters of synovial fluid serve to identify normal or pathological states of joints and diseases of connective tissue. The cellular composition of synovia can be estimated quantitatively and characterizes a joint state. Nevertheless, synovia being unique in structure, properties, and functions, is paid insufficient attention in medical literature. A Russian "Synovial Medium of Joints" monograph by V.N. Pavlova accumulates fundamental knowledge about synovia that is still topical. It was published in 1980 and became a rarity long time ago. The lack of publications explains largely why the analytical approach is rarely used in investigations of synovial fluid in orthopedic practice. Moreover, in recent 50 years surgical methods with use of endoprostheses have become the governing tendency in joint therapy all over the world.

A long-standing experience of joint endoprosthetics and impartial estimation of its results have led to increasing attention of orthopedists to conservative methods of treatment of joints at the turn of the century. The state of the joint rubbing surfaces, i.e., articular cartilage surfaces, as any friction assembly, is one the most intrinsic factors of its efficiency along with lubrication and feeding. Chondroprotection – the complex of preventive and therapeutic measures aimed to maintain physiological regeneration of the cartilage and normal exchange between joints and bloodstreams, and, hence, protecting the cartilage from destruction and wear – is an up-to-date tendency in orthopedics. Synovial fluid as a movable medium that ensures the mass exchange between joint elements and unites them into a single biophysical and biochemical system is of importance in solving this complex problem.

Since the late XX century, chondroprotection with use of artificial synovial fluids has being used intensively. The impetus was given by the cases of contradictions to joint replacement and understanding of the fact that necessity of joint replacement was caused by an insufficient attention to the tribological state of osteoarthritis-afflicted joints. Numerous substitutes of synovial fluid have appeared, first based on artificial polymers and afterwards on organic materials. Unfortunately, the foreign proteins found in these medical preparations as well as insufficient biocompatibility have caused side effects and in many cases a doubtful validity of treatment efficacy. Now, when millions of people suffer from joint diseases and lose their working ability, chondroprotection has become a global challenge attracting attention of WHO and UN organizations.

Synovial fluid has a multi-component chemical composition including low-molecular mineral and high-molecular organic substances. The combination of a variety of ions, atoms, and molecules in synovial fluid assumes a hierarchic multilevel structure of the fluid. This structure allows synovial fluid to perform its functions and actively react to the changes in the joint by reconstructing the structure at respective levels. It causes inexhaustibility of properties of synovial fluid and imparts the features of a cybernetic system to it. The system is capable of perceiving data on the state of tissues, cartilage surfaces, and pathological processes in the joint, actively respond to them by altering its structure, and exchanging information with the sympathetic nervous system centers.

Within recent decades, an extensive experimental material about new properties of synovial fluid has been accumulated, primarily concerning its sensibility to physical fields that emerge in a living organism. Electric stress arising on the cellular membrane is explained by the theory suggested by a Nobelist British physiologist A. Hodgkin. A potential difference on the membranes (resting potential) of unexcited cells results from semi-permeability of membranes and nonuniform distribution of ions between cell and its environment. Muscular and nervous fibers of a movable joint are characterized by the existence of ion streams running in both sides through the membrane. Ion currents running in the joint tissues generate magnetic or more specifically, biomagnetic fields. They can also emerge from the joint parts distinguished by magnetic receptivity, the fields of ferromagnetic particles and paramagnetic substances found in the joint tissue. As the joint moves, magnetic fields emerge in the articulating bones showing a piezoelectric effect. Therefore, synovial fluid performs its functions in the electromagnetic biofield of the joint. It comprises the structures susceptible to it.

The origin of synovial fluid from blood was revealed in the 18th century. Its base is a blood transsudate (filtrate) infiltrated through the capillary walls into the synovial membrane. Lipids, i.e., a wide group of natural organic compounds including fats and adipose matters, are its regular component. Phospholipids, i.e., complex lipids containing phosphoric acid are constituents of the erythrocyte membrane. The unique property of lipids is temperature transition within which their hydrocarbon chains existing in the crystal-like gelatinous state change to a less ordered mesomorphic state. In the 1970s, D. Chapman disclosed that cholesterol found in all biological human liquids regulated the fluidity of the mesomorphic phase of lipids at physiological temperatures In the 1980s, Belarusian scientists V.A. Belyi, B.I. Kupchinov et al. proved experimentally that the lipid-cholesterol mesomorphic phase of synovial fluid was responsible for its increased lubricity. The biophysical field of the joint regulates the synovia motion in the joint cavity and distribution of the lubricating interlayer on the cartilage surface in the optimal way to provide the lowest friction. It is possible because synovia possesses quasi-electret properties. The quasi-electret phenomenon implies that free charge carriers and electrically nonequilibrium structures of synovial fluid in the lubricating interlayer are optimally distributed in the joint space under the action of joint biofield. In such a way the wetting of cartilage with synovia and electrostatic withholding of the lubricating interlayer in the friction zone are regulated. The study of the effects of synovia as the quasi-electret mesomorphic medium that interacts with the electromagnetic field of joint is a new trend in orthopedics. It has given an impetus to consider the synovial joint as an "intelligent" friction assembly capable of responding to the variations in friction and lubrication conditions through the correction of, first, composition and structure of synovia and, second, distribution of the biophysical field on the cartilage surface and in the joint capsule tissues. The "intelligent" friction assembly is provided with a feedback system with the sympathetic centers that govern the metabolism as well as the narrowing and widening of the vessels of blood and lymphatic streams.

Nevertheless, up to recent time the blood preparations have not been used in joint therapy. Just in 2000s, chondroprotection has started developing with making use of blood serum as the basis of drugs injected in the joint cavity.

The objective of the book is to present a new understanding of the joint functioning as an "intelligent" friction assembly and of the biophysical mechanisms of interaction of synovial fluid with joint tissues through the electromagnetic biofield of the joint. These ideas have served the basis for the methodology of transfusion chondroprotection of synovial joints. Its main propositions and first encouraging results of clinical application are discussed in this book. The book can be of interest to orthopedists, physiologists, biophysists, and specialists in material science and tribology.

The authors are grateful to professor S.I. Boltrukevich, head of Grodno Traumatology and Orthopedics Center; collaborators from the Belyi Metal-Polymer Research Institute, National Academy of Sciences, Gomel, Belarus; Gomel State Medical University, Gomel regional hospital, and city hospital no. 1 involved in the experiments and clinical trials of the transfusion chondroprotection method.

Chapter 1

The Synovial Joint

Present-day arthrology – a branch of medicine studying joints and their disorders – is based on the idea of functional and morphogenetic unity of synovial fluid, synovial membrane, and articular cartilage. A general origin and functioning of joint elements as a single biophysical system is discussed in recent publications [1–3].

The set of terms and definitions to describe the interaction of synovial fluid (SF) and other joint elements is easier to systematize in terms of chronology of the development of views on biochemical functioning of joints. Therefore, the chapter is arranged in the form of interrelated paragraphs containing retrospective reviews on joint anatomy, interaction of their elements, SF functions, and joint lubrication system. Such structure, in authors' opinion, allows better understanding of the cause-and-effect relationship of basic notions of arthrology and phenomena accompanying biomechanical processes of friction, lubrication, and wear of synovial joints.

The terms defined in this chapter will be used for description of composition, properties, pathologies, and research methods of the joint medium. When constructing the hierarchy of arthrological notions the authors used the terms as defined in medical and biophysical encyclopedias.

1.1. Retrospection

The *synovia* term was introduced in arthrology by the ancient Greek physician, reformer of antic medicine Hippocrates (400s B.C.). Under synovia (it was first presented in Greek transcription) he meant an articular fluid, that is, the mucous content of the joint.

Philosopher and healer Ibn Sina who lived in the early 1000s (Latinized Avicenna) composed an encyclopedia of theoretical and clinical medicine *The Canon of Medicine*. In its *About liquors* section he described SF as "natural sweet mucus" that resembled blood. The mucus wets low-movable members and joints to avoid their drying up due to friction [4].

A French doctor and anatomist A. Vesalius, the founder of anatomy, when describing (in 1543) the conjugations of bones mentioned "glue slippery moisture resembling a lubricant" and "mucous viscous articular fluid, namely, plica synovialis" [5].

The *synovia* term was used by a German physician and naturalist Paracelsus (born Phillip von Hohenheim), one of the founders of iatrochemistry, a branch in the medicine of 16th –18th

centuries (according to which all processes that take place in an organism are chemical phenomena. He believed that joint diseases were caused by the chemical misbalance in the joint cavity.

In the Middle Ages the *synovia* term was forgotten. Anatomists called it *a limb-linking juice, a limb and joint moisture,* and *a limb mucus.*

In 1692, an English anatomist C. Havers disclosed mucous glands in the joint that, in his opinion, secreted SF. They were termed “Haversian glands”. The *synovial membrane* (SM) term was first introduced in 1763 by a Holland physician R. Bonn. Prior to him and C. Havers the membrane lining the joint cavity was named a *capsular ligament.*

In the second part of the 18th century practical physicians started considering the joint as a natural tribosystem (tribology is the science about friction, wear, and lubrication) including SM and SF. In 1758, a German surgeon J. Platner published his *Comprehensive Admonitions in Surgery* translated into Russian by a well-known anatomist M. Shein. It describes “membranous ligaments” surrounding the joint and SF is termed “a phlegm” that is similar to “protein, is salty and thickens in air”. In his opinion, its sources are: 1) the aforementioned “membranous ligaments”, 2) “large” glands where it is mixed with fat, and 3) “the ends of the smallest veins”. As for the latter, he meant blood capillaries via which the liquid phase, that is, the SF base, is filtered. Platner believed that “a part of phlegm is absorbed by blood-returning veins and dispersed in the entire body”. Thus mass exchange between joints and vessels was first mentioned [6].

By early 19th century SM was presented in anatomical and medical publications as a membranous structure with characteristic morphological and functional features. The main idea concerned the presence of the blood vessels in the membrane and, as was believed that time, mucous glands secreting “an articular juice”. In 1801, a French anatomist and histologist X. Bishat called the presence of mucous membranes in joints in question. He believed that adipose plicae were taken for them erroneously. Bishat referred synovial linings of joints to the serous (Lat. serum) membranes. After that the *synovial membrane* term has become common in anatomic terminology. SM was presented as a kind of serous membranes lining the inner cavities of a human body and producing a serous liquid that makes movements of inner organs easier and provides a protective function. All serous membranes, such as peritoneum, pleura, pericardium, etc. consist of a dense connective tissue coated by epithelium, namely, the layer of closely located cells. Undoubtedly, the SM tissue is rich in blood vessels; however, lymphatic vessels were not found in it. In the early 19th century it was found out that SM innervation (connection with the nervous system) was provided by the branches of spinal nerves. One of the greatest anatomists in that time an Austrian physician J. Hyrtle believed that the functional state of the entire joint depended on the SM state. The investigation of the chemical and cellular SM composition of cattle resulted in disclosing the dependence of its structure on the functional loading of the limb.

In the 1870s, the ideas of the synovial lining of the joint as a mucous membrane were called in question. At first, a German anatomist W. His disclosed that the cellular layer lining the joint capsule from inside differed essentially from the epithelial one. To icon the layer similar to that one lining the vessel he proposed an *endothelium* term. Then it was found out that SM did not have either epithelial or endothelial layer and consisted of connective cartilage-like tissue.

The results of the fruitful stage in joint investigation were summed up in the works (1882-83) by an eminent Russian physician O.E. Gagen-Torn. He put forward the idea that bones, cartilages, and connective tissue of joints developed from one and the same rudiment, namely, a mesoderm. In his opinion, SM of joints, tendon sheaths, and bursae is a loosened connective tissue provided by a dense layer of cells lining the surface layer. It is permeated through blood vessels, nervous fibers and contains nerve terminals. Gagen-Torn believed that shaped lymphatic vessels were absent in SM.

Nevertheless, lymphatic vessels were disclosed (1891) by a German histologist L. Teichmann. However, the first findings of the research have resulted in a mistaken idea of open connection between lymphatic vessels and joint cavity.

Persistent needs of practical medicine stimulated systematic research into morphology and physiological properties of synovial linings of joint surfaces. By the early 20th century direct experimental evidence was obtained that substances penetrated from the joint cavity into the vessels and vice versa, and an unusual SM reaction to joint pathologies was reveled. In the 1920s the long-standing ideas have come to light on the cell capability of secreting a mucous substance. It was found out that the humidity and elasticity of SM was provided by mucins, namely, glycoproteids (mucoproteids, complex proteins) comprising SF. A Holland physiologist R. Magnus proved the absence of the open communication between joint cavity and lymphatic vessels. An American surgeon J. Key, at a high for that time engineering level, performed cytological examination (1926–1932) that allowed for determining the cellular composition of SM and mechanisms of resorption of joint wear products with synovial cells. A major part of the latter is, in his opinion, microphages capable of capturing and digesting bacteria, cartilage wear particles, and other foreign to human organism particles. J. Key proved the analysis of synovia in cadavers to be unadvisable because of its after-death changes caused by the outcome of a large number of leucocytes from vessels.

Works by an Austrian surgeon E. Vaubel have become a conspicuous event in the synovial cells research. He came to a conclusion (1933) that surface synovial cells (synovioblasts, in his terminology) produced specific substances including mucin. He revealed an amusing phenomenon, namely, the SM tissue culturing is accompanied by the dissolution of its ground (interstitial) substance. The ground substance comprises the extracellular part of connective tissue and is a colloid formed by mucopolysaccharides. Vaubel believed that the similar dissolution occurred in the embryonic period of joint formation from the embryonic rudiment. In his opinion, the products of dissolution in the tissue fluid of interstitial substance and cartilage are the SF components in adults [7].

In 1935, a Golgi complex was found out in synovial cells (after the name of an Italian histologist G. Golgi), that is, an organoid (specialized structure) involved in the formation of products of vital activity of cells (secretes, lipids, collagen, etc.) and in the synthesis of glycoproteins, that is, proteins containing carbon components. It is worth mentioning that great investigations of the 1920–30s that developed the ideas on the synovial joint system belong to pathologists and clinical physicians.

A large scope of facts accumulated by surgeons, traumatologists, orthopedists, and pathological anatomists required a generalization. In 1930, a *Chirurgical Pathophysiology* book by R. Lerish and F. Policard, French surgeons and pathological anatomists, was published. The authors stressed that SM was not a serous membrane, and the joint cavity was just a fissure in the connective tissue consisting of two layers. The SM layer facing the inner part of the joint is transformed under friction and consists of flat compacted cells. It makes possible transudation (filtering) of blood serum from SM capillaries into the joint cavity, but is almost impermeable for the cavity fluid and functions as a one-way barrier. The next –

vascular – SM layer has a structure of a loose tissue in whose free volume the lymph circulates. It is this layer that gives rise to aseptic and microbe inflammations of joints. The difference between SM and cartilage structures is insignificant. SM is transformed into cartilage without a demarcation line. In these terms the mechanism of formation of chondromas, viz benign cartilaginous tumors is easy to explain. At first in the vascular SM layer a multiple focal metaplasia occurs (transformation of organism tissues into another tissue) afterwards the nods emerge in the joint cavity where calcinosis (calcification) takes place, i.e., the formation of calcium deposits in the tissue.

Simultaneously, the concepts concerning joint as a part of the human body closely interrelated with its muscular system and nervous centers have been developed. In 1937, M.M. Diterikhs, a Russian surgeon arthrologist, predicted many so far unknown properties of the joint elements experimentally substantiated much later. While noting that SM is supplied with a large number of blood vessels he denied the availability of "naked" vascular capillaries on its surface. The intercellular substance of the compacted SM layer facing the joint cavity is, in Diterikhs's opinion, the onset of the joint lymphatic system. Further the so-called "juice channels" connected with the network of lymphatic passes in the vascular SM layer are found. M. Diterikhs revealed the main mechanisms of joint regulation via clinical observations. Reflex variations in joint elements occur, first, in response to irritations from the joint itself and, second, in damages of the central nervous system, e. g., hemiplegia (paralysis), nerve cutting, etc. Among the main factors affecting the absorption of wear products from the joint one can name the structure of the substances to be absorbed (molecular or colloid solutions, suspensions); pressure in the joint cavity; the state of SM, blood and lymphatic streams, and nervous system tonus [8].

Late in the 1930s, in Great Britain complex morphological studies of SM were performed with using the tissue-staining technique. In the synovial cell cytoplasm metachromatic (whose color differed from the stain) granules that turned out to be mucin granules. Their presence in synovial cells and network structure typical of secreting cells proves the SM capability of true secretion or formation of specific products, namely, secrets that are necessary for joint vital activity. Therefore, the dual nature of SM as a specific connective tissue containing secretory elements was established.

A tremendous experience of surgical interventions in open and close injuries of joints accumulated during World War II included direct observations of SM under various conditions. Therefore, during next years almost every large work on surgery and joint pathology brought up the question about the structure and functions of the synovial lining of articular capsule. The *synovial membrane* term designated the set of tissues contained between muscles, periosteum, and articular capsule on the one hand, and the joint cavity, on the other. The outer and inner (intima) layers were distinguished in the SM structure. It was believed that the mechanical load and friction accompanying joint movement caused desquamation (peeling) of synovial cells of the SM surface layer together with the surrounding ground substance. Nevertheless, the fibrous SM elements never become "naked" in normal joint functioning.

In post-war times I.P. Kallistov, the Soviet arthrologist, studied collagen elastic SM fibers. He disclosed (1947) five layers of the membrane distinguished by the structure of connective fibers. The structural distinctions were caused, in his opinion, by rubbing the opposite layers against each other [9].

A British orthopedist D. Davies was the first [10] to state a relation between SM properties and hyaluronic acid, the main mucin component. He has found out that in contrast to common fibroblasts (the main cellular form of connective tissues), synovial cells are involved in the removal from the joint cavity of suspended particles that catalyze the peptide bond cleavage in proteins.

The system of views on the SM activity shaped in the first half of the 20th century is presented in work [11] by a British surgeon E. Gardner. In his opinion, the *synovial membrane* notion should include not only the layer of the surface cells but also the cells lying deeper, connective fibers, and vessels. He supported the hypothesis put forward in the 1930s that the regeneration of surface synovial cells occurs via the metaplasia of the connective tissue cells lying deeper.

Russian orthopedist D.A. Zhdanov formulated (1950) the idea on the interstitial SM substance as a "live colloid barrier" wherein the substances are removed from the joint cavity through the walls of lymphatic and blood capillaries. He believed the absorption of SM proteins as the substances not penetrating through the walls of blood vessels to be the main function of lymphatic vessels [12].

In the 1950s systemic research of nervous regulation of tissue permeability in the joint, joint innervation sources, and structure of nervous fibers and terminals started. The following understanding of the structure of synovial joints was set to the mid-twentieth century. SM and the cells inside the joint cavity arise from the embryonic connective tissue (mesenchyme), and have full blood supply and innervation. Any open communication between joint cavity and membrane lymphatic vessels is absent. The vital activity of both healthy and pathologically changed joints depends on the SF properties and circulation. The SF consists of proteins and polysaccharides including hyaluronic acid that govern to a large extent the structure, properties, and functions of synovia.

In the 1960–70s advances in electron microscopy as well as histo- and cytochemistry, enzymology, and immunology with application of biophysical, biochemical, and mathematical methods brought arthrology up to higher standards. This has resulted in increasing data on the structure and functioning of joints and providing a new computerized analytical level. Up to the 1980s the main directions in joint research were as follows: 1) elucidating the nature and functioning mechanisms of synovial cells in the SM surface layer; 2) setting regularities of mass exchange in synovial cavities; 3) assessment of the significance of vascular and secretory mechanisms of SM formation; and 4) setting regularities of articular cartilage effect on the joint activity. The last direction was intensively developed by D. Dowson's (English physician and tribologist) [13] tribological school.

An insufficient number of works to generalize the results of research performed by narrow specialists in different divisions of arthrology, biophysics, and biochemistry is still a shortcoming in the study of functional morphology of joints. Therefore, the publication in the 1980s of monographs [14, 15] by an eminent Russian arthrologist V.N. Pavlova having determined the system approach to joint investigation was logical. The essence of the approach is in considering the synovial joint system based on the general development and structural-functional interrelation of SM, SF, and articular cartilage. The main results of the generalizations and up-to-date experimental research performed at the junction of arthrology and physics of condensed states are outlined below.

1.2. The Synovial Medium of a Joint

Joints are unique natural friction assemblies. As mentioned above, the features of joint structure, contact interaction of movable elements, and joint lubrication as well as dynamics of their modifications in growth and vital activity of a human body are responsible for a record-low (about 0.01) coefficient of friction and wear compensation which allows the human locomotor activity for a long time. Morphological and functional integrity of the joint elements has made it possible to introduce a notion of *the synovial medium of a joint* in the late 1960s – early 1970s [14]. It has given rise to a tendency to consider friction and wear in terms of system analysis [16]. Nowadays, *the synovial medium of a joint* term unites the complex of main joint components, i.e., articular cartilage, synovial membrane, and the product of its secretion, namely, synovial fluid, which together ensure the operation of a joint as an "intelligent" friction unit. This means that the joint ensures optimal tribological conditions for sliding of articulating bones producing SF via metabolism processes between joint cavity and vessels and regulates them by feedback with the nervous center (proprioceptive afference).

The *synovial medium of a joint* term assumes the human joint to be an "intelligent" system. The concept of "intelligent" (or "smart") cybernetic systems appeared in the late 1970s [17]. "Intelligent" engineering systems adapt themselves to operating conditions by modifying their mechanical and physicochemical structure as well the stress or charge state, and regulate the degree of the adaptation by means of feedback [18]. Current engineering systems comprise elements functioning as [19] 1) a sensor reacting to environment variations; 2) an actuator through which the system affects the environment; or 3) a processor controlling the actuator activity by sensor-emitted signal. The systems comprising the pair of these elements were termed "adaptive", that is, "adapting themselves" to a varying environment and "active", viz. programmed to environment variations. An "intelligent" system comprises all three elements and therefore not only adapts itself to environment and has an effect on it, but also regulates the level of its variations depending on environment variations [20].

The idea of the synovial joint as an "intelligent" friction unit is based on the interrelation and interaction of the elements of the synovial system of joints having their common prehistory and specific structure.

1.2.1. The Origin of Synovial System Elements

The common origin of the joint synovial system elements is substantiated by the study results of the biology of embryonic and stem cells [21] as well as the morphological studies [22]. At the early stages of embryonic development, the joint rudiment is presented by morphologically homogeneous proliferating (multiplying) mesenchymal cells. Differentiation of these cells by location and design gives origin to all connective components of limbs including the joint elements. Next generations of fibroblast cells (a fibroblast is the main cell form of connective tissue) retain the capability of producing collagen (the protein proving the strength of the connective tissue) and proteoglycans (the carbon-protein component of the tissue). Differentiation of fibroblast cells in the embryonic state goes in three directions (Fig. 1.1).

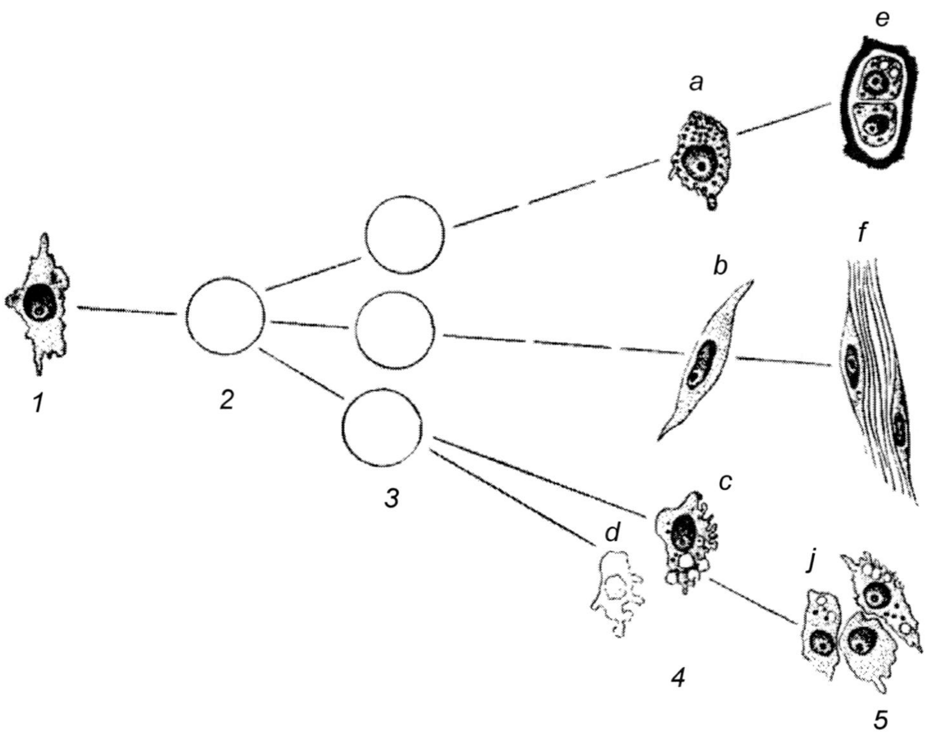

Figure 1.1. Differentiation of cells in the limb rudiment.

1 – mesenchymal cells; 2 – intermediate morphologically unrecognized cells capable of producing collagen and proteoglycans; 3 – intermediate cells separating in one of the possible directions of differentiation; 4 – morphologically recognizable division-incapable cells: *a)* chondroblast, *b* – fibroblast, *c* – synovioblast, *d* – dying cell of interchondral (cartilaginous) zone; 5 – mature functioning mitosis-incapable cells: e – chondrocytes in the isogenic group, *f* – fibrocyte of dense connective tissue, *j* – synoviocytes of A, B, and C types.

The first direction is the separation of the cells producing collagen and nonsulfated proteoglycans. As the limb rudiments, they are localized in the interchondral and parachondral zones (Latin *inter* is between, *para* is near, at). The fibroblasts lost the capability of mitotic division (mitosis is the way of cell-division providing equal distribution of genetic material and continuity of chromosomes in cell generations) are the descendants of these cells. They are main cells of all structures of the articular capsule and produce collagen and protein-polysaccharide complexes. Their differentiation results in fibrocytes, i.e., cells of the division-incapable dense connective tissue of ligaments, articular capsule, and menisci.

The second direction is the isolation of chondroblasts, i.e., the cells secreting one of the types of collagen and sulfated proteoglycans in cartilaginous rudiments of the limbs. Chondrocytes, i.e., mature cells of cartilaginous tissue with the lost capability of mitotic division are the final stage of chondroblast development. In a mature cartilage they are presented by isogenic (of common origin) groups.

The third direction of the differentiation is implemented by the cells of the central regions of interchondral zones. Some cells experience dystrophic and destructive modifications. One can see the fissure-like cavities filled with destruction products in the zone of cell destruction. At the boundaries of cartilaginous fissures the embryonic cells of synovial elements, namely, synovioblasts are subjected to structural reconstruction, that is, are transformed into synovial cells namely, synoviocytes,

The human knee joint cavity develops during 8.5–9th week of intrauterine development. Differentiation of the mesenchymal tissue results in the formation of the cartilaginous rudiments of the femur, tibia, and patella as well as rudiments of tendon tissues of the proper patella ligament. During week 11 the joint space is extended and the embryonic connective tissue arises at the boundaries of the cavities due to interstitial tissue destruction between the cartilaginous rudiments of bones. Within these terms the compacted layer of cells with oval and rounded nuclei adjacent to the joint cavity and a more loosened layer lying underneath are discernible. It serves as the onset of SM formation. Thin elastic collagen fibers appear underlying the compacted tectorial layer of the membrane at week 15. The joint cavity is enlarged as the synovial plicae arise. Within the same terms the loosened connective tissue carrying blood vessels is growing into the cartilage from the cartilaginous epiphyses. Their most intense development takes place during week 16. Nervous fibers appear in SM during weeks 14–19 and grow in the tectorial cell layer. By weeks 19–20 the joint elements are differentiated: the joint cavity is the space between the articulating cartilages restricted by the embryonic SM consisting of the dense tectorial layer and the loosened layer lying underneath wherein collagen fibers and blood capillaries arise.

Structurization, destruction, and reparation (recovering from damages) of the elements of the synovial medium of joints occur during the entire human life as the response to genetic and external effects (traumas, diseases, functional and physical loads).

The morphology and functions of the elements of the synovial medium of joints substantiate their common origin.

1.2.2. The Element Structure

The synovial membrane is the layer of connective tissue lining the inside of a fibrous capsule and binding the joint cavity. It consists of the cells of the ground substance wherein blood and lymphatic vessels, nerve terminals, and fibers are found. The SM layer bordering the joint cavity is not epithelium itself, and the structure of the tectorial layer is detected by means of histological cuts.

The SM lining is the layer of the frictionally deformed connective tissue containing cells, ground substance, capillaries of blood vessels, and nervous fibers and terminals. Its thickness in adults is 160±60 μm. Numerous villi enlarge the SM surface area. Synoviocytes of the lining are located at different levels from the SM surface and the sites of ground substance are adjacent to the joint cavity. Structure of the lining is as shown in Fig. 1.2.

SM lining cells are referred to histogenetic (stipulating the development) synoviocytes. They are fibroblast cells subjected to friction during joint operation and can be divided into two types: 1) A-cells, or enzyme-producing macrophage synoviocytes capable of phagocytosis, i.e., active capture and absorption of living cells and inorganic particles; 2) B-cells, or hyaluronic acid producing fibroblast synoviocytes. Electron microscopy of SM of animals has revealed an intermediate form of synoviocytes, namely, C-cells combining structural features of A- and B-cells. They are precursors of both macrophagocyte (A) and fibroblast (B) synoviocytes. Under extreme conditions, e.g., in aseptic joint inflammation, all cells of (A–C) types become capable of secreting hyaluronic acid. In terms of biophysics, the synoviocytes are featured by their polarity. Nuclei and organoids (specialized structures in cells) are arranged along the long axis of cells. On the SF wetted apical ends of synoviocytes numerous microvilli and vacuoles (microcavities) involved in first-stage metabolism between SF and SM are found.

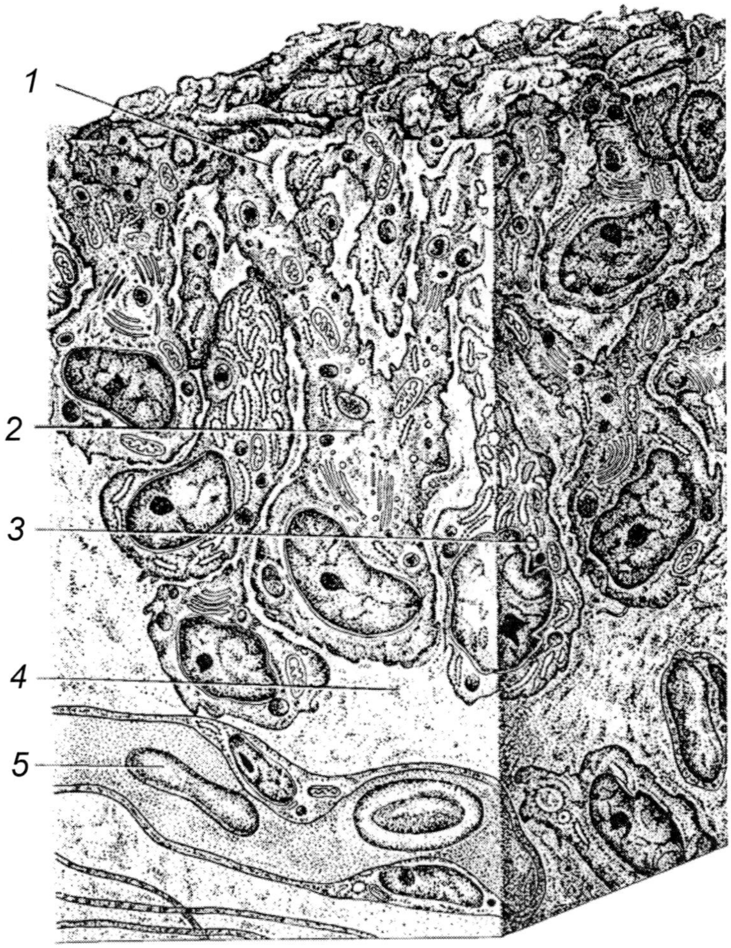

Figure 1.2. Diagram of SM lining structure [23].

1 – SM surface, 2 and 3 – cells of types A and B, 4 – ground substance, 5 – blood capillary.

The ground substance of the SM lining consists of the net of reticuline (i.e. protein similar to collagen in composition) and argyrophil (to be stained by silver salts) fibers. The net cells are filled with homogeneous protein-polysaccharide mass sometimes called a matrix. Matrix is the fine-granular semi-fluid viscous substance that fills the intracellular structures and spaces between them [24]. Matrix proteoglycans and glycoproteids have the properties of polyions. They bind the extracellular water, are capable of aggregation and have a plasticizing effect on reticuline [25]. Synoviocyte product, namely, hyaluronic acid is the matrix proteoglycan. Its content of the SM ground substance is 40–120 g/l [14].

The SM collagen elastic layer has the gradient structure. Near the SM surface the bundles of collagen fibers and net loops are ordered and oriented along the long axis of the joint and the tendon sheath. This allows extension and shifting of SM areas along with displacement of the bone elements of the joint. The thickness of the SM surface layer in adults is normally 190–300 μm. Within this layer blood and lymphatic capillaries, nerve fibers and terminals are located.

Inside SM, the fibers of the collagen complex are also ordered but oriented along the normal or at an angle to the surface layer fibers. They are woven in the fibrous (consisting of fibrous connective tissue) part of the joint capsule to provide the membrane fixation and ability to move and extend in joint motions. The ground substance and cellular elements have the same composition as the surface layer; however, at SM depth the lipid cells located along blood vessels are accumulated. The thickness of the SM ground layer is 450–750 μm.

The blood supply of SM is ensured through the artery branches that nourish the joint. The vessels penetrate into the membrane from the fibrous joint wall, reach the surface layer and ramify manifold forming dense capillary nets. SM blood vessels are separated from the joint cavity by surface layer cells and matrix as well as the proper capillary endothelium.

Lymphatic vessels are found in the whole SM bulk except for the outer layer. They are anastomosed (anastomosis is the side branch connecting vessels) and arranged in parallel to blood vessels. The ratio of the areas of lymphatic and blood streams is 1.9:1.0 [26].

The articular cartilage is the antifriction element of synovial medium that carries the main mechanical load at locomotion, i.e., human motions to provide his active movement in space.

The articular cartilage consists of the cartilaginous hyaline tissue formed by chondroblasts, chondrocytes, and matrix with collagen fibers and chondromucoproteids (a specific kind of glycoproteids). The hyaline cartilage is strong and elastic.

The hyaline cartilage has several hierarchic structural levels. According to [14, 15, 27], its formation can be presented in the following manner. Procollagen, that is, the intracellular precursor of collagen is synthesized from proteoglycans in fibroblast cells. Biosynthesis lasts 1.5–4.0 hours, then procollagen macromolecules outcome to the matrix near to the cellular membrane. The ending fragments are detached from them and collagen macromolecules arise. The latter are the basis for strand-like permolecular formations or microfibrils 3–5 nm in diameter consisting of 4–5 collagen macromolecules. Microfibrils make aggregates with glycoprotein macromolecules and are changed to fibrils 20–100 μm in diameter.

The following proteoglycans are main lipid components of cartilage governing its functional potentialities:

- hyaluronic acid, that is, a polysaccharide, high-molecular carbohydrate whose structure and properties are discussed in 2.1;
- chondroitin sulphates – complexes of high-molecular compounds (hexosamines and uronic acids) and proteins involved in water-salt metabolism, regulation of cell-division and having anticoagulation properties;

- keratan sulphate – mucopolysaccharides (complex polysaccharide, high-molecular carbon) is formed by biosynthesis from polymer antecursors and consists of oligosaccharide chains of mucin type;
- dermatan sulphate – mucopolysaccharides that contain disaccharide units in its macromolecule and in complex with proteins provides the cartilage strength.

As the result of hydroxyl group sulfation proteoglycans are able to set valence bonds with hyaluronic acid macromolecules forming typical aggregates of molecular mass 10^6 and higher. Concentration of the polysaccharides and proteoglycans in the aggregates depends on joint anatomy, load, and age. The aggregates together with collagen fibrils form the labile net structures (lability is functional mobility of tissue) to maintain the ground substance, water, and electrolytes in the cells in the same concentrations as SF and blood plasma [15]. Owing to cartilage matrix lability, metabolism occurs inside the vessel-free cartilage. Chondrocytes, viz mature cartilaginous tissue cells arising from chobdroblasts being low-differentiated division-capable matrix cells, produce the components of the articular cartilage matrix. Cartilage cells are divided into three types according to their structural and functional features [27]. Type I cells are mitotically active owing to which physiological regeneration of chondrocytes occurs. Type II cells are involved in the biosynthesis of proteins and polysaccharides. Type III cells produce proteins.

Seven layers of cartilaginous tissue are discerned by morphological features [14]. Figure 1.3 shows them on the cross section of the human articular cartilage.

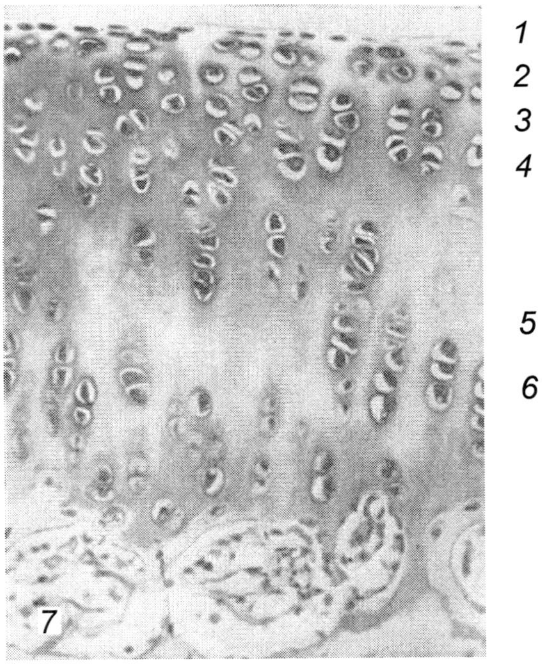

Figure 1.3. The structure of human articular cartilage.

1 – cell-free zone, 2 – surface zone, 3 – transitional zone, 4 – isogenic group zone, 5 – colony zone, 6 – hypertrophic cell zone, 7 – primary calcinosis zone.

Cell-free zone 1 is a thin proteoglycan-free membrane ~ 3 μm thick. It is directly involved in friction and enriched with liquid lubricating components.

The surface zone 2200−600 μm thick is formed by closely adjacent bundles of collagen fibers oriented in parallel to the tribosurface. Such orientation of the fibers produces a wavy and rough cartilage surface. The space between the fibers is filled with the ground substance which contains an insignificant amount of proteoglycans. Chondrocytes of the surface zone located along fibers are similar to fibroblasts in shape and structure. This zone undergoes mechanical load in friction and participates in metabolism between matrix and SF.

Transitional zone 3 is formed by the frame of collagen fibers of different diameter and ground substance filling the space between fibers. The fibers of this zone do not have any certain orientation. Cartilage cells or single accumulations are located in lacunas formed by concentrically oriented fibers. Owing to this, chondrocytes are protected against mechanical damage in cartilage compression.

Isogenic group zone 4 (structures of similar origin) is characterized by chondrocytes accumulated in lacunas. Here a great amount of collagen fibers is concentrated that form protective "perilacunar rings" around chondrocytes. The areas away from the lacunas are relatively collagen-deficient. The transitional and isogenic group zones reproduce fibroblasts and synthesize collagen and matrix polysaccharides. A friable distribution of the collagen bundles oriented in different directions is the place where the shear stress changes its direction from horizontal to vertical.

Colony zone 5 is discerned by the shape or orientation of isogenic chondrocytes groups. They are arranged perpendicularly to the cartilage surface and elongated in the form of colonies. The zone is seen the most clearly in young growing organisms. Here the synthesis of matrix components and regeneration of chondrocytes occurs.

Hypertrophic cells in zone 6 are characterized by enhanced metabolic and secreting functions. The reason of their hypertrophy is not still understood. The main versions are: enhancement of cellular nourishment which causes the true hypertrophy of cells; misbalance of aqueous and polysaccharide exchange in the matrix resulting in swelling and dystrophy of chondrocytes.

Calcinosis zone 7 is a basal one, i. e. located at the basis of the articular cartilage and arising from primary matrix calcification. Powerful bundles of collagen fibers as well as the blood vessel capillaries nourishing the cartilage at the bone side are found in this zone.

Synovial fluid is the main constituent of joint synovial medium through which all its elements interact.

The SF circulation from SM to cartilage pores provides the metabolism in the synovial system. SF is a biologically active labile polyfunctional component of synovial medium reacting delicately and fast to changes in the joint and the organism. Its structure and properties reflect the state of SM, cartilage, blood stream, and metabolism in joint tissue. The cellular composition of synovia is characterized by the presence of both living full value cells and those finishing their life cycle, dystrophically modified, and dying ones. It is believed [14] that three components take part in SF formation:

- blood transsudate containing water, electrolytes, proteins, and blood cells, i.e., lymphocytes and neutrophilic leucocytes (different types of white blood cells) as well as monocytes which function as macrophages in inflammations;

- products secreted by synovial cells of the SM surface layer, particularly, hyaluronate and proteolytic enzymes which catalyze the breakdown of peptide (–CO–NH–) bonds in proteins;
- products of cartilage wear and SM surface layer replacement – proteoglycans and glycoproteins that come to the joint cavity in the course of their normal vital activity and undergo lysis (dissolution and degradation) and resorption.

These components united in special complexes in a certain way make SF fulfill four functions in the joint's synovial system:

1) *locomotion, or tribological function* – to ensure low friction in the joint and of wear of the cartilage and SM; to damp impact loads in the joint thanks to viscoelasticity of the lubricating layer thickened by hyaluronates; to regulate the viscosity and carrying capacity of the lubricating layer depending on load and filtration rate of high-molecular weight and low-molecular weight SF components in cartilage micropores;
2) *metabolic function* – to participate, together with SM and cartilage, in mass exchange between joint contents and blood stream of the organism; transfer, inside the joint cavity, and fermentative breakdown of protein chain fragments resulted from rubbing, cells changed by dystrophy and perishing, and colloidal particles of worn cartilage; transport the products of fermentative destruction into the zone of communication between joint cavity and lymphatic channel;
3) *trophic function* – cellular feeding that ensures maintenance of structure and function of peripheral vessel-free areas of articular cartilage, which fact is evidenced by a prolonged presence and growth of free cartilaginous formations in joints;
4) *protective function* – involvement of enzymes, living cells, and immune-competent SF agents (together with active SM components) in interning (arrest and localization), inhibition (growth retardation), and dissolution of foreign cells penetrated into the joint from blood or through damaged capsule of the joint.

Having considered the synovia elements and their interaction, we can conclude that functioning of the joint as a multifactor tribological system presumes the coordinated action of its elements. It is achieved via management of the coordination by the central nervous system and availability of feedback that informs the nervous center about the current state of joints.

1.2.3. Joint as an Intelligent Friction Assembly

The joint is an anatomical friction assembly which consists of articular ends of bones covered by the layer of antifriction hyaline cartilage and enclosed in the articular capsule. It is reinforced by ligaments and lined from inside by SF-secreting SM.

Congruence of tribosurfaces of the articulated bones is achieved owing to elastic menisci, adipose pads, and SM plicae protruding from the capsule into the joint cavity and involved in friction. The space between these intra-articular elements and cartilage micropores are filled with SF. Its amount in joints is insignificant (2 to 4 ml) but under vacuum pressure in the capsule the SF lubricating film is spread uniformly in micropores and over the cartilage rubbing surfaces [14]. It provides liquid-film lubrication in a healthy joint even under heavy (but less than the ultimate strength of cartilaginous tissue) loads because in a loaded joint SF is squeezed out from cartilage micropores onto the rubbing surface directly into the zone of maximal contact stresses. In work [28] a mechanism of formation of SF lubricating layer is proposed in terms of polarization-electric interactions of the elements of synovial medium, i.e. availability, in a joint, of a biophysical field engaged in metabolism.

In that way, we may present the synovial joint structure as a tribosystem connected with the nervous center which regulates its operation (Fig. 1.4). The joint capsule has capillary vessels connected with the blood stream, and the blood serum, while piercing through the capillary walls, feeds SM. In SM the structure of complex SF compounds based on serum and hyaluronic acid occurs. SF enters the joint cavity and cartilage micropores and forms a lubricating interlayer between movably conjugated bone ends of the joint. The lubrication regime of the friction pair is automatically regulated according to the load distribution on the tribosurface by SF squeezed out from cartilage micropores onto the most heavy-duty surface areas. Cartilage debris and degradation products of SF move from the joint capsule into SM. They are consumed by enzymes and microphages available. The utilized products are removed via lymphatic and blood peri-articular vascular systems. The processes are regulated by the sympathetic center provided by the feedback systems with the blood stream (nerve impulses regulate the permeability of capillaries and have the vasodilating effect depending on biochemical parameters of blood and SF) and with SM via afferent (directed to the center) and efferent (from center to membrane) impulses. Such a tribosystem has all features of an "intelligent" system owing to which: 1) lubrication is self-regulated; 2) joints function reliably for a long time; 3) their working capacity depends on the total condition of an organism.

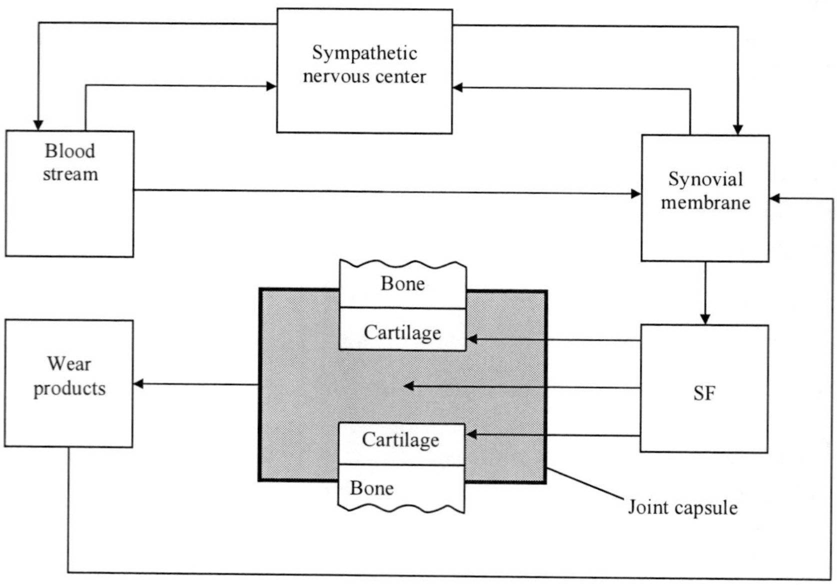

Figure 1.4. Diagram of synovial joint as an "intelligent" friction unit.

Osteoarthritis is the most widely spread rheumatic disorder which 10–12% of global population is afflicted with [29]. It is caused by deteriorating metabolism in the organism resulting in reduced lumen in the capillaries and their increased resistance to the blood current. It is responsible for decreasing filtration parameters of blood serum through the capillary walls into SM. Nutrition and membrane efficiency of SF production are getting worse. At the same time, the biochemical composition of SF is disrupted [30] and it starts performing metabolic and locomotor functions less efficiently. As the consequence, the cartilage tribosurface is damaged passing through the following stages: disappearance of the characteristic microrelief, collagen hydration, fiber deprivation of cartilaginous tissue, and degeneration of collagen fibers [31]. The broken microrelief of the tribosurface leads to a worse adherence of the SF lubricating layer to the cartilage and increasing friction in the joint [3].

In chronic joint inflammation, SF amount increases in the joint cavity, however, the joint lubrication does not improve. The cartilage under destruction the so-called proteolytic enzymes are released, which results in pathological protein fraction appearing in SF and disturbed optimal lubrication regime caused by worse carrying capacity of the lubricating layer [32]. The ultimate level of osteoarthritis is "a dry joint" characterized by the absence of lubrication because of SM cell atrophy as well as cicatrices and adhesions in the joint capsule [33].

Therefore, the main cause of joint disorder is metabolism impairment in the blood stream–SM system, which causes deficient joint lubrication and cartilaginous tissue nutrition, resulting in the damage of cartilage as a friction material. Therefore, the state of the cartilage tribosurface and its lubrication conditions are the main concern of orthopedists. Chondroprotection, namely, a complex of measures serving to support the physiological cartilage regeneration, normal metabolism between joint and vascular streams in the organism, and as a result, prevention of cartilage from destruction and wearing, is a modern tendency in arthrology [34]. The successful chondroprotection aims at satisfactory lubrication of movably conjugated joint elements.

1.3. Joint Lubrication Theories

The views on lubrication of such a perfect friction unit as the synovial joint have been developing with time before having become the system of modern conceptions. Nevertheless, the theory of joint lubrication characterized today as superlubricity is not fully understood and needs further intensive development.

1.3.1. A Historical Essay

The problem of the joint lubrication mechanism as unique kinematic pairs still occupies a significant place in the totality of arthrological and tribological issues [1, 14, 35–37]. Its solution is complicated by the variety of physicochemical processes running in the synovial medium and unique biomechanical processes inherent of its components [1, 36, 37]. Low friction in joint would be evidently impossible without SF. As early as in 1743, J. Hunter in his report to the Queen Society noted that SF was a lubricant in joints [38]. The works in this direction were developed only in the early 20th century when in 1925 a German orthopedist A. Benninghoff assumed that the cartilage elasticity was due to SF secretion and absorption [39]. However, this important conclusion stayed unnoticed during many years.

Investigation of the cartilage friction mechanisms in the early 1930s made researchers turn their attention to lubrication theories approved in engineering. In 1932, based on the hydrodynamic lubrication theory developed by an English physicist O. Reynolds, his countryman M.A. McConail put forward a hypothesis that the geometry of cartilage surfaces and synovia viscosity produced the hydrodynamic effect in joint lubrication [40]. Soon it became evident that the hypothesis could not explain extremely low coefficients of friction in joints. The sliding velocity in the joint never exceeds several centimeters per second and rated thickness of the lubricating film at this velocity calculated on the basis of the Reynolds theory which does not take into account the viscoelastic nature of cartilages, is extremely low – somewhat of cartilage roughness. The film of the similar thickness cannot produce the hydrodynamic effect. Despite the disadvantages, the McConail theory was of tremendous significance as the first attempt to use achievements in physics in arthrology and stimulated further research in this direction.

At that time, a gravitation pendulum was used to experimentally evaluate friction in joints [38]. By the kinetic dependence of its oscillation damping not only the value but also the friction mechanism in a bearing unit was judged. The linear curve of damping was characteristic of boundary lubrication and exponential curve of damping – of hydrodynamic lubrication. Under boundary lubrication, friction is governed by the properties of the thin absorption layer of the lubricant differing from its properties in volume. Hydrodynamic, or liquid-film lubrication is responsible for full separation of tribosurfaces because of the pressure arising in the lubricating layer in their movement.

In 1934, a British physicist E.S. Jones was first to experimentally measure the coefficient of friction in animal's joints. He stated that the coefficient of friction was about 0.2 in knee joints lubricated with SF or a physiological solution whereas it was larger by an order of magnitude in "dry" ones. It was noted that in the latter case the cartilage failed fast in friction. The data was supported by later investigations that proved the coefficient of friction in animal's joints to vary from 0.005 to 0.02 [41, 42]. Jones came to a conclusion that joints were characterized by mixed lubrication, that is, it is hydrodynamic in movement and boundary at starts and stops.

After that, during almost 20 years there were no new theories dealing with joint lubrication. Researchers turned their attention to investigation of SF and hyaluronic acid found in it. Only in the early 1950s, McConail assumed that owing to additional structures such as menisci and lipid bodies, convergent SF flows could be produced at low sliding velocities in the joint friction zone. The bearing capacity of these flows can separate the tribosurfaces. An English tribologist E. Gardner developed the McConail's ideas concerning the importance of hydrodynamic principles of joint lubrication, yet, like Jones, he believed that in certain situations boundary lubrication might occur.

Soon it became evident that the Reynolds hydrodynamic lubrication theory assuming the rigidity of contact bodies can only partially explain the lubrication of joints whose cartilages are easily deformed under dynamic contact conditions. These limitations were removed in 1949 by a Russian tribologist A.N. Grubin who took into account elastic deformations of rubbing bodies in his calculations. He theoretically substantiated that the thickness of the lubricating film was larger in this case and, consequently, hydrodynamic lubrication was possible under conditions where just boundary lubrication was assumed. In 1959, D. Dowson and G.R. Higginson applied Grubin's theory to describe friction in joints and proposed an *elastohydrodynamic-lubrication* term. In their opinion, the friction unit under lubrication can theoretically function in different lubrication regimes – from boundary to mixed and from elastohydrodynamic to hydrodynamic depending on load, velocity, temperature, tribosurface geometry, characteristics of lubricant, and tribosystem carrying capacity.

The calculation results of SF viscosity and thickness of the lubricating film by means of the equations of classical hydrodynamics were discussed elsewhere [43]. Analysis of the discrepancy between calculated and experimental data has shown the elastohydrodynamic model of joint lubrication to be more validated. Nevertheless, the theory failed to become universal. It was shown theoretically [44] that joint lubrication may occur not only in elastohydrodynamic conditions.

In the late 1950s, a British orthopedist, founder of prosthetic arthroplasty J. Charnley called in question the data obtained Jones on exponential damping of pendulum oscillations testifying to the liquid-film lubrication mechanism in the inter-phalangeal joint. He conducted his proper experiments using the ankle joint as a supporting unit. The kinetic dependence of pendulum oscillation damping turned out to be linear rather than exponential, which proved the boundary lubrication mechanism. As has been found, Jones conducted his experiments with integral joints rather than cut ones, when friction was accompanied by deformation resistance of connective tissue. It was justified by a series of experiments with dog's ankles [45]. With ligaments and tendons undamaged, the kinetic dependences of pendulum amplitude were exponential and once the ligaments were cut, the dependence became linear. Charnley noted that the low coefficient of friction in joints retained until ceasing motion and believed that it only could be under boundary lubrication.

Later on a lot of contradictory results were obtained indicating that lubrication conditions might transform in synovial joints. Comparison of the joint with the hydrostatic bearing operating under liquid-film lubrication [46] has shown their identity. The authors of work [47], while investigating human joints by a pendulum tribometer, have come to a conclusion that friction depends linearly on load, yet the relationship typical of boundary lubrication, is distorted when the thickness of the lubricating layer increases and SF starts presenting viscous resistance to friction. A British tribologist S.A.V. Swanson has shown theoretically [48] that SF viscosity should be by 2–3 orders higher than its measured value to explain most of the experimental results in studying friction in natural joints. He believed that joint lubrication was largely boundary with an insignificant share of liquid-film lubrication regime. The opinion was not shared by the researchers who used reciprocate friction machines in their experiments and believed that liquid-film lubrication prevailed in human and animal joint operation [38].

To eliminate the contradictions, new theories of joint lubrication were put forward with account for specific structure of cartilage as a friction material.

It has been noted that 60–80% of the cartilage matrix volume is occupied by SF. Therefore, in cartilage deformation, SF is squeezed out from cartilaginous tissue micropores in the friction zone and once the load is relieved SF is squeezed in the pores [39]. The idea was enthusiastically supported by a British arthrologist K. McCutchen. While investigating a cartilage-glass friction pair he has shown that after each period of SF squeezing, the coefficient of friction dropped essentially in the pair. With decreasing fluid content of the cartilage the coefficient of friction increased up to 0.35. McCutchen named such a lubrication mechanism *a weeping-lubrication* and assumed that SF circulated between the lubricating film squeezed by rubbing cartilages and cartilaginous tissue micropores (Fig. 1.5). The theory explained the causes of low friction in joints in motion and at the moment of start of motion (the so-called static friction).

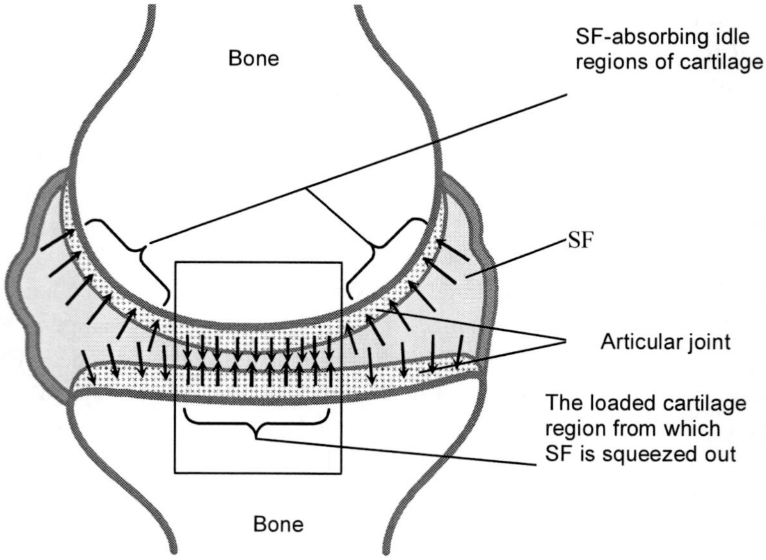

Figure 1.5. Diagram of the *weeping-lubrication* mechanism [38]. The arrows show the SF flow directions.

In the 1960s, the cartilage was examined by scanning electron microscopy, which allowed up-to-date concepts on the structure of cartilaginous tissue to develop [49]. The morphological distinctions of cartilage surface layer mentioned in 1.2.2 uninvolved in friction were revealed [50]. A hypothesis was put forward that the cartilage surface layer, along with tribological functions, plays the role of a membrane [51]. It is highly permeable for water and organic nutrients of a small molecular weight and less permeable for high-molecular weight compounds. This makes it possible to regulate the feeding of cartilaginous tissue and damping of impact loads [52, 53].

The research of the physicochemical interaction of SF and cartilage performed in the late 1960s has given impetus to development of new theories of joint lubrication. The following findings served as a basis for the theories:

- disclosure of hyaluronate adsorption on the cartilage surface that forms the layer to prevent the cartilage against overloads in friction;
- disclosure of SF viscosity as a function of shear rate and pressure;
- determination of the lubricating film thickness that ensures maximum approach of elastic cartilages and the possibility of separating rubbing surfaces via this film.

Hyaline cartilages dried by freezing were examined by the scanning electron microscopy technique. A regular microrelief was detected on the rubbing surface [54], permitting maintenance of the SF film between 0.25 and 10 μm thick in the friction zone. The rated SF viscosity in the lubricating layer turned out to be higher than that one measured by the viscosimetry method, which was confirmed by the witty comparative experiment [55]. It was concluded that the SF layer squeezed between cartilages was saturated with high-molecular compounds at the cost of low-molecular SF components flowing in the cartilage micropores. It improves the stability and load-carrying capacity of the lubricating layer. This kind of lubrication was named *boosted-lubrication* [56] (Fig. 1.6).

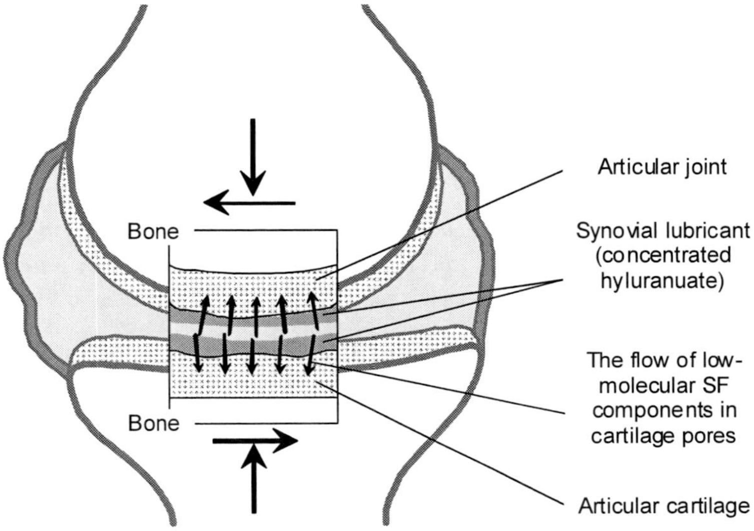

Figure 1.6. Diagram of the boosted lubrication mechanism of the joint [46]. The arrows show the directions of low-molecular SF component flows and forces acting in joint motion.

Nevertheless, experimental data obtained the late 60s – early 70s proved the insufficiency of these theories. It was revealed that the lubricity of viscous SF was much higher than that of fluid physiological saline [47]. Enzymatic decomposition of hyaluronic acid was initiated in SF, which resulted in the loss of SF viscosity with the lubricity remaining the same [57]. To adequately describe deformation and strength characteristics of the cartilage a model shaped as a three-layer microporous structure filled with a fluid proved to be the most suitable [58]. SF circulation in a joint is presented as the result of displacement of compression stress front in the cartilaginous tissue because of which SF is condensed and squeezed out from the micropores. After passing the stress front, the phase occurs when the cartilage absorbs SF from the articular cavity [59]. Clearly pronounced rheological properties of SF caused certain friction regularities in joint models under applied impact loads [60]. It was an attempt to take into account many factors governing friction in joints with making use of the theory of *living friction* [61]. The authors used the term to define the specific distribution of load in the cartilage contact zone between, first, contact spots separated by the boundary SF film and, second, load-carrying SF microvolumes being under all-round squeezing. Unfortunately, the theory could not help understand joint lubrication mechanisms.

1.3.2. State of the Art

As there was no single theory of joint lubrication, the researchers had to study the cartilage structure assuming it a dynamically changeable system that readily interacts with SF. A new stage in the research started when protein-polysaccharide complexes consisting of hyaluronic acid and protein molecules were discovered. There were two points of view concerning their formation [62]: 1) protein molecules were assumed to serve a linking unit which allows macromolecules of hyaluronic acid to be adsorbed on the cartilage surface; 2) proteins favor adsorption of hydrogen onto disaccharide chains of hyaluronic acid, which causes the macromolecules to combine into complexes through hydrogen bonds. Protein-polysaccharide complexes are found in SF in the form of spherical structures 100–1000 nm in diameter, as it was detected by the scanning electron microscopy technique [54].

In the 1980s, aggregates of similar globules were found on the rubbing surfaces of articular cartilage and menisci. Their concentration depends on the age of the cartilaginous tissue; the globules were of protein nature and formed from SF and metabolic products of cartilaginous tissue [63]. Their density was higher than that of SF and they remain spherical at surface tension. A lubrication model was proposed with protein globules to function as rolling elements in joints.

The model outlined in 1.2.3 of boundary lubrication in a joint based of hydrophilic property of cartilages and adsorption, on their surfaces, of thin films of water and glycoproteins looks more convincing [28]. Figure 1.7 shows how such films are formed.

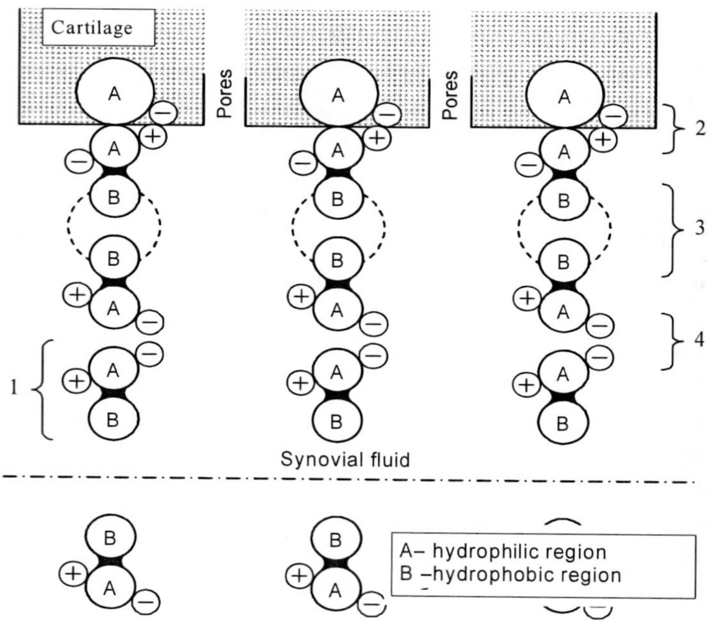

Figure 1.7. Boundary lubrication model of articular cartilages: *1* – lubricating glycoprotein subunit; *2* – zone of electrostatic attraction of glycoprotein hydrophilic areas to the cartilage hydrophilic areas; *3* – zone of attraction of hydrophobic areas of glycoproteins (high shear resistance); *4* – zone of attraction of hydrophilic areas of glycoproteins (low shear resistance) [28].

Glycoprotein identified in SF by the authors of work [64] exists as subunits (permolecular formations) having both hydrophilic and hydrophobic regions. A monolayer of glycoproteins is attached to a negatively charged rubbing cartilage surface by the mechanisms of electrostatic adsorption (Fig. 17, zone 2). Another subunits layer is strongly attached with its hydrophobic zones to the hydrophobic "ends" of high surface energy belonging to the adsorbed complexes (zone 3). This zone is characterized by high shear resistance. Another subunits layer is attached to the complexes immobilized on the cartilage through weak bonds arising between lyophilic regions (zone 4). Cartilage sliding causes these bonds of low shear resistance to break. Therefore, easy separation of rubbing surfaces in a joint results from adsorption, on the cartilage, of protein boundary layers and from electrostatic repulsive forces.

Simultaneously, alternative points of view were advanced concerning the mechanisms of formation of lubricating monolayers on rubbing cartilage surfaces; those hypotheses excluded electrostatic interactions [65].

In the 1980s, an hypothesis was advanced to attribute the extremely low friction in joints to the liquid-crystal condition of the SF lubricating layer [66]. Liquid crystals show properties of both liquid (fluidity) and those of solid crystals (anisotropy of properties) and, in the degree of molecular arrangement, occupy the intermediate position between solid crystals with a long-range order and liquids which do not have it. That is why, the liquid-crystal state is often called mesomorphous state or mesophase (*meso*… is a part of compound words meaning *occupying a medium-intermediate position*). Liquid crystals exist in a temperature range between the melting temperature of solids and so-called clearing temperature when they change to an isotropic liquid (when turbid samples become transparent). One kind of liquid crystals, nematic crystals, whose molecular long axes have fixed orientation but their gravity centers are randomly disposed. The cholesterol-type crystals most often result from cholesterol compounds whose macromolecules are arranged in a layer-to-layer manner: in every layer like in nematic crystals, but the axis direction of the macromolecule deviates by some angle of rotation from the axis direction. As a result, the direction vectors in the layers are arranged in a spiral with the pitch depending on the macromolecule origin. The structure is easily modified by heating, under mechanical stresses, electric or magnetic fields, which modify physical properties of liquid crystals. Numerous biological fluids of living organisms involved in metabolism are found in the liquid-crystalline state [67–69].

The SF is a selective blood dialysate; 60–80% of cholesterol in it is etherified [14]. The liquid-crystal lubrication theory of joints presumes that cholesterol ethers cause the liquid-crystal state of the SF lubricating layer separating the cartilage tribosurfaces [3]. The latter have the ordered microrelief corresponding to the regular arrangement of collagen fibers in the cartilaginous tissue [54]. Microgrooves on the cartilage surface increase its adhesion to the lubricating layer. The diagram of the liquid-crystal structure of the lubricating layer of joints is shown in Fig. 1.8.

In zone I of the collagenous fiber contact, the SF layer has a minimal thickness making half of the pitch of the spiral structure of a cholesterol crystal ($s/2 \sim 200 \div 550$ nm) [70]. In the vicinity of the contact area of fibers (zone II) a larger layer thickness is also a multiple of $s/2$. The molecular interaction between layers of $s/2$ thickness is much weaker than in the depth of the layer. This structure is similar to Solid-film lubricants. When a joint is in motion, shear is localized between layers of the cholesterol lubricating interlayer that results in easy sliding and low friction in the joint. The liquid-crystal theory of joint lubrication relies upon the conceptual understanding of physics that is true for dynamically contacting solids of any nature and therefore, is a general theory. The application of this theory in tribology is justified by the following facts:

- it is established [7] that the liquid-crystal state of SF arises at physiological temperatures if the mesogenous compounds of cholesterol are present;
- model lubricating substances containing a cholesterol mesophase ensure as low friction in cartilage-cartilage and cartilage-glass pairs as SF does [72];
- lubricity of the synthetic analogs of SF can be improved by using cholesterol compounds [73].

The results agree with the present-day conceptions of the phenomenological theory of liquid crystals [74].

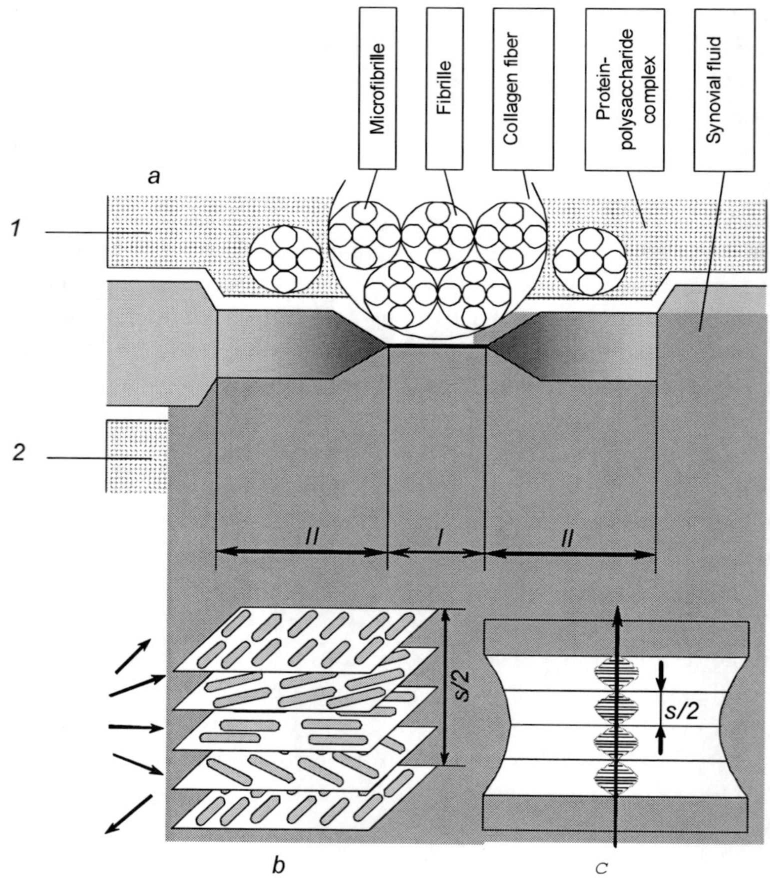

Figure 1.8. Liquid-crystalline model of joint lubrication [1]: *a* – diagram of contact interaction in the "cartilage 1 – SF – cartilage 2" system; I and II – zones of contact of collagen fibers and approach of cartilage surfaces; *b* and *c* – structures of the liquid-crystal film in zones I and II.

The present-day understanding of boundary lubrication in joints assumes formation on the cartilage surface of adsorbed hydrophobic layers of natural brush polymers, first of all, surface-active phospholipids generated by B-lymphocytes of SF [75]. Lipids are found in all living cells where they make an energy reserve and participate in development of water-proof linings, in transfer of nervous impulses, etc. They consist of three basic components, namely, cholesterol, triglycerides, and phospholipids found in the largest amounts (up to 61%) in lipids [76]. Phosphatidylcholines (PC) – the main component of phospholipids –show high surface activity. PC (or lecithins, choline phosphoglycerids) belong to complex lipids whose molecules consist of alcohol, high-molecular weight fatty acids, and some other components.

In a healthy joint, PC molecules are adsorbed on the rubbing cartilage surface that carries negative charge [77]. A diagram of the adsorbed layer is shown in Fig. 1.9. The positively charged end of the PC molecule (the end groups of quaternary ammonium) [78] "looks for" air, neutral lipids or a hydrophilic surface *2*. Mobile cations *3* neutralize negatively charged phosphate ions in PC molecules providing high cohesive strength of the adsorbed molecule layer; the molecules are strongly (adhesionally) connected with the cartilage. This results in high load-carrying capacity of the adsorbed layer which provides a boundary lubricating film in a cartilage–cartilage friction pair. Neutral hydrocarbon chains *4* of fatty acids make densely packed "tails" of the PC molecules. Such arrangement makes the hydrophilic phase of proteoglycans a hydrophobic surface in the surface cartilage layer. It is this layer of adsorbed phospholipids that ensures lubrication of joint endoprostheses after they have been implanted [79].

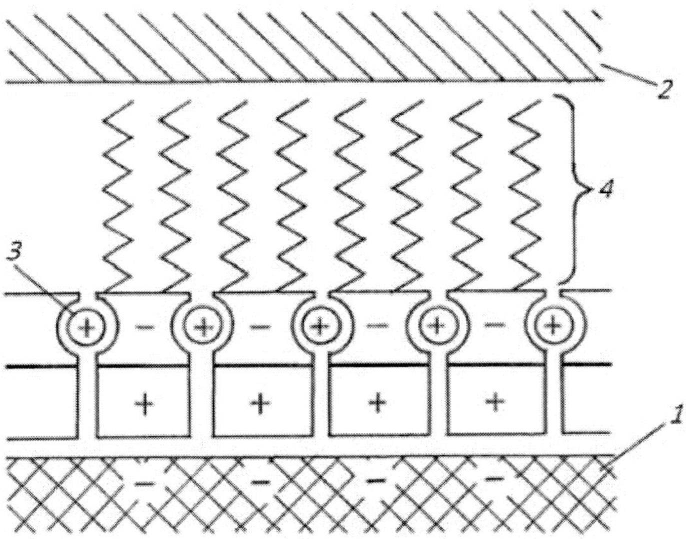

Figure 1.9. Diagram of adsorption layer of PC molecules on the cartilage tribosurface [75]: 1 – cartilage surface under wetting; 2 – less wetted surface, 3 – Ca^{2+}, 4 – hydrocarbon chains of fatty acids.

Another theory of joint lubrication [80] that does not contradict the aforesaid implies formation, on the cartilage surface, of specific lubricating structures secreted by fibroblasts and chondrocytes. Biophysicists and rheumatologists paid attention to the fact that boundary lubrication occurs even in arthrosis-damaged joints where SF has lost its natural viscosity maintained by hyaluronic acid. A British tribologist D. Swan extracted, from SF, glycoproteid of molecular weight (MW) = 227 and proposed the term *lubricin* to denote the glycoproteid-containing lubricating layer on the cartilage surface [81]. Glycoproteids (mucoproteids) are complex proteins containing hydrocarbon components $C_m(H_2O)_n$. The group of glycoproteids also includes proteins of blood plasma. In the postgenomous period of molecular biology, lubricin became an object of biotribologists' interest as a substance forming, in the joint, a lubricating layer of nano-sized thickness.

The method of biochemical extraction was employed to get a protein of MW = 345 from a nanolayer of cartilage surface; this protein is the main component of lubricin [82]. While making attempts to grow cartilage *in vitro* by cultivating chondrocytes on a molecular substrate, Flannery et al. [83] discovered that chondrocytes excreted lubricin. The level of lubricin is lower in joints afflicted with traumatic synovitis [84]. The lubricin concentration adequate for boundary lubrication has become an important biophysical marker in cartilaginous tissue engineering [75]. In the course of tribological investigations carried out *in vitro* with making use of atomic force microscopy it was established that molecules of hyaluronic acid molecules adsorbed on the rubbing surface synergetically improve the lubricin lubricity [85].

Thus, these two models of boundary lubrication of joints imply:

- that SF, being a natural lubricant of joint always ensures boundary lubrication of cartilages;
- a possibility of liquid-crystal state of the lubricating layer which contains lipids, particularly cholesterol;
- participation of blood serum components in joint lubrication.

The recent understanding of synovial joint lubrication agrees with the superlubricity concept which has been widely used in tribology in recent years [86]. A Japanese tribologist Motohisa Hirano was the first to use the word *superlubricity* to describe a theoretical sliding regime in which friction or resistance to sliding completely vanishes. In this regime, the extent of physical and/or chemical interactions is extremely small or essentially absent, and hence the surfaces can slide over one another without causing much friction. The synovial joint as an intelligent system shows superlubricity that provides a long-duration functioning of joints within a period commensurable with human life span.

ACKNOWLEDGMENTS

The historical aspects of arthrology considered above indicate the unity of the elements of the synovial medium of the joint. SF functions as a mobile agent whose motion is responsible for mass exchange and initiates metabolism in a joint. It is a unique type of condensed medium having the properties if both a liquid and a solid that is found in liquid-crystal state in the boundary lubricating layer. Lubrication of joints is a multifactor biophysical process with all the elements of synovial medium of the joint involved. Tanks to its multilevel hierarchical structure, unique physical and chemical properties, and variety of the functions SF plays a major role in joint operation as an intelligent-friction assembly.

REFERENCES

[1] Humphrey, ID; DeLange, S. *An introduction to biomechanics*. Berlin: Springer, 2004.

[2] Bruce, N; Gamboa-deBuen, I; Rodriguez-Villatuerte, M. *Medical physics*. Amsterdam: Elsevier, 2003.

[3] Ermakov, SF; Rodnenkov, VG; Beloenko, ED, Kupchinov, BI. *Liquid crystals in engineering and medicine*. Minsk: Asar, Moscow: CheRo, 2002.

[4] Chikin, SYa. *Philosophers doctors*. Moscow: Medicine, 1990.

[5] Vesalius, A. *De humani corporis fabrica epitome (Russian Translation)*. Moscow: Medicine, 1974.

[6] Sorokina, TS. *A handbook for students of medical universities. 3rd ed.* Moscow: Academia, 2004.

[7] Vaubel, E. The form and function of synovial cells in tissue culture. *J. Exp. Med.* 1963, N 58, 63–83.

[8] Diterikhs, MM. *An introduction to clinics of joint disorders*. Moscow: Medgiz, 1937.

[9] Kallistov, IP. *Age-related features of joint synovial membrane. In: Age-related features of the composition of joint synovial membrane*. Kiev, 1951, 141−153.

[10] Davies, DV. Properties of synovial fluid. *Proc. Inst. Mech. Eng.* 1967, Vol 181, 3J, 25–29.

[11] Gardner, E. Physiology of movable joints. *Physiol. Rew.* 1950, Vol 30, N 2, 127–177.

[12] Zhdano, DA. *General anatomy and physiology of lymphatic system*. Moscow: Medgiz, 1952.

[13] Dowson, D. Lubrication and wear of joints. *Physiotherapy.* 1973, Vol 59, N 4, 101–106.

[14] Pavlova, VN. *Synovial medium of joints*. Moscow: Medicine, 1980.

[15] Pavlova, VN; Kop'eva, TN; Slutskii, LI; Pavlov, GG. *The Cartilage*. Moscow: Medicine, 1988.

[16] Czichos, H. Systemanalyse und physic tribologischer vorgange. 1 – Grundlagen, 2– Anvendungen. *Schmiertechnik Tribologie.* 1975, Vol 22, 126–130; 1976, Vol 23, 6–12.

[17] *Smart materials and structures*. Ed. Friend, CM. London: Chapmen and Hill, 1994.

[18] Chung, DDL. *Composite materials: functional materials for modern technologies.* NY: Springer, 2003.

[19] Wallace, GG; Spinks, GM; Taesdale, PR. *Conductive electroactive polymers: intelligent materials system*. Lancaster: Technomic Publishing Co, 2002.

[20] Motyl, E. *Space charge in solid dielectrics analysis of measurement methods and investigation*. Dr Sci Thesis, Wroclaw, 2000.

[21] Kozlov, VA. Comparative aspects of biology of embryonic and blood-producing stem cells. *Immunology*, 2006, Vol 28, N 1, 60−64.

[22] Wassilew, W. Electronmicroscopische und histochimische Untersuchungen zur Entwicklung des Kniegelenkes der Rate. *Z Anat. und Entwicklungsgesch.* 1972, Bd 137, N 2, 113–117.

[23] Barland, P; Janis, R; Sandson J. Immunofluorescent studies of human articular cartilage. *Ann. Rheum. Dis.* 1966, N 25, 165–185.

[24] *Encyclopedic dictionary of medical terms in 3 vol.* Ed. Petrovskii, BV. Moscow: Soviet Encyclopedia, 1983, Vol 2.

[25] Slutskii, LI. *Biochemistry of normal and pathologically changed connective tissue.* Moscow: Medicine, 1969.

[26] Pavlova, VN; Fradkin, AR. *Modern evaluation of haemotissue relations in joint synovial membranes, in lymphatic and blood streams.* Novosibirsk, 1976.

[27] Modayev, VP; Ankina, MA. On the composition of the outer part of articular cartilage. *Arch. Anat.* 1978, Vol 74, N 4, 57–62.

[28] Davis, WHJ; Lee, SL; Socoloff, L. A proposed model of boundary lubrication by synovial liquid: structuring of boundary water. *Trans. ASME J. Biomech. Eng.* 1979, Vol 101, N 3, 185–192.

[29] Tsurko, VV. Oosteoarthrosis: A geriatric problem. *Russk. Med. Zh.* 2005, Vol 13, N 24, 1627–1631.

[30] Gerasimov, AM; Furtseva, LN. *Biochemical diagnostics in traumatology and orthopedics.* Moscow: Medicine, 1986.

[31] Mironov, SP; Omel'yanenko, NP; Sherepo, KM; Karpov, IN; Semenova, LA; Kurpyakov, AP. Morphology of tissue components of hip joint in experimental animals in osteoarthrosis simulation. *NN Priorov Vestnik traumatol. and orthop.* 2006, N 1, 57–63.

[32] Plyatsko, VV; Levenets, VN; Stavinskii, YuA. Changes in synovial medium in deforming gonarthrosis. *Orthop. Traum. Prosth.* 1990, N 5, 24–28.

[33] Chichasova, NV. Treatment of osteoarthrosis: the effect of various anti-inflammatory drugs on cartilaginous tissue. *Russk. Med. Zh.* 2005, Vol 13, N 8, 539–543.

[34] *Selective lectures on clinical rheumatology.* Ed. Nasonov, VA; Bunchuk, NV. Moscow: Medicine, 2001.

[35] Persson, BNJ. *Sliding friction: physical principles and applications.* Berlin–Heidelberg–NY: Springer-Verlag, 2000.

[36] *Biomechanics of diarthrodial joints.* Ed. Mow, VC; Ratcliffe, A; Woo, SL-Y. – NY–Berlin–Heidelberg–London: Springer-Verlag, 1990, Vol 1.

[37] Pinchuk, LS; Nikolaev, VI; Tsvetkova, EA; Goldade, VA. *Tribology and biophysics of artificial joints.* London: Elsevier, 2006.

[38] Brand, RA. *Joint lubrication. Ch. 13.* In: The Scientific Basis of Orthopaedics, 2nd Edition. London: Elsevier, 1987, 373–386.

[39] Beninghoff, A. Form und Bau der Gelenkknorpel in ihrem Beziehungen zu Function. *Zeitschr Zellforsch.* 1925, N 2, 783–862.

[40] Mow, VC. Role of Lubricant in Joint Biomechanics. *Problems of Friction-and-Lubrication: Trans. ASME.* 1969, N 2, 131–141.

[41] Unsworth, A; Dowson, D; Wright, V. Some new evidence on human joint lubrication. *Ann. Rheum. Dis.* 1975, Vol 34, 277–281.

[42] Mansour, JM; Mow, VC. On the natural lubrication of synovial joints: normal and degenerate. *Trans. ASME*. 1977, Vol F99, N 2, 163–173.

[43] Tanner, RI. An alternative mechanism for the lubrication of synovial joints. *Phys. Med. Biol*. 1966, Vol 11, 119.

[44] Marnell, P; White, RK. Quantitative analysis of joint lubrication. *Wear*. 1980, Vol 61, 203.

[45] Barnett, CH; Davies, DV; McConail, MA. *Synovial joints*. London: Elsevier, 1968.

[46] Clarke, IC; Contini, R; Kenedi, RM. Friction and wear studies of articular cartilage: a scanning electron microscope study. *Trans. ASME*. 1975, Vol F97, N 3, 358–368.

[47] Unsworth, A; Dowson, D; Wright, V. The frictional behavior of human synovial joints. Part 1. Natural joints. *Trans ASME*. 1975, Vol F97, N 3, 369–376.

[48] Swanson, SAV. *Friction, wear and lubrication. In: Adult Articular Cartilage*. London: Pitman. Publ. 1979, 401–414.

[49] Muir, H; Bullough, P; Maroudas, A. The distribution of collagen in human articular cartilage with some of its physiological implications. *J. Bone Joint Surg*. 1970, Vol 52B, 554–563.

[50] Lipshitz, H; Etheredge, R; Climcher, MJ. In vitro studies of the wear of articular cartilage. The wear characteristics of chemically modified articular cartilage when worn against a highly polished characterized stainless steel surface. *J. Biomech*. 1980, Vol 13, 423–436.

[51] Weiss, C; Rosenberg, L; Helfet, AJ. An ultrastructural study of normal young adult human articular cartilage. *J. Bone Joint Surg*. 1968, Vol 50A, 663.

[52] Maroudas, A; Bullough, P; Swanson, SAV; Freeman, MAR. The permeability of articular cartilage. *J. Bone Joint Surg*. 1968, Vol 50B, 166.

[53] Jaffe, FF; Mankin, HJ; Weiss, C; Zarins, A. Water binding in the articular cartilage of rabbits. *J. Bone Joint Surg*. 1974, Vol 56A, 1031.

[54] Walker, PS; Sikorski, J; Dowson, D; et al. Behavior of synovial fluid on surfaces of articular cartilage: A scanning electron microscope study. *Ann. Rheum. Dis*. 1969, Vol 28, N 1, 1–14.

[55] Walker, PS; Gold, BL. Comparison of the bearing performance of normal and artificial human joints. *Trans ASME*. 1973, Vol F95, N 3, 333–341.

[56] Dowson, D; Unsworth, A; Wright, V. Analysis of boosted lubrication in human joints. *J. Mech. Eng. Science*. 1970, Vol 12, 364–369.

[57] Wright, V; Dowson, D; Kerr, J. The structure of joints. IV. Articular cartilage. *Int. Rev. Connect. Tissue Res*. 1973, Vol 6, 105–124.

[58] Mow, VC; Mansour, JM. The nonlinear interaction between cartilage deformation and interstitial fluid flow. *J. Biomech*. 1977, Vol 10, N 1, 31–39.

[59] Torzilli, PA; Mow, VC. On the fundamental fluid transport mechanisms through normal and pathological articular cartilage during function: The formulation. *J. Biomech*. 1976, Vol 9, N 8, 541–552.

[60] Unsworth, A; Dowson, D; Wright, V; Koshal, D. The frictional behavior of human synovial joints. 2. Artificial joints. *Trans. ASME*. 1975, Vol F97, N 3, 377–382.

[61] Prokhorova, TA; Oganesyan, OV; Mikhailov, VK. On the problem of low friction mechanism in articular cartilages. *Friction, Wear and Lubricants. Proc. Int. Conf.* Moscow: 1985, 15–16.
[62] Seller, PC; Dowson, D; Wright, V. The rheology of synovial fluid. *Rheol. Acta.* 1971, Vol 10, 2–7.
[63] Pavlova, MN; Kumanin, BN. Ultrastructure of rubbing surfaces in a joint. *Arch. Anat. Gistol and Embriol.* 1983, N 8, 38–42.
[64] Swann, DA. *Macromolecules of synovial fluid. In: The joints and synovial fluid.* Ed. Sokoloff, L. NY: Dekker, 1978, 374.
[65] Gvozdanovic, D; Wright, V; Dowson, D. Formation of lubricating monolayers at the cartilage surface. *Ann. Rheum. Dis.* 1975, Vol 34, 100–106.
[66] Kupchinov, BI; Rodnenkov, VG; Ermakov, SF; et al. On the problem of the joint performance mechanism as a rubbing unit. *Dokl. AN BSSR.* 1985, Vol 29, N 5, 463–465.
[67] Usol'tseva, NV. Chemical characteristic, biological and medical value of lyotropic liquid crystals. *J. DI Mendeleev All-Union Chem. Soc.* 1983, Vol 28, N 2, 36–45.
[68] Khalatov, SS. *Cholesterol disease.* Moscow: Medgiz, 1946.
[69] Brown, G; Wolken, D. *Liquid crystals and biological Structures.* Ed. Varshavskii, YaM; translated from English by Vedenov, AA. Moscow: Mir, 1982.
[70] Beloenko, ED; Kupchinov, BI; Ermakov, SF; Rodnenkov, VG; Eismont, OL. Liquid-crystal state of joint synovial lubricating medium. Experimental substantiation. *Acta of Bioeng and Biomech.* 2001, Vol 3, 24–32.
[71] Beloenko, ED; Ermakov, SF; Kupchinov, BI. Synovial Fluid as a Liquid-Crystalline Biological Medium. *Orthop. Traumatol. Prosth.* 1997, N 3, 40–41.
[72] Kupchinov, BI; Ermakov, SF; Rodnenkov, VG; Beloenko, ED; Eismont, OL. Some results of studies of liquid-crystalline state of synovial lubricant in joints. *J. of Friction and Wear.* 2002, Vol. 23, N 3, 310–317.
[73] Beloenko, ED; Eismont, OL; Pashkevch, LA; Shved, IA; Ermakov, SF. Effectiveness of a drug based on cholesterol-nematic bioactive substance in treatment of experimental arthrosis-arthritis. *Vesti NAN of Belarus. Med. Sci. Ser.* 2005, N 1, 5–8.
[74] Sonin, AS. *An introduction to physics of liquid crystals.* Moscow: *Nauka,* 1983.
[75] Hills, BA; Crawford, RW. Normal and prosthetic synovial joints are lubricated by surface-active phospholipid. A hypothesis. *J. of Arthroplasty.* 2003, Vol 18, N 4, 499–505.
[76] Rabinowitz, JL; Gregg, JR; Nixon, JE. Lipid composition of the tissues of human knee joints. II. Synovial fluid in trauma. *Clin. Orthop. Rel. Res.* 1984, Vol 190, 292–300.
[77] Glosh, P. *Anti rheumatic drugs and cartilage. In: Bailliere's clinical rheumatology.* Ed. Brooks, P. London: Bailliere, 1988, 310–333.
[78] Hills, BA. *The biology of surfactant.* Cambridge: Cambridge University Press, 1988.
[79] Bell, J; Tipper, JL; Ingham, E; et al. The influence of phospholipid concentration in protein-containing lubricants on the wear of ultra-high molecular weight polyethylene in articular hip joints. *Proc. Inst. Mech. Eng.* 2001, H, 215–259.
[80] Jay, GD. Lubricin and surfacing of artificial joints. *Current Opinion in Orthopedics.* 2004, Vol 15, 355–359.

[81] Swann, DA; Silver, FH; Slayter, HS; et al. The molecular structure and lubricating ability of lubricin isolated from bovine and human synovial fluids. *Biochem. J.* 1985, Vol 225, 195–201.

[82] Schumacher, BL; Block, JA; Schmid, TM; et al. A novel proteoglycan synthesized and secreted by chondrocytes of the superficial zone of articular cartilage. *Arch. Biochem. Biophys*. 1994, Vol 311, 144–152.

[83] Flannery, CR; Hughes, CR; Schumacher, BC; et al. Articular cartilage superficial zone protein (SZP) is homologous to megakaryocyte stimulating factor precursor and a multifunctional proteoglycan with potential growth – promoting, cytoprotective and lubricating properties in cartilage metabolism. *Biochem. Biophys. Res. Comun.* 1999, Vol 234, 535–541.

[84] Jay, GD; Khaled, EA; Zack, J; et al. Lack of chondroprotection occurs among emergency department patients with knee joint synovitis. *J. of Rheum.* 2004, Vol 31, 557–564.

[85] Tadmor, R; Chen, N; Israelishvili, J. Normal and shear forces between mica and model membrane surfaces with absorbed hyaluronan. *Macromolecules.* 2003, Vol 36, 9516–9526.

[86] *Superlubricity*. Ed. Erdemir, A; Martin, J-M. Amsterdam, Oxford: Elsevier, 2007.

Chapter 2

Composition and Properties of Synovia

Synovial fluid is a viscous liquid found in the cavities of synovial joints. Its circulation is responsible for the metabolic processes between synovial medium and blood streams in a joint. Therefore, its composition and properties have an essential effect on the physiological state of joints, physical activity, and, in a way, general state of a human organism. SF reacts to damages of joint functions by varying its composition and properties, which bear primary information necessary to diagnose a joint disease. Checking of biochemical and biophysical SF parameters allows determination of pathology in joints, cartilages, and connective tissue.

The chapter reports the data that reveal a dual nature of SF, first, its origin from blood plasma and, second, the presence of components produced in the synovial medium of a joint, i.e., hyaluronates, enzymes, and synoviocytes. SF contains cellular forms involved in immune reactions and functions as a chondroprotector decreasing the cartilage wear and supporting the metabolism of cartilage tissue. Numerous SF components make complex chemical compounds structurally associated with synovial cells and products of their secretion. Consideration of SF as a condensed medium of short-range order makes it possible to evaluate in a different way the mechanisms used by SF to perform its functions as an intelligent friction assembly. SF is a quasi-electret (quasi - almost, close to) liquid-crystal biological medium. Biophysical mechanisms of SF spread on the cartilage surface and reducing friction in the joint are governed to a large degree by electret and mesomorphic states of the SF lubricating layer that comprises protein-polysaccharide macromolecules and cholesterol compounds united in complexes.

A hierarchic multilevel structure as well as unique biophysical and physiological properties of SF causes a variety of research methods for joint pathologies and technologies for medication control of the joint synovial medium.

2.1. Biochemical Composition

The biochemical basis of SF is the blood filtrate seeping in tissue cavities of SM from capillaries and venules (fine veins arising in capillary confluence). All aggressive effects onto the joint cause the respective reaction of SF. Synovium reacts to aggression by varying its biochemical composition. Recording of the variation is a source of valuable information for differential diagnosis at early stages of joint synovium diseases.

Up to now of importance are the fundamental research of the biochemical composition of SF first implemented by the representatives of the English arthrological school M. Ropes, D. Davies [2], J. Lever and E. Ford [3], E. Jebens and M. Monk-Jones [4], and A. Ogston [5]. Afterwards, these results were supported by the experiments carried out at a higher methodic level by V.A. Dulyapin [6], S.M. Bychkov [7], British researchers J. Fessler [8], P. Walker [9], W. Wright [10], French researcher R. Medicis [11], German researcher V. Horn, and American L. Sokoloff [13]. In the 1970–80s owing to the works by Russian arthrologists V.N. Pavlova [14], S.V. Zubryakov [15], O.A. Latyshev [16], V.N. Luzgin [17], and A.R. Fradkin [18], modern views on biochemical characteristics and biophysical parameters of SF took shape. They are presented in Table 2.1 wherein the chemical compositions of SF and blood plasma are compared.

Table 2.1. Comparative chemical composition of SF and blood plasma

Component	Medium	
	SF	Blood plasma
Total protein, g/l	2.5–31.5	65–85
Albumins, %	63	54–65
Globulins, %	37	35–46
α_1	7	2–5
α_2	7	7–13
β	9	8–15
γ	14	12–22
Hyaluronic acid, g/l	2.45–3.97	not found
Glucose, mmol/l	4.95	3.3–5.5
Fibrinogen, g/l	not found	2.0–4.0
Cholesterol, mmol/l	3.8±0,4	3.63–8.03
Na^+,mmol/l	130–157	130–157
K^+, mmol/l	3.4–5.3	3.4–5.3
Ca^{++}, mmol/l	2.0–2.5	2.0–2.5

We can comment the data presented in Table 2.1 in the following way.

Glucose and cholesterol having a small molecular mass are easily filtered through the walls of blood capillaries and therefore found in SF in the same concentrations as in blood plasma. The longer protein macromolecules and the larger protein globulins are, the fewer blood protein components ingress into the joint cavity. Protein macromolecules of a molecular mass more than 160000 do not penetrate into the joint and, consequently, are not contained in SF. In turn, globular proteins (enzymes, antibodies, hormones, etc.) found in the joint with polypeptide chains rolled in compact spherical structures more than 100 μm in size are deprived of opportunity to pass from joint cavity to bloodstreams.

SF proteins are identical with plasma proteins in electrophoretic (electrophoresis is the motion of particles suspended in a liquid under the effect of external current) and immunological parameters. Nevertheless, the total protein and the ratio of its fractions in SF and blood plasma are different. The total protein in normal SF is 3 times lower than in plasma. In blood plasma and SF albumins (A), namely, simple proteins, and globulins (G) or proteins soluble in diluted salt solutions but insoluble in water are contained. The ratio of A/G concentrations is 3–4 in SF and 1 in plasma. Penetration of high-molecular G fractions through the vessel walls is impeded and therefore, their content of SF is lower than in plasma. Fibrinogen (also called factor I) is the blood protein transforming into insoluble protein or fibrin in blood coagulation. Fibrinogen macromolecules have a large molecular mass and therefore are absent in SF. A specific SM-produced proteoglycan is found in SF and absent in blood. It is the product of extracellular ground substance of the connective tissue of cartilage and SM, namely, hyaluronic acid.

Hyaluronic acid (hyaluronate) is a linear polymer referring to mucopolysaccharides whose macromolecule consists of alternating monomers of N-acetylglucosamine and D-glucuronic acid:

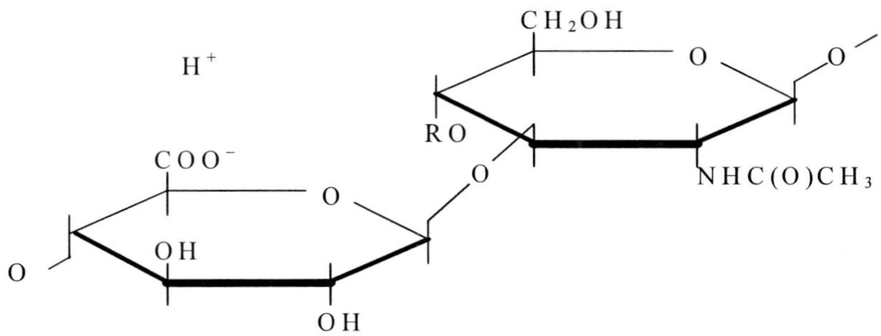

The molecular mass of hyaluronic acid in healthy SF is 10^6, the value depending on joint pathology. In SF, its macromolecules are geometrically shaped as a loose glomus 150−140 μm in radius and their volume is by an order of magnitude larger than that of proteoglycan globules. In aqueous electrolytes the macromolecules of hyaluronic acid form complex (coordination) compounds binding water macromolecules. Hyaluronic acid forms with SF proteins coordination-bound spatial structures known as mucin. In joint inflammations, SF is nourished by hyaluronidases or enzyme found in the membranes of pathogenic bacteria and catalyzing the hydrolysis of the macromolecules of hyaluronic acid to be decomposed into short constituents. The electrolytic compositions of SF and blood plasma characterized by ions Na^+, K^+, and Ca^{++} are identical.

2.2. Synovia Cells

A cell is an elementary living system consisting of a nucleus and cytoplasm and capable of independent existence, self-production, and development. SF comprises the cells that origin from blood and SM. Blood cells are presented in SF mainly, by lymphocytes and to a lesser degree by monocytes and neutrophils (leucocytes capable of phagocytosis, i.e., active capture and absorption of fine foreign particles and destruction of devitalized tissues). The SM cells found in SF are synoviocytes (cells of connective tissue capable of phagocytosis). Other cellular elements in SF are occasional and changeable. The ratio of the tissue cells and blood cells in SF is 51:49. The cell concentration in SF is low and varies within 13−180 in 1 mm^3 [6]. 150 years ago, a German arthrologist F. Frerikh established that SF of an intensively operating joint comprised manifold more cells than SF of a joint at rest [19].

A differential quantitative accounting of cellular elements in SF aims to objectively assess the joint state. It is conventionally executed by means of a synoviocytogram or a table presenting the data about the composition and content of cells in synovia. The following technique is used to draw it up.

SF cells are found in a joint at different stages of their lifecycle, viz. some of them are viable and others are under decay. The viable and dying cells can be differentiated by their capability to accumulate the particles of a neutral red dye in cytoplasm. Intensively phagocizing viable cells after staining have bright and clear zones of dye-stuff accumulation whereas their nucleus and shell do not stain in the cytoplasm. Macrophagal synoviocytes (A-cells) are the most capable of active rapture of the dye. The cells that are incapable of accumulating the dye are considered as decomposing and dying. The nuclei of the dying cells are dense and size-reduced (shrunk) looking like swollen and shapeless microparticles. They both stain insignificantly, their cytoplasm is vacuolated, i. e., contains cavities filled with a liquid. The features of dying blood cells found in SF taken from a healthy joint are given in Table 2.2.

Table 2.2. Characteristics of healthy SF-contained leucocytes

Appearance	Lymphocytes	Monocytes	Neutrophils	
			sticknuclear	segmentonuclear
Cell size, μm	8–10	15–20	10–15	10–15
Nucleus: shape	Rounded or bean-like	Polymorphic: rounded, bean-like with impressions	Narrow elongated shaped as a stick	Narrow, consists of 4–5 segments
Structure	Heterogeneous block-like	Homogeneous reticular	Heterogeneous block-like	
Color	Dark-violet	Light-violet	Dark-violet	
Cytoplasm	As a narrow ring, sometimes a wide blue zone	Profuse light-blue or grayish	Pink	
Granulosity, its color and nature	Rare individual violet granules	Inconstant sometimes fine pale violet	Profuse, fine, pale violet	

Analysis of the data of Table 2.2 shows that the SF cells can be identified by morphological analysis with a high validity. Comparison of the characteristics presented in Table 2.2 of SF cells and blood leucocytes [20] proves their identity.

Table 2.3 presents the SF synoviocytogram taken from a healthy human joint [14]. Its analysis allows the following conclusions to be drawn.

Synoviocytes have the highest concentration in SF among SM tissue cells. They are characterized by large size (within 10x20 μm), a coarse oval or rounded nucleus with clearly seen chromatin inclusions (blocks) (chromatin is a complex compound of protein and nucleic acids) and a well contoured nucleus membrane. In the cytoplasm of some synoviocytes methachromatic (i.e. acquiring a color other than a dye) spots are revealed which are non-sulfated proteoglycans or hyaluronic acid.

Histiocytes (tissue macrophages) are present in SF in a lesser amount than synoviocytes. They have the rounded compact nucleus and fine-grainy cytoplasm. Histiocyte size and shape are various.

Table 2.3. Normal cellular composition of SF

SM cells, %		Blood cells, %			Unclassified cells, %
Synoviocytes	Histiocytes	Lymphocytes	Monocytes	Neutrophils	
34.2–37.8	8.9–12.5	37.4–42.6	1.8–3.2	1.2–2.0	8.3–10.1

Blood cells are presented in SF largely by lymphocytes whose concentration is higher than that of any other cells. Only 1/5 of SF lymphocytes are involved in immune reactions.

Monocytes, the most active phagocytes of peripheral blood are found in SF to a lesser extent (by an order of magnitude). They are cells 12–20 μm in diameter with granular protoplasm and the eccentrically located polymorphic (existing in several morphological variants) nucleus having loose inclusions of chromatin.

Neutrophils are found in SF in the least amount. They are one of the forms of granular leucocytes (granulocytes) 9–12 μm in diameter. Neutrophils are responsible for phagocytosis of wear products resulting from joint operation. Determination of the neutrophil content is one the most informative tests that allow inflammatory joint diseases to be differentiated with a high validity.

Up to 10% of SF cells are so-called unclassified cells. Morphological features of these cells are not typical but their content of SF is sufficiently stable, which allows us to isolate them as an individual group. According to data [14], unclassified cells are damaged ones in testing and ultimately degenerated SF cells.

2.3. Immunogenic Properties

Immunology is the science about protective capabilities of organism, his immune system, in other words, the organism ability to resist the effects of damaging agents. Immunogenetics is a branch of immunology dealing with genetic responsibility of immune system factors, tissue compatibility or incompatibility.

Before we start evaluating immunogenic properties of SF we will specify the terms under usage in this discipline.

2.3.1. Terminology

Agents damaging the synovial medium of joints are the substances that are perceived by joint tissues as foreign and cause a specific immune response. They form antibodies or globular proteins of blood plasma. Foreign substances are neutralized by immune reactions, i.e., biochemical interaction of antibodies with respective antigens. The cells responsible for immune response are called immunocytes. They include immune-competent cells and phagocytes. Immune-competent cells are capable of specific interaction (i. e., via immune reactions) with antigens. Phagocytes actively trap foreign living objects (bacteria, cell fragments) and solid particles, e.g., cartilage wear products. With SF involvement the humoral regulation of synovial medium occurs. Humoral regulation is one of the mechanisms of metabolism coordination in the organism that is executed via fluids by means of active substances secreted by cells and tissues. SF provides humoral regulation of the cell protective mechanism in the joint and mass exchange between SM and articular cartilage.

SF immunocytes are derivatives of the hematopoietic system and synovial medium.

Immune-competent cells are presented in SF by lymphocytes of T- and B-types. They arise from stem hematopoietic cells by differentiation. Stem (cambial) cells are parent cells in renewing human tissues. Differentiation is the transformation of identical stem cells into specialized tissue cells in the course of organism development. B-lymphocytes (bone marrow lymphocytes) are formed from stem cells in the bone marrow and involved in immediate immune reactions incipient at the moment of antigen and lymphocyte contact. T-lymphocytes (thymus gland, lymphocytes, thymus-dependent), after their maturation in the bone marrow, are differentiated under the effect of thymosin. T-helpers, T-suppressors, T-killers, T-effectors, and T-amplifiers are distinguished. These names are given according to whether they initiate or inhibit the functions of other cells or act independently [21]. T-lymphocytes participate in delayed immune reactions. Both kinds of immune reactions are the interrelated chains of immune response of synovial medium to antigens.

Phagocytes are macrophages of SM as well so-called activated B-lymphocytes synthesizing immunoglobulins. Immunoglobulins are proteins (glycoproteins) (see below) that possess antibody's activity.

Active substances produced by SM and SF immunocytes are globulins, complement proteins, enzymes, and reactive proteins.

Globulins are simple proteins whose polysaccharide chains are curled up in compact spherical or ellipsoidal structures. SF globulins are bonded to carbons and lipids and insoluble in water. They amount to the third of all proteins found in SF. Most (~ 2/3) SF globulins are gamma-globulins. This globulin fraction is characterized by low electrophoretic mobility in the joint biofield and is a carrier of anti-bacterial and anti-viral antibodies. Gamma-globulins include immunoglobulins. The fragments of the immunoglobulin molecular chain are able to easily rotate relative each other around "hinges" to induce a variety of molecule conformations.

A complement is the system of proteins of fresh blood serum consisting of 9 components, 11 proteins included. Joining the antigen-antibody complex the complement protein produces active substances that cause irreversible damages (lysis) of cellular membranes. Thus the elimination of pathogenic bacteria and cells in the synovial medium is accelerated.

Enzymes are biological catalyzers found in all living cells. In numerous biochemical reactions running in cells, a great number of various enzymes are involved. The International Classification [22] enumerating the working names of most enzymes regulates their hierarchy. SF is characterized by the following kinds of enzymes: adaptive ones accelerate immune reactions with lymphocytes involved; regulatory – their activity is regulated by chemical compounds differing from the substances whose transformations they catalyze; flavoproteides or enzymes of redox reactions; constituents - permanently existing in macrophages; and proteolytic ones that catalyze the proteolysis and peptide lysis.

Reactivity is the property of a living organism to react in a way to environment factors. The reaction of joints to the effects inducing inflammations of synovial medium manifests in specific protein found in SF namely, C-reactive protein included in acute-phase protein group. This protein being an inflammation marker serves an index in diagnosing arthritis of different genesis. Interacting with SF polysaccharides C-reactive protein activates the formation of immune complexes and accelerates antigen-antibody reactions.

2.3.2. Immunological Causes of Diseases

Joint disorders are caused by so-called immunological tolerance, i.e. incapability of synovial medium of ensuring immune response to a certain antigen while maintaining immunological reactivity to other antigens. A disease-inducing antigen is brought by infectious agents, such as bacteria, viruses, and microplasma (bacteria deprived of the cellular wall). In many cases, which are to be further understood, synovial medium does not give a traditional immunological response to a disease-inducing antigen appearing in the joint. Instead of this, SF starts accumulating pathological antibodies that are specifically bonded to the macromolecules of SM proteins and proper joint cartilage similar to antigen molecules. Activation of SF B-lymphocytes precedes the production of these antibodies. Protein content of SF increases owing to globulins and fibrin, a water-insoluble protein absent in normal SF and transforming to fibrinogen. Modified SF composition and structure are responsible for its pathological aggressive character relative to joint tissues. An uncontrollable process of occurrence of immune complexes starts: a pathological antibody found in SF is bonded to the antigen being the protein of proper joint tissues. This results in chronic autoimmune inflammation of joint that is differentiated as rheumatoid arthritis including juvenile, Bekhterev's disease, and diffuse diseases of connective tissues.

Diagnostics of autoimmune joint inflammation needs a laboratory SF analysis to register an increased amount of immunoglobulins, which is detected in SF earlier than in blood. Rheumatoid arthritis is characterized by the presence of rheumatoid factor in SF, namely, antibodies to one of the fragments (a Fc-fragment) of the G-group (Ig G) immunoglobulin. The Fc-fragment governs the passage of antibodies through cell membranes as well a capability of binding the complement and fixing in protoplasm. Ig G is one of five immunoglobulin classes consisting of so-called effector molecules, i.e., molecules containing effector centers. The latter are responsible for protein binding and activation of antibody metabolism.

In rheumatoid arthritis, a synoviocytogram of effusion shows an increased concentration of microphages and polynuclear (containing several nuclei) cells. This indicates the activation of humoral and cellular forms of immune response in the joint. In 95% of joint rheumatoid arthritis, rhagocytes are revealed in SF. They are phagocytes (granulocytes) with the cytoplasm filled with grape-like clusters of granules including rheumatoid factor. Their function is to entrap and digest foreign particles, primarily, bacteria, and be involved in immunological reactions. In the leucocytes of SF taken from arthritis-affected joints the following substances demonstrate an increased activity:

- Immunoglobulins G and M; the latter consists of effector molecules serving receptors for B-lymphocytes, which causes an early anti-infectious response of SF;
- Chromatin or the matter of the cellular nucleus containing genetic material.

Other signs of SF leukocyte activation in rheumatoid arthritis are as follows: eccentric arrangement of the cell nuclei and their consolidation; manifestation of endoplasmatic net, namely, a system of cytoplasm channels in which biosynthesis of active substances occurs; increasing concentration of lysosomes, namely, cellular enzyme-containing organelles, and mitochondria or organelles that provide leucocytes with energy.

In autoimmune joint inflammation, the aggregates (rosettes) of immune complexes such as lymphocytic antigen–macrophagal antibody are formed in SF cell protoplasm. Further elimination of antigens initiates the immune response of joint synovial medium as delayed- or immediate-type allergic reactions. During first months of immune joint inflammation T-lymphocytes prevail, then the ratio of T-and B-cells becomes a norm. Fibroblasts transform to ovular cells with coarse nuclei and several small nuclei (dense components of a cell nucleus) provided with cilia, which indicate their metabolic and secretory activity.

Reliable signs of autoimmune inflammation in joint are as follows:

- cytosis or an increased cellular element content of SF;
- neutrophilosis or an increased concentration of neutrophilous granulocytes;
- occurrence of rhagocytes;
- an increased amount in SF of proteoglycans of acid phosphatases, i.e., enzymes that regulate the exchange of phosphates in the joint.

Therefore, autoimmune joint inflammation is an uncontrollable process of occurrence of immune complexes that consist of pathological antibodies and are perceived as antigens of the proteins of the proper joint.

2.3.3. Group Types of Synovial Fluid

The up-to-date level of prophylaxis and treatment of degenerative joint diseases is governed by, first, conservative treatment (by medication including chondroprotectors, i.e., drugs that prevent the cartilage from destruction and wear) and, second, surgery (arthroplasty or joint replacement). Search for SF substitutes (the stages are described in Chapter 5) identical to synovia and biocompatible with human organism assumes the treatment of joints using donor SF. As mentioned above, SF is based on blood dialysate. Therefore, the problem of the substitute tissue compatibility is the key problem in chondroprotection with donor SF.

Blood groups discovered in 1900 by K. Landsteiner, a Vienna physician and Noble prize winner (1930), formed the grounds of immune hematology – a section in medicine dealing with the study of immune mechanisms of blood diseases and methods for their diagnostics, treatment, and prophylaxis based on immunological reactions. It has resulted in new therapeutic methods and development of [23]:

- transfusiology, a division of clinical medicine that studies the problems of transfusing blood and its preparations including blood- and plasma-substituting fluids;
- transplantology, a division of biology and medicine that studies the problems of transplantation and develops methods for organ and tissue conservation, production, and application of artificial organs;

- transfusion immunology studying the genetic conditionality of organism state that may occur in intravenous injections of fluids.

An individual nature of tissues and fluids in the human organism is governed by their antigens. Presently, more than 250 antigens of blood groups are known. They are united in 25 systems localized on the surface of complex proteins and polysaccharides of the erythrocyte membrane [24]. The molecules on the erythrocyte surface are recognized as antigens by the immune system of people who do not have such structures on their erythrocytes. Modern medicine uses the system of blood groups AB0 according to which there are four main structural types of polysaccharide precursor chains to form antigens A or B. The variant of group 0 does not carry antigens owing to short inactive protein macromolecules.

Rhesus antigens are localized in the erythrocyte membrane in the form of macromolecular loops piercing it through. A physiological role of rhesus system proteins is not fully understood although the rhesus factor takes an important part in transfusiology: heteroimmunization with the rhesus factor, namely, production of anti-rhesus antibodies in recipient's organism (a man who receives blood from a donor) with positive erythrocytes contained in the donor blood may cause hemolysis (decomposition) of erythrocytes and recipient's death. As a rule, such reaction occurs in the repeated contact of the rhesus-negative organism with rhesus-positive erythrocytes.

Group antigens A and B were revealed in biological fluids, that is, saliva, gastric juice, sperm, and blood including its erythrocytes and plasma [25]. Evidently, SF also must have a group, however, the data is absent in modern medical literature. Below the results of the pioneer experimental study of SF groups and compatibility are presented.

The SF for the experimental studies was taken during diagnostic punctures or operations on knee joints from patients (with their consent) with a traumatic pathology and non-immune synovitis. In standard clinical-laboratory examination, the rhesus-factor and AB0 blood groups of the patients were determined (using the set of standard hemagglutinating sera). There were studied the SF samples taken from the patients having I–IV blood groups and both positive and negative rhesus (Rh+ and Rh–) were studied. Erythrocyte masses of I–IV blood groups with Rh+ and Rh– rhesus factors produced for transfusion at the blood transfusion station were used as test antigens.

In order to determine the group of SF a technique similar to blood group determination was used. It consists in direct hemagglutination on the surface with standard hemagglutinating sera. Instead of sera, the SF samples taken from patients having I–IV blood groups and Rh+ and Rh– were used. 2–3 drops of the SF sample were placed in the grooves of the white plate, and then 0.01 ml of erythrocytes of the blood under testing was added after which the fluids were mixed. Mixing was complicated by high SF viscosity. To reduce it, 2–3 drops of isotonic (0.9%) sodium chloride solution were added and once mixed, the reaction in the samples was observed.

The compatibility of SF and erythrocytes by rhesus factor, is determined using the 33% solution of Polyglucinum (the compatibility of donor's erythrocytes and recipient's blood serum is determined in a similar way [26]). The drops of SF, Polyglucinum, and blood of different groups and rhesus were placed in a test tube. Upon mixing, an isotonic sodium chloride solution was added to the mixture and then the reaction of component compatibility was estimated. All the experiments were executed at a room temperature of 18–22 °C.

Table 2.4 shows the results of immunological reactions of SF with erythrocytes of different blood groups. Ac positive reaction occurred in the form of erythrocyte agglutination. Agglutination is the gluing and precipitation from homogeneous suspensions of antigen-carrying cells under the action of specific antibodies, namely, agglutinins. In mixing SF and erythrocytes, the reaction was considered negative if the test looked like a sediment-free homogeneous fluid uniformly colored in red.

Table 2.4. The result of SF reaction of the patient group under study with erythrocytes of I–IV blood groups Rh+ and Rh–

Erythrocyte mass (antigens)		Synovia (antigens)							
		0 (I), αβ		A (II), β		B (III), α		AB (IV), 0	
		Rh+	Rh–	Rh+	Rh–	Rh+	Rh–	Rh+	Rh–
0 (I)	Rh+	–	–	–	–	–	–	–	–
	Rh–	–	–	–	–	–	–	–	–
A (II)	Rh+	+	+	–	–	+	+	–	–
	Rh–	+	+	–	–	+	+	–	–
B (III)	Rh+	+	+	+	+	–	–	–	–
	Rh–	+	+	+	+	–	–	–	–
AB (IV)	Rh+	+	+	+	+	+	+	–	–
	Rh–	+	+	+	+	+	+	–	–

Note: «+» and «–» are positive and negative reactions.

The agglutination on mixing of SF with erythrocyte mass differs from that of erythrocytes with serum because the agglutinates in SF are of small size (of a 10–100 μm order) and look like fine sand particles in contrast to flocculent agglutinates of erythrocytes in serum.

As follows from Table 2.4, the reactions of SF with erythrocytes are similar to the reactions of standard hemagglutinating sera with erythrocytes of different groups. In order to initiate agglutination of erythrocyte mass of a certain group SF should contain antibodies against the antigens of these erythrocytes. The fact that group II erythrocytes are agglutinated by the synovia belonging to people with blood groups I and III indicates the presence of antibodies in their SF – α-agglutinates – against antigen A. The agglutination of group III erythrocytes with the synovia of people with blood groups I and II points to the presence in SF of β-agglutinins against antigen B. Hence, in SF of people with group I blood there are α- and β-agglutinins, in the people having group II blood – β, and in the people having group III blood there are α-agglutinins. The presence of α or β antibodies (or α and β) in SF of groups I, II, and III causes the positive reaction with erythrocytes of group IV blood containing A and B antigens. The synovia of the people having group IV blood that gives the negative reaction with erythrocytes of all groups, the same as plasma, does not contain antibodies to antigens A and B. A long-term reaction (up to 10 min) of SF antibodies with erythrocyte antigens is primarily due to a higher SF viscosity as compared to serum.

Identical reactions of Rh+ and Rh– erythrocytes of each blood group are detected in the people with the same blood groups but different rhesus-factors. Consequently, the rhesus of SF and erythrocytes does not affect the results in the groups. The cause is that SF being a blood dialysate with the positive rhesus factor does not contain anti-rhesus antibodies, therefore on mixing with both Rh+ and Rh– erythrocytes the SF reaction to the rhesus antigen must be negative. On the other hand, SF of the people with the negative rhesus factor also does not have anti-rhesus antibodies, which resulted in a negative reaction of SF of the people with Rh+ blood. One can assume that only in the case of previous immunization of a Rh– person with Rh+ blood his/her SF (the same as in blood serum) will contain anti-rhesus antibodies, and only in this case one may expect a positive reaction of Rh– SF with Rh+ erythrocytes in the same blood group. The Polyglucinum test confirmed the absence of anti-rhesus antibodies in the tested SF samples.

In the SF – erythrocyte compatibility test by Rh-factor, the samples were compatible in all cases, that is, the fluid in the test tube was bright-red free of sediment and flakes, uniformly colored, and opalescent.

The findings reported indicate that human SF has the same set of group antibodies as blood serum and similarly to serum it can be involved in the tissue immune response. Four AB0 groups of SF identical to four blood groups were set. It is shown that a human SF group corresponds to a blood group. The tissue (group) compatibility of donor's and recipient's synovia can serve an evidence of the biocompatibility of human SF-based chondroprotectors and of the possibility of using donor SF in joint treatment.

2.4. The Spatial Structure

SF has a multicomponent chemical composition including aqueous solutions of salts, proteins (albumins, globulins, and polysaccharides) hyaluronate, up to 30 names of enzymes, urea, lipids, and glucose [1, 2, 5, 6, 11, 14, 19]. As shown above, the SF functions are so various that they hardly could be performed by mechanical mixing of the above-mentioned components. Even the existence itself of such mixture is hardly probable in terms of classical and colloidal chemistry. In the liquid phase the dissimilar components will interact physically and chemically forming Van der Waals, hydrogen, covalent, and some other chemical bonds. In arthrological literature there are a lot of data on the ordered distribution of the SF components at different structural levels.

Thus, hyaluronate can be found in SF as long (molecular weight 10^7) and shorter (10^6) chains with positively charged groups distributed along the chain [14]. This assumes possibility of electric interactions during SF structure formation. The conformation of hyaluronic acid molecules is mainly a loose ball 300–800 nm in diameter. However, in the 1960s the idea was advanced [27] that the SF macromolecules are cross-linked and form spatial "cell" binding water in great amounts. Hyaluronic acid forms a complex compound with albumins known as mucin. The division of strong molecular mucin aggregates into components meets serious methodological difficulties [28]. This protein-polysaccharide complex is negatively charged and tends to spherical configuration in solution.

The structure of the lubricating SF layer that separates the cartilage surfaces in the joint becomes three-dimensional and therefore has a highly elastic gel consistency [9]. In its formation protein-polysaccharide globules that form a spatial net are involved [29]. The availability of the SF structures bound physicochemically is supported by the results of spectrophotometry of synovial effusion samples [30]. Variations in optical density of SF proteins make it possible to differentiate pigmented villonodular synovitis and synovitis of traumatic and rheumatoid etiology.

Nevertheless, the monitoring of SF structure has not been introduced in clinical practice mainly because of methodological reasons. Standard techniques of SF analysis aim to determine the chemical and cellular composition of synovia whereas techniques to control the structural SF state have not been developed. In work [31] the idea is put forward to measure 11 characteristics of SF (lymphocyte number, rheumatoid factor, protein fraction, etc.) as an alternative to the structural investigation of SF. Then the data are processed and analyzed by a computer. Qualitatively new concepts about the SF structure emerged during late 1980s – mid-1990s upon revealing liquid crystalline phase in it [32] that combines the structural order of solid and mobility of liquid. Initially, the liquid crystal phase was recorded with temperature variation of the dried SF films, which allowed a temperature range for a mesophase to be set [33]. Afterwards, it was confirmed through heating SF samples placed between crossed microscope polaroids and measuring the intensity of the light stream passing through.

Physically, all fluids have a certain degree of order of atomic-molecular structure. The closest neighbors of each fluid molecule are placed in an order so that their number and mutual arrangement are averagely identical in all molecules. This means that fluids are characterized by short-range order. Crystals are characterized by long-range order in particle arrangement: a probability of an atom to be found outside the lattice node is close to zero, i.e., almost all atoms are found in fixed positions. In a fluid, an atom can be found at different distances from other atoms with lower or higher probability. Away from the boiling temperature, the heat motion of particles refers to irregular oscillations at a mean frequency close to particle oscillations in crystals and amplitude governed by the fluid "free volume". SF has an individual structure irregular for low-molecular fluids. This allows combination of the properties of solids (elasticity, low viscosity, significant carrying capacity of the lubricating layer) and fluids (fluidity). The multilevel hierarchic structure makes it possible to perform the functions listed in 1.2.2 that are characteristic of a living mulicellular organism to a larger degree than of fluid filling the joint cavity. The similar structure is to a certain degree characteristic of all biological fluids (blood, lymph, gland secrets, etc.). This formed the grounds for appearance in the 1990s of a discipline called "mechanics of biological fluids" [35]. It is a division of biology wherein concepts, methodology, and tools of hydromechanics are applied to study biological phenomena. Hydromechanics is a division of mechanics to study equilibrium and motion of fluids.

Therefore, SF is a unique liquid medium characterized by not only a short- but also long-range order to a certain degree. SF consists of complex (coordination) chemical compounds associated in supermolecular aggregates that form several stages of the spatial structure. The multilevel SF structure makes it low-informative when applying the methods of experimental physics to study atomic-molecular structure of the liquid phase including X-ray structural analysis, electronography, and neutronography. These highly specialized methods are inefficient when dealing with the physicochemical SF structure and retrieving data at each hierarchic level. Besides, their wide application in clinical practice is still unachievable.

The properties of SF as a medium with unusual biophysical properties protecting the cartilage from mechanical damages and demonstrating liquid-crystal order substantiate the hypothesis of the unique chemical, physical, and biological nature of this condensed body. Below they will be discussed in detail.

2.5. Synovia as a Chondroprotector

According to present-day views on the synovial medium, joint motion causes the circulation of the liquid phase found in cartilage pores [32, 36, 37] thus ensuring its normal biochemical functioning. It is mixed with SF and again absorbed by the cartilage. The process is of importance for maintaining the life of cartilage tissue since the fluid to be absorbed contains nutrients necessary for chondrocytes. The concept was supported by the experimental findings *in vivo*, during which the synovial joint underwent a permanent compressing load for a long time. As reported elsewhere [37] the permanent compression of the joint not only prevents the delivery of SF to the friction surface but also stops the diffusion of the liquid phase in the intercellular substance of cartilage matrix. As a result, chondrocytes die and the liquid phase substance degenerates since the cartilage deformation breaks down the normal transfer mechanism of fluid. In osteoarthritis, limitation of joint movement can lead to similar degenerative processes of articular cartilage. Early sites of tissue degeneration are observed in those joint regions that did not undergo mechanical effects arising in body movement [36, 38].

In line with recent views [14, 39], SF functions as a chondroprotector owing to a load-depending origin of the viscosity of its lubricating layer on the cartilage surface. This happens because SF is a complex compound containing hyaluronic acid along with protein (see Table 2.1). The following experiment indicates that hyaluronic acid is responsible for SF viscosity. In heating, the SF sample was mixed with tripsin, that is, a proteolytic enzyme catalyzing the hydrolytic proteolysis and decomposition of peptides (organic substances consisting of peptide-bound amino acid residues). If the SF viscosity were only governed by the properties of protein macromolecules, it would decrease essentially upon such treatment. However, the mixture viscosity remained at the same level. The similar experiment was repeated with adding hyaluronidase, that is, the enzyme mentioned in 2.1 that catalyzes hydrolysis of hyaluronic acid. This resulted in a sharp decrease in SF viscosity becoming close to that for water [40]. The experimental findings are presented in Fig. 2.1., *a*.

As has been found earlier [38, 41], the viscosity of original SF exponentially decreases with increasing shear rate (*a*) from a *max* value. A similar dependence is characteristic of SF depolymerized by hyaluronidase as well, but in this case the viscosity is by an order and a half lower indicating that this is hyaluronic acid that makes SF a pseudo-elastic thixotropic medium (thixotropy is a capability of disperse systems of recovering their original structure broken down under mechanical effects).

In the 1950s, orthopedists related a high SF lubricity to thixotropy. Low friction in joints was attributed to formation of thixotropic adsorption layers on the cartilage surface similar to the SA surface layers [10, 13]. However, the tribotest results of the SF-lubricated cartilage–glass pair shown in Fig. 2.1, *b* [42] demonstrate an insignificant influence of hyaluronic acid on cartilage friction. As shown previously, the purified hyaluronic acid does not display any significant lubricity [43]. This means that the function of the SF protein – polysaccharide complex is not just being a lubricating medium in synovial joints.

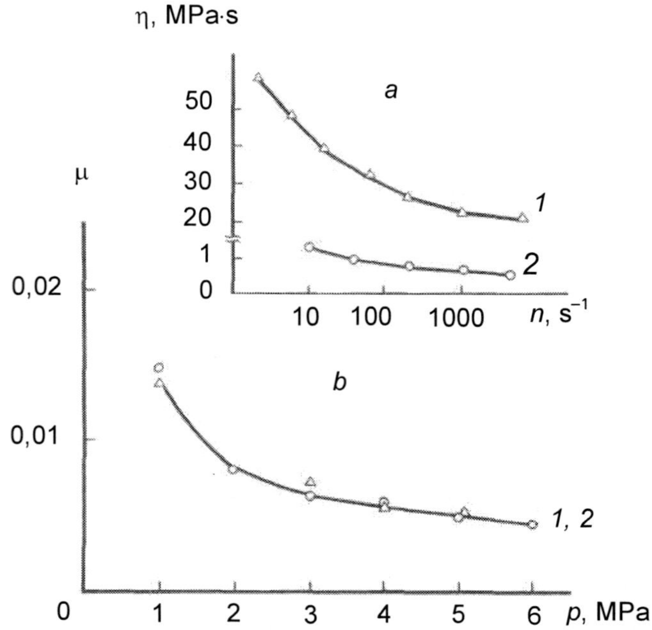

Figure 2.1. SF viscosity vs. shear rate (*a*) and coefficient of friction vs. load *(b)*. 1 – original SF; 2 – SF mixed with hyaluronidase.

Thus a hypothesis put forward in the 1960s was supported that the macromolecular complexes of hyaluronic acid and proteins were responsible for SF viscoelasticity and absorbing effect of its lubricating layer. It is supported by the experimentally revealed three-dimensional networks consisting of protein–polysaccharide globules that interact with each other making SF gelatinous under static conditions [39, 44]. The rheological properties of the structure can be described using the Kelvin-Voigt model, namely, the simplest model of a viscoelastic polymeric body (Fig. 2.2). It consists of a spring with rigidity module G and a connected in parallel damper filled with a fluid of viscosity η [45]. Displacement of points *A* and *B* in the model along the normal simulates deformation γ of the SF layer and force *F* applied to the model is analogous to stresses τ arising in the SF layer. The rheological equation of model state and model-simulated SF layer state has the following form

$$\tau = G\gamma + \eta(d\gamma/dt),$$

where t is time. Under instantaneous loading with constant stress τ = const the deformation in the layer occurs with delay by the law

$$\gamma = \gamma_0(1-e^{-t/\theta}),$$

where $\gamma_0 = \lim\gamma = t/G$ при $t \rightarrow \infty$, and $\theta = \eta/G$ is the so-called delay time. If γ = const, then τ = const, that is, the stress relaxation time in the SF layer remains infinitely large. At alternating layer deformations the phase difference between τ and γ increases with increasing oscillation frequency or delay time. Upon removing external load F the parameters of the SF layer are recovered elastically without irreversible deformations.

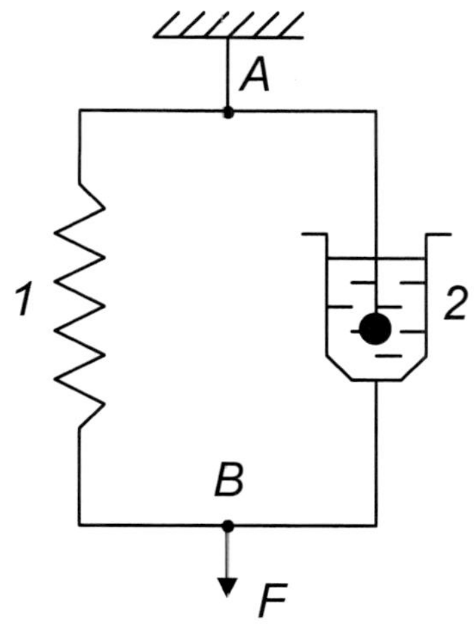

Figure 2.2. Kelvin-Voigt model. *1* – spring; *2* – damper.

Hyaluronic acid molecules are adsorbed on the cartilage surface and form a surface layer to protect the cartilage against mechanical damages. Increasing load to the joint causes the filtration of low-molecular SF components in the cartilage micropores. The lubricating layer that separates the cartilage surfaces is enriched by hyaluronate owing to which the three-dimensional structure occurs in the gelatinous layer of a fairly high carrying capacity [46]. The layer in combination with elastically deformable cartilage provides the congruency of the friction surfaces in the loaded moving joint. Thus the biomechanical function of SF is ensured that protects the cartilage against excessive loads and deformations.

SF with the broken rheological properties is evidently incapable of executing the functions of chondroprotector. This occurs in rheumatoid arthritis and osteoarthrosis deformans. In pathogenesis of the latter increased loads to joint play the crucial role since they cause the depolymerization of proteoglycans of cartilage matrix which results in decreasing cartilage elasticity and breaking normal running of diffusion [47, 48]. SF with the modified rheological properties flows out from the cartilage micropores and is incapable of providing chondroprotection and damping. Joint functioning is accompanied by microtraumatization of cartilages that become low-elastic, dry, and less wear-resistant [49]. Pathogenesis of rheumatoid arthritis includes an increase in the catabolic phase of metabolism (catabolism is the set of biochemical reactions of formation of simple substances from more complex ones), activation of proteolytic enzymes, accelerated decomposition of cartilage proteoglycans, depolymerization of hyaluronic acid, and reduction of its concentration in SF [43, 50], after which SF loses most of its protective functions.

2.6. Biophysical Properties

Biophysics deals with physical and physicochemical phenomena in living organisms, structure and properties of biopolymers, and influence of physical factors on living systems. Fundamental findings by I.M. Sechenov, S.P. Botkin, I.P. Pavlov as well next generations of physiologists, primarily, Noble winners A.F. Huxley, A.L. Hodgkin (England), and J.C. Eccles (Australia) concerned the electromagnetic regulation of physiological processes ensuring the coordinated activities of all organism systems and their adaptation to changing environmental conditions. Functioning of joints, their adaptation to changing environmental conditions and treatment are regulated by proper biophysical fields in the organism that are much faster than the streams of biological fluids in tissues.

Joint tissues as any biological system perceive and generate electromagnetic fields [51]. The electromagnetic fields have an energetic effect on the synovial medium and govern biophysical mechanisms according to which SF performs its specific functions in the organism. This is possible because SF possesses specific properties responsible for its susceptibility to bioelectrical potentials and magnetic field of the joint. The latter is produced by magnetic moments of protein molecules and movement in the tissue structures of biological fluids referring to electrolytes [52].

2.6.1. The Main Concepts

Susceptibility of synovial medium to biophysical fields is characterized by the following parameters.

Electric conductivity is the ability of SF and tissues to conduct an electric current owing to movable charged particles (current or charge carriers) available in them. In SF the charge carriers are, first, electrolyte ions that are associated in a healthy joint physically and chemically with protein structures forming complex compounds, and, second, polar molecules of proteins, polysaccharides, hyaluronates, enzymes, urea, and glucose. Polarity is orientation of organism structures in space resulting in morphological distinctions at the opposite ends (sides) of cells, tissues, and organs. Most polar macromolecules are associated in permolecular agglomerates that, although carrying a nonequilibrium electric charge, have a limited mobility in disperse SF due to large sizes and mutual physicochemical bonds. The specific electric conductivity of organism fluids including SF is within σ = 0.5–2.0 cm/m. This means that SF refers to semiconductors occupying a region of 10^{-8} cm/m < σ <10^{6} cm/m with dielectrics from the left (σ <10^{-8} cm/m), and conductors from the right (σ>10^{6} cm/m).

Dielectric permeability ε is a measure showing how many times force of cooperation of two electric charges in an environment is less than that in vacuum. Dielectric polarization is characterized by dielectric permeability. Polarization is the displacement of electric charges in a dielectric under exposure to electric field. It occurs owing to shear of ions relative each other or orientation of electric dipoles existing in the substance in the absence of electric field. Electric dipole is a set of two point electric charges equal in value and opposite in sign and located at a distance from each other. Dipole moment is a physical measure to characterizes dipole properties. Dielectric susceptibility is the proportionality coefficient χ between polarization P of a medium (dipole moment of unit volume) and intensity E of external electric field: $P = \chi E$. Electrets are dielectrics that maintain polarization for a long time arising in their hardening in a powerful electric field. Some molecules that make up electrets have dipole electric moments. The external field orients them and the substance hardening fixes the orientation of the dipoles. At first sight, this reasoning does not refer to SF since it, first, does not belong to dielectrics and, second, exists in the liquid phase. However, below we will show that this is far from being true.

The magnetic moment is a vector value characterizing a substance as a source of magnetic field. Magnetization is the ratio of magnetic moment M of the substance to its volume: $J = M/V$. In the course of magnetization, magnetization J of the substance increases with increasing intensity H of external magnetic field. Magnetic induction B is the mean resulting magnetic field in the substance: $B = \mu_0(H+J)$, where μ_0 is magnetic constant or magnetic permeability of vacuum. Magnetic permeability of substance (or medium) characterizes the relation between magnetic induction B and magnetic field intensity in a substance: $\mu = B/(\mu_0 H)$. Magnetic susceptibility of substance is $æ = J/H$. Magnetic permeability is related to magnetic susceptibility in the following way: $\mu = 1 + æ$. Organism tissues and fluids are diamagnetic, i.e., they possess negative magnetic susceptibility $æ<0$. This means that they are magnetized weakly in the external magnetic field (æ of SF is of order minus 10^{-6}–10^{-5}) in the direction being opposite to the field direction. Magnetic permeability of a healthy SF is $\mu = 0.99995$ [53]. Magnetic properties and magnetic fields produced by SF and other biological objects are called biomagnetism. The magnetic field of a living organism has an effect on SF and other biological systems to be found in it. These effects are studied in magnetobiology, a division of biophysics.

Alternating electromagnetic fields produce oscillations of ions and displacements of SF dipole molecules with the polarization proportional to the electric field intensity and depending on its frequency and molecule size. As the alternating current is transmitted through organism fluids its strength advances the stress applied [51]. This means that the capacitive impedance of SF (it characterizes the resistance of SF electric capacity to alternating current, i.e. its capability of holding electric charge) is larger than its inductive impedance. Inductive impedance characterizes the impedance of SF inductivity, i.e., its magnetic properties, to alternating current. Therefore, SF is a medium having the properties of both a conductor (electrolyte) and a dielectric. Polarization of a dielectric in the external electric field is time-dependent. Electric properties of such substances are simulated by means of so-called equivalent electric circuits that consist of resistors characterized by active resistance and condenser or the carriers of capacitive impedance. The equivalent electric circuit shown in Fig. 2.3 can serve a SF model [51]. Relaxation, i.e., equilibrium setting in current impulse transmitted through the chain is described by the relations identical to those used for the relaxation of mechanical stresses in the model shown in Fig. 2.2.

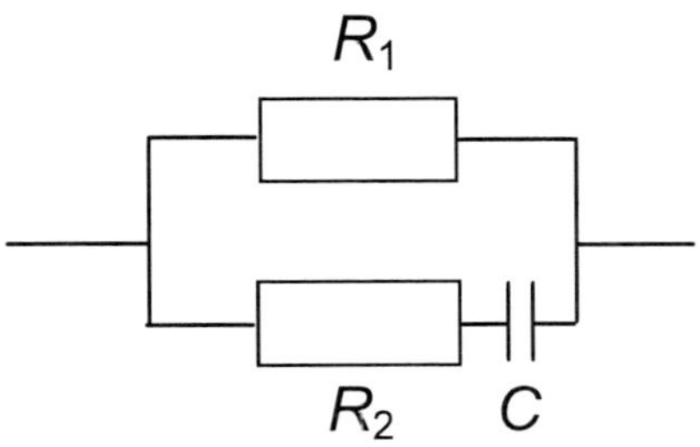

Figure 2.3. Electric model of SF. R1 and R2 are resistors, C is a condenser.

Dependence of the full electric impedance (Z) on frequency (ω) of electric current corresponds to the similar experimental dependence obtained on the SF samples. Analysis of the dependence Z(ω) for the model shows that its electrical capacity and, hence, dielectric permeability and polarization are constant only at ω = const and in a general case decrease with increasing frequency. The same regularities are characteristic of SF as well. This is natural regarding that the SF polarization delay relative to variations in the electric field intensity is governed by the polarization mechanism. In SF, water molecules and unbound ions of a low mass are polarized most quickly. Protein macromolecules are polarized more slowly and permolecular complexes consisting of several macromolecules are polarized even more slowly. With increasing ω less and less SF structures will react to variations in the electric field and polarization P will be progressively less. Respectively, dielectric permeability ε and electric capacity C decrease, which cause the growth of capacitive impedance and full electric resistance of SF.

The listed regularities indicate that the biophysical field of the joint is responsible for essential variations in the parameters of SF component interaction and, consequently, tribological, trophic, metabolic, and barrier functioning in the joint. The joint biofield exerts an influence on SF physicochemical structure at different hierarchic levels as well as its enzymatic activity [53].

2.6.2. Electromechanical Aspects of Synovia Circulation

Sliding of bone articular ends leading to cartilage deformation is accompanied by electromechanical processes [54]. One of them is occurrence of a so-called current potential in circulation of anion-containing SF in the cartilage tissue micropores carrying the negative charge. Mainly Na^{+} and Ca^{++} ions are involved in the electrodynamic process. The next process is electrostatic interaction on the molecular level between the polar components of the cartilage tissue, that is, proteoglycan–proteoglycan and proteoglycan–collagen. Kinetics of these electromechanical processes depends on the structure of porous cartilage system and governs the parameters of SF transportation in it.

The bioelectrical properties of cartilage were for the first time studied in the USA by a biophysist A. Maroudas who put forward a hypothesis about cartilage functioning as an ion-exchange membrane [55]. Current potential ΔE arises in the cartilage matrix carrying the polarization charge due to movement of ions in micropores in the SF convective flow. Its experimentally measured value is from 0.4 to 0.6 mV in human cartilage at SF pressure difference Δp = 0.1 MPa. Afterwards it was found that the current potential linearly depends on the pressure difference and at Δp = 1.72 MPa ΔE = 5.4 mV [56]. Maroudas determined that cartilage permeability was in inverse proportion to its charge density [57], i.e., it was in line with the classic formula [58]:

$$\Delta E = \frac{FkC}{\partial \ell} \Delta p ,$$

where F is Faraday constant, C is the density of negative charge in cartilage; æ is specific conductivity, and k is cartilage permeability. In the course of the experiments, the cartilage sample carrying polarization charge was compressed to increase the charge density. Later on, the technique was used as a tool to study the charge density distribution in tissues.

Occurrence of ΔE causes a "reverse current" of SF in cartilage micropores. The calculation reported in [56] shows an increase in SF current potential to cause decreasing cartilage permeability by 50 % at high pressure differences of physiological solution. The dependence of ΔE on pH and ion strength of the solution indicates that the current potential mainly refers to electrokinetic parameters [59].

Once the cartilage is immersed in the electrolyte, tensile stresses arise in micropore walls [60] from transformation of double electric layer at the cartilage-electrolyte boundary and repulsion forces between them. This happens because of ion diffusion into the cartilage matrix, predominantly into proteoglycan components of the collagen matrix that swallows and undergoes tensile stresses. Swallowing depends on the concentration and valence of ions in the electrolyte. Diffusion is responsible for the transformation of the double electric layer, since ions screen the charged groups of molecules on the micropore walls. Ion H^+ diffusion into the cartilage-modeling collagen film is described by the following equation [61]:

$$\frac{dC_{H^+}}{dt}\left[1+\frac{KB}{\left(K+C_{H^+}\right)^2}\right]=D_{H^+}\left(\frac{d^2C_{H^+}}{dx^2}\right), \tag{2.1}$$

where C_{H+} is concentration of diffused ions H^+ in the film, K is a constant, B is the number of ion bonds with the film, $D_H^{\ +}$ is a diffusion coefficient. When deriving the equation we assume that ions H^+ are in equilibrium with polar COO^- and $NH_3^{\ +}$ groups fixed in the film.

Fourier transforms was used to find the time Eq. (2.1) upon which the steady-state diffusion occurs in the film:

$$\tau = D_{H^+}\left[1+\frac{KB}{\left(K+C_{H^0}\right)^2}\right]^{-1}, \tag{2.2}$$

where $C_H^{\ 0}$ is the concentration of neutralized ions H^+ in the film. From Eq. (2.2) we can derive K, $D_H^{\ +}$, and concentration of the bonds arising in the films that are able to dissociate.

In work [60] this approach was used to evaluate the binding of ions Ca^{++} in the cartilage. Unfortunately, Eqs. (2.1) and (2.2) do not comprise the values of sample deformation and parameters of the bulk fluid flow in it. A correct electromechanical theory of SF circulation in cartilage does not still exist. Presently, the rational approach to studying these systems is in performing plain experiments on differential investigation of electromechanical and physicochemical phenomena accompanying the flow of biological fluids in microcappilaries and in creating a biophysical model for their description. This in combination with the quantitative control of biophysical modifications in the tissue remains the major problem in understanding the nature of normal and pathological states of cartilage and arthritis etiology [54].

2.6.3. Quasi-Electret State of SF

The method for electret-thermal analysis (ETA) has emerged in the physics of dielectrics to determine mechanisms and parameters of electric polarization of solids. The technique for registering the nonequilibrium distribution of electric charges in polymer films is regulated by the Russian State Standard [62]. In solid samples of tissues and frozen blood, the quasi-electret effect has been revealed as a characteristic of such biological substances as collagen, polysaccharides [63], hemoglobin, and myoglobin [64]. The effect is similar to the electret effect. The quasi-electret effect is displayed by the human blood found in the liquid phase [65].

The ETA method was used to examine SF taken from conditionally healthy people with no knee joint pathology detected during diagnostic arthroscopy. The idea of the experiment was as follows. A SF drop was placed between the couple of electrodes so that the SF layer wetted and separated them. In heating of this cell, the SF structures found at different hierarchic levels were broken. First weak van der Waals bonds were broken down that provided intermolecular cooperation of the permolecular SF structures. With temperature elevation, stronger coordination bonds in permolecular structures were broken, and finally – strong covalent and ionic bonds existing in the macromolecules of proteins, peptides, and hyaluronate went. Breakage of each type of bonds occurs, first, at a definite temperature characteristic of just this bond, and second, is accompanied by the liberation of charge carriers, whose number and polarity also correspond to a type of bond. At the potential difference in the cell available, the charge carriers move to electrodes and the current flows in the external circuit closing the electrodes. The temperature dependence of the current is a spectrum of thermostimulated currents (TSC). Analysis of TSC spectra provides information about the mechanisms responsible for the development of quasi-electret effect in SF samples. The ETA technique is described in more detail in 4.8.

The TSC spectrum taken from the arthritis-affected joint SF was first presented in [66]. In Fig. 2.4 the spectrum of “a conventionally healthy” SF is shown. It has two peaks corresponding to the breaks of three types of bonds in the synovia structure [67].

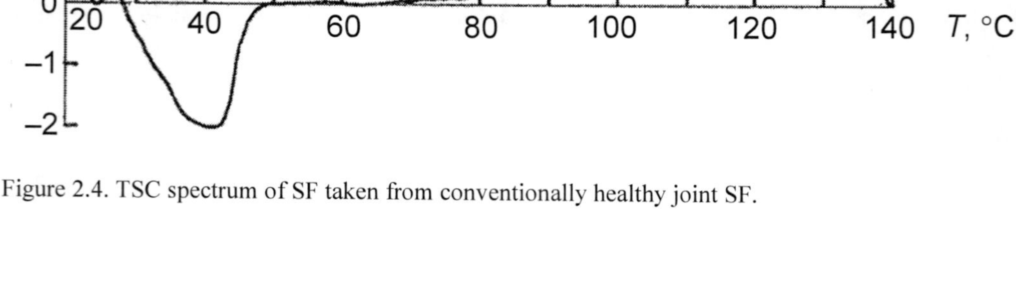

Figure 2.4. TSC spectrum of SF taken from conventionally healthy joint SF.

The low-temperature peak of negative charge relaxation is located within T = 35–50 °C. It corresponds to thermally stimulated breaking of coordination structures that consist of protein structures surrounded by hydrate membranes. The latter arise from associating water molecules with polar fragments of macromolecules via hydrogen bonds [63]. Activation energy of the charge relaxation corresponding to the peak was found by the Garlic-Gibson method [68] by the slope of the initial part of the curve $I(T)$. It is W = 0.25–0.45 eV, which coincides with the breakage energy of hydrogen bonds. As shown elsewhere [66], the charges are liberated within the same temperature range to accompany the heat rearrangement of SF liquid-crystal structures based on cholesterol derivatives [40].

The medium-temperature peak (T = 80–100 °C) of positive charge relaxation seemingly corresponds to the destruction of protein-polysaccharide complex compounds, permolecular protein structures, and irreversible changes in tertiary and in part secondary structure of protein macromolecular spirals not accompanied by the rapture of the polypeptide chain. The activation energy of charge relaxation corresponding to this peak essentially coincides with the activation energy of the above-said processes and falls within W = 0.5–0.7 eV [69, 70].

The most intensive peak corresponds to 110–120 °C. It is in part overlapped by the medium-temperature peak forming a double peak and corresponds to the phase transition in the SF protein component giving rise to solid phase [70]. The thermooxidative destruction of protein macromolecules is followed by the charge liberation responsible for the appearance of the peak.

In friction, mechanical loading of the lubricating layer results in the destruction of the initial SF structure at all hierarchic levels. This is supported by the lowered peaks on the synovia TSC spectrum taken from the friction zone of the pendulum tribometer upon 2-hour operation [71]. The macromolecules and permolecular masses of protein structures are damaged most of all whereas the specific layer-to-layer structure of the mesophase is maintained in friction. It can be judged by an insignificant lowering of the low-temperature peak.

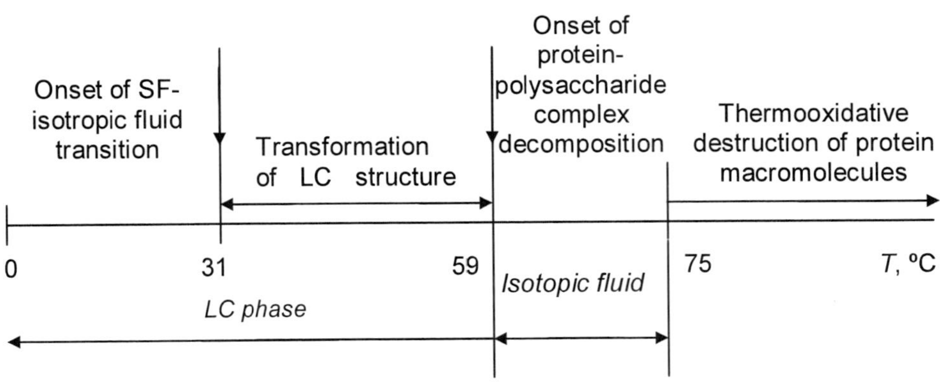

Figure 2.5. Diagram of temperature transitions in synovial.

Based on the analysis of the TSC spectra and study results of phase transitions in the cholesterol mesophase [34] the temperature variation in SF structure due to rearrangement of the liquid-crystal SF phase and thermodestruction of protein macromolecules can be presented in the following way (Fig. 2.5). At $T \sim 31$ °C – clarification temperature - the mesophase starts melting and the LC component is transformed into a common isotropic fluid. The process lasts up to T ~ 59 °C, namely, the onset of destruction of protein-polysaccharide complexes. Beginning from T = 75 °C thermodestruction of protein and polypeptide macromolecules occurs and the SF structure is totally broken at all levels.

Within the range of physiological temperatures of a human body, SF is an anisotropic liquid-crystal quasi-electret colloid system that in this proper state can perform locomotion, metabolic, trophic, and barrier functions in a joint ensuring its operation as an "intelligent" friction assembly in a human organism. These general findings are specified in the next paragraph devoted to the study of SF mesophase.

2.7. Synovia as a Liquid-Crystal Medium

Liquid-crystal state provides ideal conditions for numerous biochemical reactions and reproductive functions of biological structures. It is inherent to cellular membranes and organoids (cytoplasmatic cell structures), photoreceptors of retina, myofibrils, (muscular tissue structures), collagen fibers, nucleic acids, and other natural objects [72−75]. This is common knowledge that complex ethers of cholesterol and fatty acids contained in blood plasma are found in the liquid-crystal state [76]. Cholesterol ethers prevent arteries from damages under the effect of blood pressure [77]. SF because of its origin from blood plasma is of similar chemical composition (Table 2.1). Liquid-crystal compounds of cholesterol were first found in it experimentally in the early 1980s [78].

2.7.1. Liquid-Crystal Components of SF

The SF taken from cattle (15 samples) and people was studied. The patients were 28 men and 18 women (aged 11−80 years) suffered from rheumatoid arthritis, traumatic synovitis, psoriatic arthritis, deforming osteoarthrosis, and infectious gonitis. The SF samples were dried during 10 days at negative temperature to exclude protein destruction. Cholesterol and its compounds content was determined by the Liberman-Burkhard reaction (L. Liberman, the Hungarian biochemist and H. Burkhard, the German chemist). This is a quantitative color reaction to cholesterol based on green coloring in its interaction with sulfuric acid in the presence of acetic anhydride (see 4.2).

The experiments show the total cholesterol content of animal SF to be 1.0±0.2 mmol/l (0.04–0.06 wt %) and that of human SF to be 3.8±0.4 mmol/l (0.16–0.20 wt %). Varying concentration of cholesterol in human SF is evidently due to differences in articular pathology-ies as well as age-related and individual features of the organisms to be studied. Nevertheless, a plausible dependence of these variations on nosological aspects (nomenclature and classification of diseases) was not revealed.

The composition of the SF lipid fraction was studied by the method of thin-layer chromatography. The SF chromatograms of the patients suffered from villonodular synovitis and traumatic synovitis are presented in Fig. 2.6. Their analysis confirms the presence of cholesterol ethers in SF. By depositing free cholesterol with a special reagent (digitonine) it was found that the share of cholesterol ethers in cholesterol was 25−35 wt %.

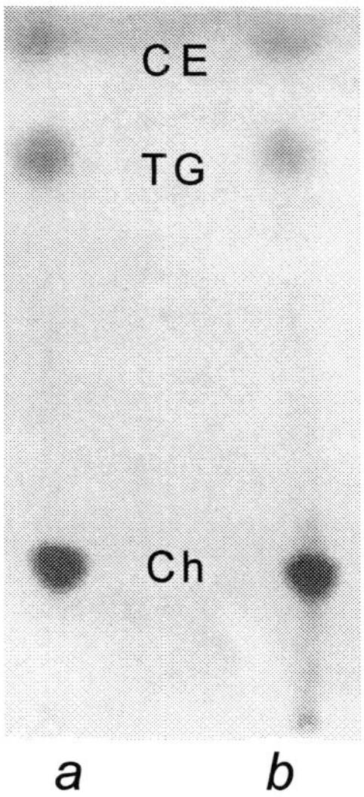

Figure 2.6. Chromatograms of synovial fluids: *a* – pigmented villonodular synovitis; *b* – traumatic synovitis. CE – cholesterol ethers, TG – triglycerides, Ch– cholesterol.

Since cholesterol ethers are optically active, the dried SF samples were examined by means of polarization microscopy using a heating table. At crossed polaroids, active inclusions in SF are seen as luminous points or regions varying their color and light emission intensity in sample rotation. Individual luminous points are radial--beam aggregates similar to spherical crystallites observed in blood plasma [79]. In sample heating up to 40–43 °C the lighting disappeared, which corresponded to the mesophase transition into isotropic state. Subsequent cooling caused reverse transition of isotropic substance into crystalline phase. Figure 2.7 shows one of these luminous inclusions located at the crack boundary formed in the sample in drying. Heating up to 24–26 °C resulted in melting of the luminous substance and its spread in the crack, causing the luminescence of its edges. At $T > 43$ °C the luminescence at the edges disappeared and appeared again when the sample was cooled down to 40–43 °C. Next heating-cooling cycles resulted in appearance and disappearance of luminescence, respectively. This allows us to conclude that the sample is optically active over a temperature range of 25–41°C and behaves as a thermotropic liquid-crystal compound.

Cholesterol and its etherized forms and a matter mesomorphic at the temperature of a living organism found in SF indicate that liquid-crystal components of SF refer to complex cholesterol ethers.

The authors of [40] reported the results of chromatographic analysis of the general fraction of cholesterol ethers extracted from synovia with help of chloroform-ethanol mixture. It turned out that complex ethers of cholesterol and some other acids enter SF (Table 2.5): palmitic (21.8–27.3%), palmitooleic (1.0–4.3%), stearinic (7.9–13.1%), oleic (21.1–25.8%), linoleic (28.8–34.4%), and arachidonic (5.2–9.5%). As seen from Table 2.5, the SF cholesterol ether fraction is based on the cholesterol ethers of oleic, palmitic and linoleic acids.

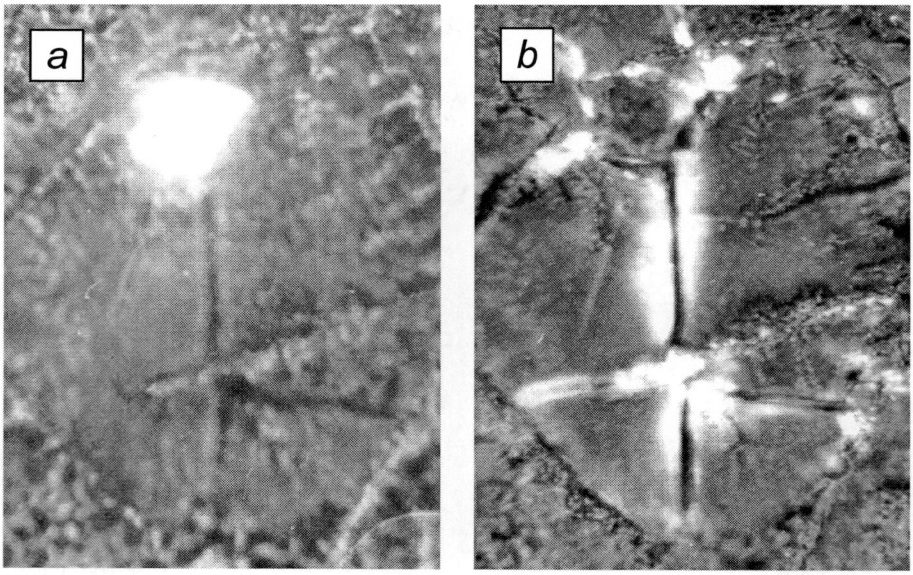

Figure 2.7. Optically active fragments of dried SF samples prior (*a*) and upon (*b*) heating. The area under examination is 240×330 mcm. Crossed polaroids.

Table 2.5. Composition of cholesterol ethers identified in SF

Cholesterol ethers	Molecular weight, arbitrary units	Average ether content in arthritis of different etiology ($M \pm m$, %)		
		Pigmented illonodular (n = 9)	Rheumatoid (n = 3)	Traumatic (n = 4)
Cholesteryl palmitate	624	25.1±1.9	26.2±1.1	24.1±2.3
Cholesteryl palmitoleate	622	1.5±0.5	2.1±0.1	3.4±0.9
Cholesteryl stearate	636	10.5±2.6	9.1±0.3	8.7±0.8
Cholesteryl oleate	650	22.0±0.9	23.6±2.0	25.1±0.7
Cholesteryl linoleate	649	32.0±1.2	32.1±1.9	31.6±2.8
Cholesteryl arachidonate	672	8.9±0.7	6.9±0.3	7.1±1.9

n is the number of examined patients.

Thus, the natural lubricating film of joints comprises the mixture of cholesterol ethers. The latter are known as thermotropic liquid-crystal compounds having mesophase intervals within a wide temperature range and structural organization of cholesterol type [72–75]. Therefore, it is natural to assume that at optimal ratio they form a liquid-crystal mixture having the mesophase interval within a physiological temperature range and, hence, the articular lubricant itself has the liquid-crystal state at the same temperatures.

2.7.2. The Mesophase Temperature

The results of experimental determination of thermodynamic transitions in the SF liquid-crystal phase were first reported in works [40, 80–82]. Below, the generalized description of the ideology and techniques of the complex research is cited.

Thermodynamic transitions accompanied by the formation and destruction of the mesophase of cholesterol ethers can corroborate their belonging to liquid-crystal substances. Temperature boundaries of mesophase existence were determined by differential scanning microcalorimetry (DSC) and probe fluorescence. The SF taken from the patients suffered from rheumatoid, pigmented villonodular and traumatic synovitis was studied. Since cholesterol is contained in SF in small amounts (0.16 – 0.20 wt %) it should be solved how to concentrate it in the samples. As known [73], cholesterol and its ethers are part of lipids contained in all living cells of fat-like substances that are insoluble in water but soluble in organic fluids. Some lipid phases soluble in water form lyotropic liquid crystals whose molecules are well oriented under exposure to the magnetic field [72]. Therefore, cholesterol and its ethers were concentrated by extracting the lipid phase of SF by the technique [83]. Liposomes or spherical particles ($d<10$ μm) made up from the biomolecular lipid layer were extracted from the suspension of lipids by means of an ultrasonic generator. A number of experiments on finding the temperature limits of mesophase existence in SF were conducted at these concentrations of cholesterol.

The results of differential thermal analysis of SF and the lipid fraction extracted from it are presented in Fig. 2.8. The y-axis corresponds to the difference of temperatures Θ of the SF sample in study and the reference that does not experience any transformations in heating. The temperature values of SF samples heated at a rate of 10 °C/min are put at the x-axis. "Exo" and "endo" correspond to heat release and absorption, respectively, by the SF samples. It is seen that the first phase transition in SF (*a*) occurs at T_1 = 63–64 °C, the second – at T_2 = 70–73, and the third one – at T_3 = 86–88 °C. These temperatures differ by 2–3 °C depending on the nosological form of articular pathology. Bearing in mind the presence of lyotropic liquid crystals in SF resulting from the dissolution of cholesterol in water in the presence of phospholipids [83] this is natural to assume that T_1 and T_2 are the boundaries of the region of the liquid crystal-isotropic fluid transition. The temperature T_3 corresponds apparently to DNA molecule destruction whose structure governs the sequence of amino acid chains in the polypeptide protein chain [32]. Analysis of the thermogram in Fig. 2.8, *b* indicates that within a range of physiological temperatures SF lipids demonstrate the peak of thermal absorption at $T \sim 29$ °C. Phase transition of lipid suspension to the mesomorphic state apparently occurs at this temperature.

Fluorescence is a short-time luminescence (lighting excessive over heat radiation) damping during 10^{-9}–10^{-8} s upon ceasing excitation. Fluorescent analysis is commonly used to quantitatively and qualitatively analyze biologically active compounds. A fluorescent probe, namely, 8-aniniline-1-naphtylsulfonate (ANS) was introduced in the samples of SF and liposome and lipid suspensions. Its molecules are adsorbed on lipid cholesterol-bearing structures. Quantum emission of ANS fluorescence depends on the environment molecule polarity. Thus, ANS fluorescence maximum at the input corresponds to frequency λ = 360 nm. On adding ANS in the samples in question the maximum is shifted to the region of high frequencies λ_p = 485–490 nm, which indicates the nonpolarity of probe environment.

Figure 2.9 shows the temperature variation of fluorescence ANS intensity *I* in SF and its lipid and cholesterol components. The value of *I* characteristic of the samples at 20 °C is taken 100%.

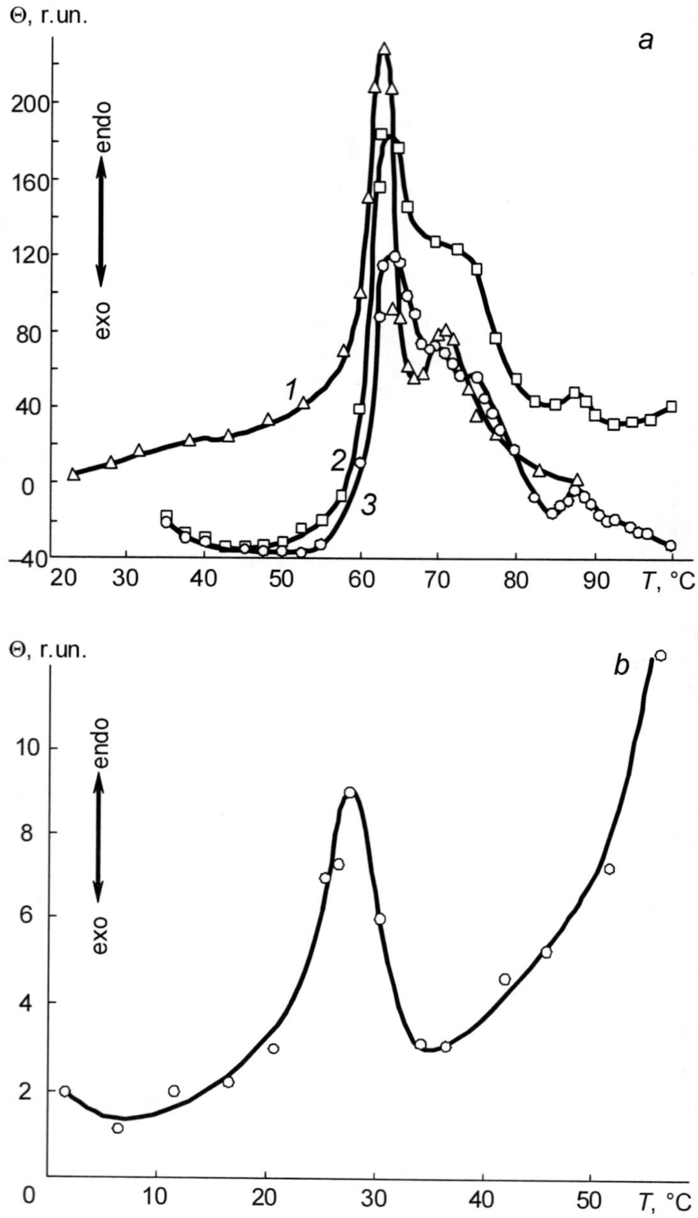

Figure 2.8. Thermograms of SF (*a*) and lipids (*b*). Synovia is taken from synovitis-affected patients: 1 – rheumatoid, 2 – traumatic, 3 – pigmented villonodular synovitis.

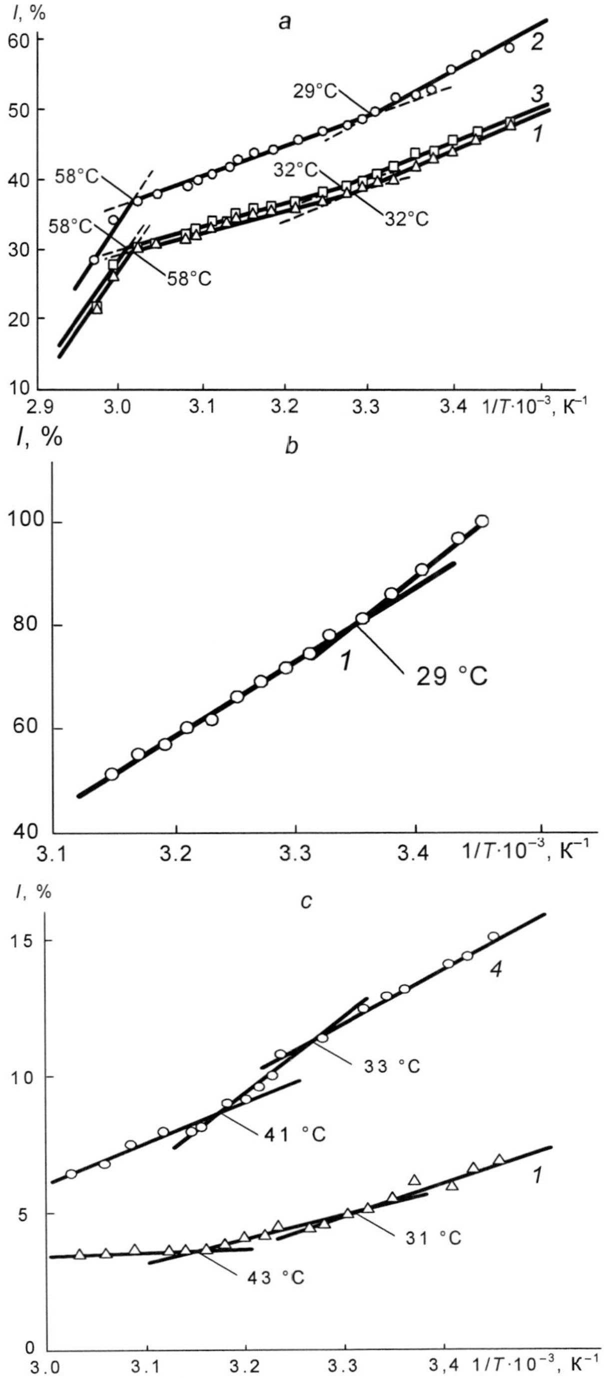

Figure 2.9. Fluorescence intensity of ANS introduced in SF and its components vs. reverse temperature: *a* – SF, *b* – liposomes, *c* – general choelsterol fraction. SF is taken from sunovitis patients: 1 and 3 – rheumatoid, 2 – traumatic, 4 – pigmented villonodular synovitis. The number at the plots correspond to the temperatures of break points of linear dependences.

It is seen that all linear dependences $I(1/T)$ have breaks corresponding to some critical temperatures. For SF (*a*) it is T_1 ~ 29–32 °C and T_2 ~ 58 °C. Inconsistence of temperatures T_1 within 2–3 °C is due to the fact that SF is a multicomponent system and concentration of its components is different in different individuals and varies in diseases. The temperatures correspond to the phase transitions of lipids and cholesterol ethers contained in SF. Thus, the temperature of the phase transition of the SF lipid fraction revealed by DSC (Fig. 2.8 *b*) is close or coincides with the lowest temperatures of the break at the plots (Fig. 2.9 *a*, *b*, and *c*). At the plots of Fig. 2.9, *c* corresponding to the general cholesterol fraction, the second break at T = 41–43 °C is characteristic of only this group of compounds among with (Table 2.5) liquid-crystal cholesterol ethers prevail. Consequently, the cholesterol liquid crystal–isotropic fluid transformation occurs at this temperature.

Critical temperatures of phase transitions in SF obtained by three independent methods are shown in Table 2.6.

Table 2.6. Variation temperatures of physical state of SF and extracted components

Examination method	Critical temperatures, °C, of phase transitions in media			
	SF	lipids	liposomes	cholesterol fraction
Thermopolarization microscopy	25 41	–	–	–
DSC	62–64 70–73 86–88	28–29	–	–
Probe fluorescence	29–32 58–59	–	29	31–33 41–43

Analysis of the data of Table 2.6 allows us to draw the following conclusions.

A. Phase transitions at 25–33 °C occur in SF and its components – lipids, liposomes, and cholesterol fraction. However, cholesterol and artificial SF are characterized by two phase transformations (the latter at T = 41–43 °C) corresponding to the appearance and disappearance of liquid-crystal phase in them. In lipids and liposomes just one phase transition is recorded in heating. This indicates that liquid-crystal cholesterol ethers are found in the bound state in them and do not demonstrate in a full measure the mesophase properties.

B. Phase transition at T = 25–33 °C is not revealed in SF by DSC due to insufficient susceptibility of the method at temperatures lower than 50 °C. The phase transition in SF (recorded by probe fluorescence at 58–59 °C) is reliably recorded by DSC at 62–64 °C. The difference can be attributed to the dissimilar technologies of sample preparation, first of all, by specific effect of lipid structures onto fluorescence of ANS molecules adsorbed on them.

C. Close critical temperatures of SF and its components recorded by the independent methods correspond to the transformations of liquid-crystal phase contained in synovia.

2.7.3. Friction Reduction

Works [80, 82, 84] experimentally corroborate the hypothesis about liquid-crystal cholesterol compounds as the main antifrictional component of SF.

Figure 2.10 presents the data on the effectiveness of the different lubricants of the pig's shoulder joint mounted in a pendulum tribometer. It is seen that the addition of liquid-crystal cholesterol with the mesophase within the physiological temperature range to the pseudo-synovial fluid (aqueous solution of Na-carboxymethyl cellulose, Na-CMC [82], curve *3*) ensures the same friction as SF with the minimal amount of general cholesterol (curves *5b*). The SF with the higher cholesterol amount (curve *7*) enlarges the pendulum damping period. Friction significantly decreases even when the joint is lubricated by a silicon-organic fluid containing a liquid-crystal additive (curve *4*).

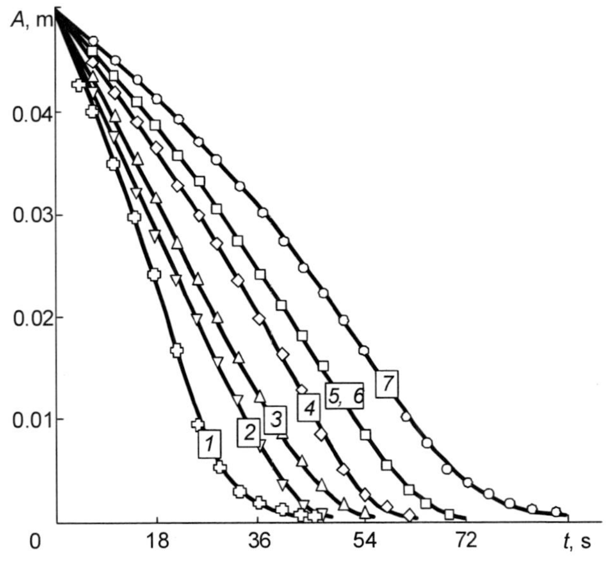

Figure 2.10. Kinetic dependences of pendulum oscillation amplitude under lubrication by different substances: *1* – distilled water; *2* – silicon-organic fluid; *3* – pseudo-SF; *4* – silicon-organic fluid with addition of 2 wt % LC; *5* – pseudo-SF with addition of 2 wt % LC; *6* – SF with cholesterol amount 0.9 mmol/l; *7* – the same 4.09 mmol/l.

The lubricity of SF and pseudo-synovia (PS) based on aqueous solution Na-CMC 1 was compared by means of an end-face friction machine to test a cartilage--glass tribopair at a sliding velocity of $v = 0.1$ m/s [86]. The experimental results are presented in Fig. 2.11. They indicate that the addition in PS of liquid-crystal compounds results in its improved lubricity and reduced coefficient of friction of the tribopair under study. Dependence $f(p)$ for PS with addition of LC practically coincides with natural SF [87]. Low friction of the articular cartilage under these conditions results from the liquid-crystal state arising in the cholesterol ether-containing lubricating layer, which is similar to the state of SF in synovial joints.

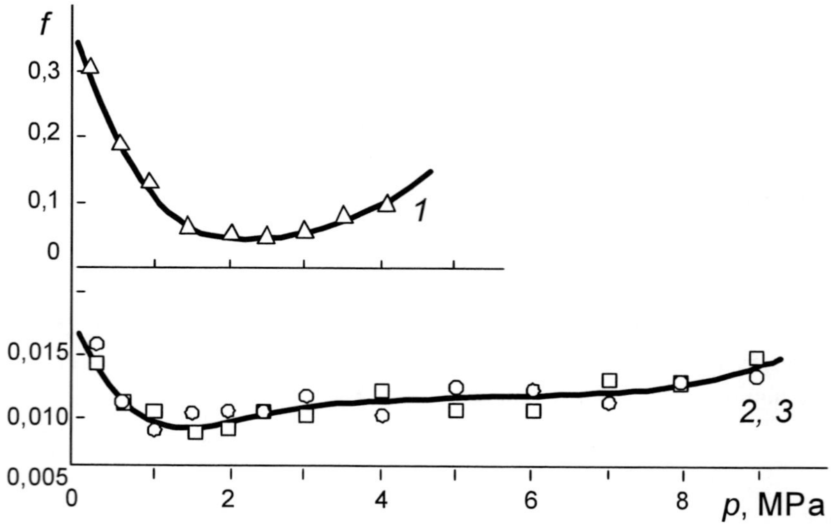

Figure 2.11. Coefficient of friction vs. load in the cartilage–glass tribopair under lubrication with: *1* – PS; *2* – SF (□), *3* – PS + 2 wt % LC (○).

A relation exists between regular microrelief of the solid surface and structure parameters of liquid-crystal contact layers [88]. The force of cohesion of the cholesterol ether molecules with the solid surface is maximal if the area of the microrelief grooves is commensurable with the sizes of these molecules having an order of 1–10 μm. The surface of articular cartilage meets the condition [36], owing to which its cohesion to aqueous solutions of cholesterol ethers is enhanced and formation on the cartilage surface of lubricating layers with the structure oriented along the grooves is provided. In movement of articular cartilages the shear is localized in the layers between the layers of the liquid crystal whose intermolecular interaction is insignificant. Therefore, in the synovial joint an extremely low friction is realized.

For a long time arthrologists has believed that hyaluronic acid is the main SF lubrication component [5, 6, 9–11, 13, 14, 19, 29]. Spiral molecules of the biopolymer are characterized by chirality, which means that they are not identical to their image in an ideal flat mirror. Therefore, aqueous solutions of hyaluronic acid demonstrate natural optical activity [89] and a particular structure order. Upon having found that depolymerization of hyaluronic acid does not affect significantly SF lubricity [40, 42, 43], the views on the functions of hyaluronic acid in SF have changed. This is due to "host–guest" effect [88]. As shown in [89], the addition of low-molecular liquid crystals has an essential effect on the structure of chiral polymers similar to hyaluronic acid. Cholesterol ethers included in SF can be such compounds. With a high degree of probability one can assume involvement of hyaluronic acid in the formation of lithotropic liquid-crystal lubricating layer in the joint [34].

These findings form the scientific grounds for a new trend in the study of physicochemical lubrication mechanisms of synovial joints and in the development of drugs containing liquid-crystal components [90].

ACKNOWLEDGMENTS

Synovial fluid is a unique condensed medium having multilevel colloidal structure characterized by the properties of liquid semiconductor but showing quasi-electret and liquid-crystal states. At the same time, SF is a living cell-containing tissue in which metabolic processes occur. It is characterized by a wide spectrum of immunological properties. As a condensed body, SF reacts to the biophysical field of the joint by variations in its structure. This allows regulation of the mobility and motion of its structural units, physical properties of the lubricating layer in a joint, and physicochemical SF characteristics as a transport medium responsible for mass exchange in the joint cavity. As a cellular culture, SF is involved in metabolic regulations in joint tissues and in protective reactions of synovial medium via antibody accumulation. A unique complex of physical, chemical, and biological properties makes SF susceptible to the signals coming to the joint from the vegetative nervous center and allows it to perform a set of functions comparable to inherent functions of an intelligent organism.

REFERENCES

[1] Ropes, MW; Bauer, W. *Synovial fluid changes in joint disease*. Cambridge: Royal Soc of Chemistry, 1953.

[2] Davies, DV. Cell content of synovial fluid. *J. Anat.* 1945, Vol 79, N 2, 66–77.

[3] Lever, JD; Ford, EMR. Histological and electron microscopic observation on synovial membrane. *Anat. Rec.* 1958, N 132, 525–540.

[4] Jebens, EM; Monk-Jones, ME. On the viscosity and pH of synovial fluid and the pH of blood. *J. Bone and Joint Surg.* 1959, N 41B, 388–400.

[5] Ogston, AG; Stanier, JE. On the state of hyaluronic acid in synovial fluid. *Biochem. J.* 1950, N 46, 364–376.

[6] Dulyapin, VA. Synovial fluid and significance of its study in joint disease diagnostics. *Vopr. Rheumat.* 1974, N 4, 72–76.

[7] Bychkov, SM; Kharlamova, VN. Study of hybrid protein-chondrotin-sulphate. *Biochem.* 1968, N 33, 4–14.

[8] Fessler, JH. Structural function of mucopolysaccharide in connective tissue. *Biochem. J.* 1960, N 76, 124–132.

[9] Walker, PS; Sicorski, J; Dowson, D; et al. Feature of the synovial fluid film in human joint lubrication. *Nature.* 1970, Vol 225, 956–957.

[10] Wright, W. Joint mechanics. *J. Physiotherapy.* 1972, Vol 11, 367–370.

[11] Medicis, R; Reboux, JF; Lussier, A. Le liquide synovial revue de la literature de 1972–75. *Pathol. et Biol.* 1976, Vol 24, N 9, 641–656.

[12] Horn, V; Bozdech, Z; Horky, D. Die rasterelectronenmicroskopische untersuchung der Gelenkhohraumzellen. *Z. Ortoped.* 1972, Bd 110, N 3, 331–336.

[13] Socoloff, L. *The joints and synovial fluid.* NY: Acad Press, 1978.

[14] Pavlova, VN. *Synovial medium of joints.* Moscow: Medicine, 1980.

[15] Zubraykov, SV; Prokhorova IM. *On the synovia cell capability of active metabolic processes. In: Adaptation of Man and Animals in Norm and Pathology*. Yaroslavl': YAMI, 1974, 172–174.

[16] Latyshev, OA. *Materials and characteristics of articular inflammation in patients suffered from infectious non-specific polyarthritis and primary osteoarthrosis deformans*. PhD Med Diss, Yaroslavl', 1971.

[17] Pavlova, VN; Luzin, VN. *Functional activity of synovial membrane cells under norm and extreme conditions. In: Modern biochemical problems of connective tissue.* Novosibirsk: HMU, 1977.

[18] Pavlova, VN; Fradkin, AR. *Modern evaluation of the features of hemotissue relations in joint synovial membranes. In: Lymphatic and blood paths*. Novosibirsk: MNI, 1976, 124–135.

[19] Frerichs, FT. *Synovia. In: Wagner's Handwörterbuch der Physiologie*, 1846, 463–487.

[20] Chirkin, AA; Okorokov, AN; Goncharik, II. *Diagnostic reference book for a physician.* Minsk: Belarus, 1994.

[21] Novikov, D K. *Medical immunology*. Minsk: Vysheishaya shkola, 2005.

[22] *Nomenclature of enzymes. English Translation*. Moscow: Mir, 1979.

[23] Zotikov, EA. Karl Landsteiner and His Heritage. *Hematol. Transfusiol.* 2001, Vol 46, N 5, 25–28.

[24] Olovnikova, NI; Nikolaeva, TL. Antigens of human erythrocytes. *Hematol. Transfusiol.* 2001, Vol 46, N 5, 37–45.

[25] Donskov, SI. Blood groups in human biology – facts and assumptions. *Hematol. Transfusiol.* 2001, Vol 46, N 5, 32–33.

[26] *Transfusion of donor blood and its components*. Instruction on application N 118-1103 MH RB, December 12, 2003.

[27] Ogston, AG; Preston, BN. The exclusion of protein by hyaluronic acid measurement by light scattering. *J. Biol. Chem.* 1996, N 241, 17–19.

[28] Hammerman, D; Rosenberg, L; Schubert, M. Reviev article diarthrodial joints revisiter. *J. Bone and Joint Surg.* 1970, Vol 52, 158–171.

[29] Mow, VK. Role of lubricant in joint biomechanics. *Probl. of Frict. and Lubr: Proc. ASME.* 1969, N 2, 131-141.

[30] Beloenko, ED; Slobozhanina, EI; Kozlova; NM. Spectrophotometric study of synovial effusion in differential diagnostics of pigmented villous synovitis. *Orthop. Traumatol. Prosth.* 1990, N 5, 32–34.

[31] Gerasimov, AM; Furtseva, LN. *Biochemical diagnostics in traumatology and orthopedics*. Moscow: Medicine, 1986.

[32] Ermakov, SF; Rodnenkov, VG; Beloenko, ED; Kupchinov, BI. *Liquid crystals in engineering and medicine*. Minsk: Asar, Moscow: CheRo, 2002.

[33] Beloenko, ED. *Optimization of orthopedic–surgical treatment of rheumatoid arthritis based on the methods of biophysical control of antifrictional characteristics of joint synovial medium (clinical experimental study). Doct. Med. Sci. Diss*. Kiev, 1992.

[34] Ermakov, SF. *Tribophysics of liquid-crystal materials in metal- and biopolymer pairs. Doct. Eng. Diss. Gomel.* 2001.

[35] *Bio-fluid mechanics*. Ed. Power, H. Southampton: CMP, 1995.

[36] Pavlova, VN; Kopyeva, TN; Slutskii, LI; Pavlov, GG. *Cartilage*. Moscow: Medicine, 1988.

[37] Jay, GD. Lubricin and surfacing of articular joints. *Current Opin. in Orthop.* 2004, Vol 15, 355–359.
[38] Mansour, JM; Mow, VC. On the natural lubrication of synovial joints: normal and degenerate. *Trans. ASME.* 1977, Vol F 99, N 2, 163–173.
[39] *Biomechanics of diarthrodial joints*. Ed. Mow, VC; Ratcliffe, A; Woo, SL-Y. NY: Springer-Verlag, 1990, Vol 1.
[40] Kupchinov, B; Ermakov, S; Rodnenkov, V; Bobrysheva, S; Beloenko, E. Role of luquid crystals in the lubrication of living joints. *Smart Materials and Structure.* 1993, N 2, 7–12.
[41] Lipshitz, H; Etheredge, R; Climcher, MJ. In vitro studies of the wear of articular cartilage. The wear characteristics of chemically modified articular cartilage when worn against a highly polished characterized stainless steel surface. *J. Biomech.* 1980, Vol 13, 423–436.
[42] Kupchinov, B; Ermakov, S; Rodnenkov, V; Bobrycheva, S; Beloenko, E. The effect of luquid crystals on joints lubrication. *Wear.* 1994, Vol 171, 7–12.
[43] Rejholec, V. Long term studies of antiosteoarthritic drugs: an assessment. *Sem. Arthritis Rheumatism.* 1987, Vol 17, N 2, 35–53.
[44] Ermakov, SF. Modern conceptions on biomechanics of human synovial joints. *Mechanics of Composite Materials.* 1992, N 4, 539–556.
[45] Chauser, MG. *Kelvin's model.* In: Encyclopedia of polymers, 1972, Vol 1, 1015-1016.
[46] Brand, RA. *Joint lubrication. Ch. 13.* In: The scientific basis of orthopedics. 2nd Ed. Los Altos: WB Saunders, 1987, 373–386.
[47] Fulkerson, JP; Edvards, CC; Christman, OD. *Articular cartilage. Chapter 12.* In: The scientific basis of orthopaedics. 2nd Ed. Los Altos: WB Saunders, 1987, 347–371.
[48] Vyrva, OE. Artificial synovial fluid in treatment of knee joint pathology. *Orthop. Traumatol. Prosth.* 2000, N 2, 146–150.
[49] Vasilenkaitis, VV. Artificial synovial fluid for joints. *Orthop. Traumatol. Prosth.* 1989, N 10, 11–15.
[50] Altman, RD; Howell, DS; Cottlieb, NL. Introduction: new directions in therapy of osteoarthritis. *Sem. Arthr. Rheum.* 1987, Vol 17, N 2, 1–2.
[51] Remizov, AN; Maksina, AG; Potapenko, AY. *Medical and biological physics: a university handbook.* Moscow: Drofa, 2003.
[52] *Biophysics*. Ed. Antonov, VF. 2nd Ed. Moscow: VLADOS, 2003.
[53] Bogolyubov, VM; Ponomarenko, GN. *General physiotherapy: VUZ handbook.* 3rd Ed. Moscow: Medicine, 1999.
[54] Mow, VC; Lai, WM. Recent developments in synovial joint biomechanics. *SIAM review.* 1980, Vol 22, N 3, 275–317.
[55] Maroudas, A. Physicochemical properties of cartilage in the light of ion exchange theory. *Biophys. J.* 1968, N 8, 575–595.
[56] Gordon, SS. *Permeability and streaming potential of normal and trypsin treated articular cartilage.* M S thesis, Rensselaer Polytechnic Inst, Troy, NY, 1978, 1–79.
[57] Maroudas, A. Biophysical chemistry of cartilaginous tissues with special reference to solute and fluid transport. *Biorheology.* 1975, N 12, 233–248.
[58] Helfferich, F. *Ion exchange.* NY: McGraw–Hill, 1962.

[59] Grodzinsky, AJ; Eisenberg, SR. Double layer mediated energy conversion with a protein membrane using an imposed fregnency and warelength. *J. Electrostatics.* 1978, N 5, 33–50.
[60] Grodzinsky, AJ; Roth, V; Fox, P; Mow, VC. The influence of electromechanical transduction on matrix interactions in articular cartilage. *Trans 25th Ann. Meeting Orthop. Res. Soc.* San Francisco, CA, 1979, Vol 4, 141.
[61] Hussbaum, JH; Grodzinsky, AJ. H^+ binding and diffusion-reaction rates in collagen electromechanics. Ed. Ostrander, LE. *Proc 7th New England (Northeast) Bioengineering Cong.* 1979, 61–64.
[62] Russian State Standard No. 25209-82. *Plastics and Polymer Films. Methods for estimating surface charge of electrets.*
[63] *Electrets.* 3rd Ed. Vol 1. Ed. Sessler, GM. Morgan Hill: Laplacian Press, 1999.
[64] Capeletti, R; Bridelli, MG. TSDC as a tool to monitor the electret state induced by water in biomolecules. *Proc Int Symp on Electrets, 10th.* Delphy, Athens, 1999, 159–166.
[65] Pinchuk, LS; Goldade, VA; Sessler, GM; et al. Electret-thermal analysis of blood. *Med. Eng. Phys.* 2002, Vol 24, 361–364.
[66] Kadolich, ZhV. *Physical simulation of polymer-metal joints to increase their wear resistance based on simulation of biophysical properties of natural joints.* PhD Diss Eng, Gomel, 2002.
[67] Pinchuk, LS; Cherniakova, YuM; Kadolich, ZhV; et al. Investigation of structural variations in synovial fluid by the method of electret-thermal analysis. *NN Priorov Vestnik traumatol. and orthop.* 2005, N 3, 57–61.
[68] Van Turnhout, J. *Thermally stimulated discharge of polymer electrets.* Amsterdam: Springer-Verlag, 1975.
[69] Knorre, DG; Myzina, SD. *Biological chemistry: A handbook for medical and biological universities.* 2nd Issue. Moscow: Vysshaya shkola, 1998.
[70] Stepanov, VM. *Molecular biology. Structure and functions of proteins. A textbook for biological universities.* Moscow: Vysshaya shkola, 1996.
[71] Tsvetkova, EA. Physical properties of synovial fluid as joint lubricating medium. *Biophysics,* 2005, Vol 20, N 2, 341–347.
[72] Usol'tseva, NV; Okopova, OB; Bykov VV; Smirnov, AI; Pikin, SA. *Liquid crystals: discotic mesogens.* Ivanovo: IGU, 2004.
[73] Brawn, G; Wolken, D. *Liquid crystals and biological structures.* Ed. Varshavskii, YaM; translated from English Vedenov, AA. Moscow: Mir, 1982.
[74] Sarma, AV; Powell, GL; LeBerge, M. Phospholipid composition of articular cartilage boundary lubricant. *J. Orthop. Res.* 2001, Vol 19, 671–676.
[75] Hills, BA. Surface-active phospholipids: a Pandora's box of clinical applications. Part II. Barrier and lubricating properties. *Int. Med. J.* 2002, Vol 32, 242–251.
[76] Sidorenko, GI; Tsapaev, VG. Diagnostic value of phase transition temperatures of cholesterol in blood serum in atherosclerosis. *Cardiology.* 1983, Vol 23, N 10, 92–95.
[77] Patsak, J. *Organic chemistry.* Ed. Butin, KP; Czech Translation. Moscow: Mir, 1986.
[78] Kupchinov, BI; Rodnenkov, VG; Bobrysheva, SN; et al. On the mechanism of joint functioning as a rubbing body. *Dokl. AN BSSR.* 1985, Vol 29, N 5, 463–465.
[79] Khalatov, SS. *Cholesterol disease.* Moscow: Medgiz, 1946.

[80] Beloenko, ED; Kupchinov, BI; Ermakov, SF; Slobozhanina, EI, Rodnenkov, VG; Kozlova, NM; Eismont, OL. Experimental substantiation of liquid-crystal state of synovial medium of joints. *Vesti NAN Belarus Ser. Medicobiol. Nauk.* 2001, N 1, 79–85.

[81] Kupchinov, BI; Ermakov, SF; Beloenko, ED; Suslov, AA. *Liquid crystalline components of synovia and their role in the joint tribology.* I Sympozjum "Inzynieria Ortopedyczna i Protetyczna –IOP 97", Bialystok, 1997, 125–131.

[82] Beloenko, ED; Kupchinov, BI; Ermakov, SF; Rodnenkov, VG; Eismont, OL. Liquid-crystal state of joint synovial lubricating medium. Experimental substantiation. *Acta of Bioeng and Biomech.* 2001, Vol 3, Supl 1, 24–32.

[83] Folch, J; Lees, M; Sloane-Stanley, GH. A simple method for isolation and purification of total lipids from animal tissue. *J. Biol. Chem.* 1967, Vol 226, 497–509.

[84] Kupchinov, BI; Ermakov, SF; Rodnenkov, VG; Beloenko, ED; Eismont, OL. Some Results of Investigation of Liquid-crystal State of Lubrication Joint Synovial Medium. *J. Friction and Wear.* 2002, Vol 23, N 3, 310–317.

[85] Patent N 1391577 USA, Int Cl C 08L 1/28, A 61K 317/15. *Pseudosynovial plastic body fluids and method of preparing some.* Homsy, CA. N 11352/73. Filed 08.03.73. Complete specification published 23.04.75.

[86] Ermakov, SF; Beloenko; ED; Eismont; OL; Shuldykov, RA. Influence of liquid crystals on biological mechanisms of reducing intra-articular friction. *Mater Tekhnolog. Instrum.* 2006, N 1, 42–47.

[87] Ermakov, SF; Beloenko, ED; Eismont, OL. The role of liquid crystals in tribomechanical properties of articular cartilages. *J. Friction and Wear.* 2004, Vol 25, N 5, 486–491.

[88] Sonin, AS. *Introduction into physics of liquid crystals.* Moscow: Nauka, 1983.

[89] Volokhina, AV; Godovskii, YuK; Kudryavtsev, GI; et al. *Liquid-crystal polymers.* Ed. Plate, NA. Moscow: Khimiya, 1988.

[90] Beloenko, ED; Eismont, OL; Pashkevich, LA; Shved IA; Ermakov, SF. Effectiveness of preparation based on cholesterol-nematic liquid-crystal biologically active substance at rubbing of experimental arthrosis-arthritis. *Vesti NAN Belarus Ser. Med. Nauk.* 2005, N 1, 5–8.

Chapter 3

PATHOLOGICAL CONDITIONS

Disorders of the synovial medium can be due to joint traumas and certain rheumatic diseases based on systemic (referring to all joint tissues) or local lesions of connective tissue. They are most often expressed as joint pains sometimes accompanied by a moderate atrophy of surrounding muscles and dystrophy of articular surfaces. Therefore, basic rheumatic and orthopedic diseases are included in chapter XIII "Diseases of Musculoskeletal System and Connective Tissue" of the International statistic classification [1]. Unfortunately, the classification does not give us an idea about the pathogenic and diagnostic interrelation of individual diseases. In this relation, the working classification and nomenclature adopted in December, 1988 at the plenary session of the National (former USSR) Society of Rheumatologists are handier to use. They are based on clinical and pathogenic symptoms of joint diseases that are divided into 13 rubrics. The first seven rubrics include proper inflammatory rheumatic diseases part of which is united in groups by etiologic principle (diffusive diseases of connective tissue, systemic vasculitis). The most widely spread and practically significant diseases such as rheumatism and rheumatoid arthritis are isolated into independent rubrics. Degenerative joint and spine diseases and nosological forms of inflammatory-degenerative nature (microcrystalline arthritis) are presented separately. Diseases of extra-articular soft tissues and bones also form an individual rubric. The rubrics of classification [2] are presented in Table 3.1.

For practical purposes, it is convenient to divide the diseases of joints by signs of their onset and by mechanism of disease development. As for the signs of pathological process, the diseases can be classified as traumatic, inflammatory, degenerative-dystrophic and oncological. The authors of [2] believe it to be advisable to systematize arthritis in terms of etiology, i.e., by the causes of disease onset thus dividing arthritis into three groups:

1. Infection-related or parasite invasion–related arthritis:

a) arthritis caused directly by the pathogen-induced damage to the synovial membrane;

b) immune-pathological arthritis caused by the action of infectious and parasite antigens on the organism.

2. Arthritis related to non-infectious factors (paraneoplastic arthritis, arthritis due to blood diseases, microcrystalline arthritis, allergic arthritis, etc.).

3. Arthritis and systemic rheumatic diseases of an unknown etiology (rheumatoid arthritis, seronegative spondylarthropathy, diffusive disease of connective tissue, etc.).

A key moment in differential diagnostics of articular syndrome is the distinction of traumatic and inflammatory diseases (arthritis) from chronic degenerative-dystrophic diseases (arthrosis, osteoarthritis). The principle moment in disease treatment is the diagnosis of inflammation etiology, aiming to specify its either immune or non-immune genesis.

Table 3.1. Classification and nomenclature of rheumatic diseases

Rubric No.	Disease group
I	Rheumatism (rheumatic fever)
II	Diffusive diseases of connective tissue
III	Systemic vasculitis (angiitis, arteritis)
IV	Rheumatoid arthritis
V	Juvenile arthritis
VI	Bekhterev's disease and other forms of arthritis together with spondylarthritis
VII	Infection-induced arthritis
VIII	Microcrystalline arthritis
IX	Osteoarthritis and similar diseases
X	Other joint diseases
XI	Diseases of extra-articular soft tissues
XII	Bone, cartilage diseases and osteochondropathies
XIII	Arthropathies in nonrheumatic diseases

3.1. Traumatic Pathology

Traumatic pathology of the synovial system can be referred to the injuries of joint capsule, tendons, and menisci located in the articular cavity, as well as to breaks in the cartilage or bone integrity within the joint that are accompanied by hemorrhage into the articular cavity or accumulation of a large volume of synovial effusions. Posttraumatic hemarthrosis (hemorrhage into the articular cavity) and synovitis are as a rule mono-articular, i.e. arise in one joint. Patients report a clear connection between a trauma and joint dysfunction. In differential diagnostics, a number of clinical symptoms are assessed [3] (Table 3.2).

Table 3.2. Clinical symptoms of synovial effusions

Clinical symptom	Effusion nature in diseases	
	Hemarthrosis	Acute posttraumatic synovitis
Effusions	Within an hour after trauma	6 hours and more after trauma
Pain	Intensive, occurs immediately, then sensation of arching	Unpleasant sensations, then pain grows
Joint palpation	Upper torsion dense, tense and painful	Upper torsion elastically tense
Local and general reaction	Local and general temperature elevation up to 38.5 °C	Not marked

Joint aspiration takes a decisive part in determining a degree of joint structure lesion. The blood can confirm the damage of blood-supplied structures such as capsule, tendons, fatty bodies, and pericapsular meniscus zones. Fat drops detected in blood point to fractures of condyles of femur and leg, intercondylar eminences, and patella. Synovial effusion in the joint is typical of damages of vessel-free structures such as meniscus cartilages and isolated damages of the articular cartilage.

Posttraumatic changes in the joint are due to, first, anatomostructural disorders caused by mechanical factors and, second, reactive processes localized in articular or para-articular tissues that run in the form of acute traumatic arthritis or are developed in the entire organism.

Hemarthrosis is accompanied by an increased volume of the articular cavity by 80–100 ml due to extension of SM torsions and the blood filling the joint as well as elevated intra-articular pressure. In addition to possible disorders of soft-tissue, cartilage and bone joint structures, hemarthrosis itself is the cause of marked pain syndrome and dysfunction of both the joint and the entire extremity. As SF is substituted with blood, the tissue exchange processes are broken in the joint and the tribological function deteriorates. The break of the hemosynovial barrier results in the stress experienced by SM and cartilage when contacting erythrocytes as antigen carriers.

The reaction of the joint elements to the autologous fresh blood has been experimentally studied [4]. In hemarthrosis, during first hours after trauma, typical inflammation-related modifications in the joint are absent. Erythrocytes of autologous blood penetrate in the SM depth on the interstitial substance of the lining layer and then enter the lymphatic stream. Within 4–5 hours, a significant part of erythrocytes is accumulated in the hollows between the membrane plicae (torsions). The lining SM layer becomes loose, and both intact erythrocytes and their fragments are revealed in the interstitial substance between the cells and desquamated cells are found on the membrane surface. Erythrocytes form clots in the articular cavity that are further subjected to lysis by SM macrophages and enzymes. These latter are liberated from the damaged blood cells and accumulated in the joint effusions. Hemolyzed effusion is red or bright-orange, does not contain any clots, and its viscosity is comparable to that of blood serum. Within 12–36 hours, reactive variations increase in the places of erythrocyte accumulations: neutrophils from the bloodstream infiltrate in SM and desquamated cells appear on its surface and numerous mitoses (mitosis is the main form of cell division that ensures an identical distribution of genetic material between daughter cells) in its deeper layers. Reactive changes in the membrane are clearly seen within 60–72 hours. The entire SM surface is covered by numerous oval cells of the lining layer and mononuclear leucocytes comprising erythrocytes and their fragments in the cytoplasm. Along the blood vessels numerous macrophages with erythrocyte inclusions are found. 3-4 days later, the effusion color becomes light-orange. After 8–9 days, fibrin threads and accumulations of desquamated cells swollen and under decay are revealed on the membrane surface and at the sites of blood localization.

Acute traumatic synovitis manifests as the accumulation of effusions in the joint cavity caused by increasing permeability of SM for low-molecular blood components. Joint effusion is a fluid soaking from SM, fine capillaries and veins to the joint cavity in inflammation. Such reaction of SM does not exclude the adaptive compensatory nature of a disease at early stages, i.e., increasing pressure in the joint cavity results in decreasing mechanical load to the traumatized cartilage surfaces thus favoring slippage. Metabolic processes between the cartilage, SF, and SM bloodstreams are accelerated because of a lower viscosity of the effusion compared to a healthy SF, which supports the homeostasis of synovial medium of the joint. Homeostasis is relative dynamic stability of the composition and properties of the internal medium and steadiness of main physiological functions of the organism. However, transition of posttraumatic synovitis to the acute phase after 1−3 months and its chronization (duration of posttraumatic synovitis for more than 3 months) causes persistent pathological biochemical, structural, and functional modifications in the joint elements.

Irrespective of the symptoms of joint effusion and a kind of intra-articular damage, the posttraumatic reaction in the form of acute traumatic arthritis always occurs although the degree of its manifestation can be different. In contrast to the traumas of other body parts, the joint trauma is distinguished by the processes running within a cavity limited by rigid tissues (hypertonic and low-extensible), which can result in inflammation chronization.

Acute traumatic arthritis leads to variations in the joint that occur at both macrolevel (organism and tissues) and microlevel (cellular and molecular) [5]. The disorders concerning the organism and tissues are anatomic defects (sprain and rapture of the intercellular substance, vessels, and nerves; broken sympathetic regulation of vessel drainage; joint capsule sprain; disorder of hemo- and lymphocirculation). The disorders at the cellular and molecular levels include enzymatic aggression, macromolecule destruction, local hypoxia (lowered oxygen content in tissues), disorder in substance transporting, accumulation of catabolites (products of enzymatic splitting reactions), etc. Three phases can be distinguished in acute traumatic arthritis [6]: the 1st one is the most pronounced destruction of synovial structures; it occurs during first 3 days; the 2nd one is characterized by the onset of decreasing inflammation (from 4th to 10−12th day); and the 3rd one is a persistent intensity of inflammatory reactions occurring 10−12 days after a trauma. The volume of the joint effusion serves a criterion of the acuteness of posttraumatic synovitis. A number of classifications by this sign are suggested [5] each of which includes three degrees of synovitis with different effusion volumes at equal degrees. In terms of practical medicine, the classification suggested by a Russian traumatologist V.A. Redin is advisable. According to it, the 1st degree is characterized by an effusion volume of up to 20 ml, the 2nd one – 20-60 ml, and the 3rd one – 60 ml and more. Synovitis of the 2nd and 3rd degrees is commonly accompanied by the joint dysfunctions and needs aspiration and fluid withdrawal from its cavity. At the 3rd degree, orthopedic treatment in the form of limb immobilization with plaster bandage is used to functionally relieve the joint.

Analysis of the biochemical composition of effusion shows an increased amount of the substances responsible for the destruction of protein macromolecules. In traumatic arthritis the level of activity of proteolytic enzymes, hyaluronidase, lysozyme, acid phosphatase increases in the synovial effusion. The cells of decaying tissues such as chondrocytes (protease, collagenase, and aminopeptidase), neutrophilic leucocytes (elastase, collagenase, catepsine, collagenpeptidase, and aminopeptidase), and synoviocytes (protease, catepsine, collagenopeptidase, and aminopeptidase) are the sources of proteolytic enzymes of synovial effusion. Enzyme spectrum of effusion depends on the damage localization. According to the data of [7] the level of activity of proteolytic enzymes of the intra-articular fluid decreases down to normal to the end of the 2nd week after a trauma. During first posttraumatic days, pH of the synovial effusion decreases down to 7.0, it reaches its normal level to the end of the 2nd week (7.3−7.6), but further it increases up to 8.2.

During first three post-traumatic days the protein concentration in effusion increases 1.5−4 times. The amount of albumins decreases down to 45% and the level of α_2, β, and γ-

globulins increases. The protein and protein fraction amount is approaching the protein blood spectrum due to hemarthrosis and enhanced exudation of the liquid blood constituent into the joint cavity. With due regard for the SF dilution with exudate, namely, a protein-rich fluid containing blood enzymes, which comes from fine veins and capillaries, the protein concentration in SF becomes uninformative and the evaluation of whole protein in effusion is more advisable. Thus, the whole protein amount in normal SF is 0.04 g and during first 3 days after trauma it increases up to 1.31±0.05, after 10–12 days it is 0.77±0.02, and after 19–21 days – 0.27±0.01 g. Dynamics of protein amount indicates its 5–30-fold increase of the joint effusion in acute traumatic arthritis [5].

During first three posttraumatic days the concentration of hyaluronic acid in SF decreases six-fold. However, with due regard for SF dilution with exudate and other biological fluids, the total amount of hyaluronic acid increases twice during the first 2 days, increases even more to the 7–9th day, and then gradually decreases remaining increased twofold to the 30th day. The accumulation of hyaluronic acid in the effusion is found despite periodic joint aspirations. The following relationship is derived between hyaluronic acid concentration and whole protein in the effusion: the lower pH the higher whole protein amount and hyaluronidase activity. The viscosity of synovial effusion during first posttraumatic days is lower than its normal measures tens folds, and afterwards it rises gradually but does not reach normal values even to the 30th day of arthritis.

The concentration of the markers of the acute phase of disease (sialic acids, hexosamines, hexose glycoproteids) and enzymatic activity in the soluble cell fraction increase 1.5–2 times within 2 posttraumatic weeks and decrease down to normal values to the 30th day. Activity of alkali phosphatase (the enzyme catalyzing hydrolysis of phosphoric acid ethers and thus involved in phosphate exchange in the organism) varies twice: the first peak of its increase occurs at the 1st week and the second one – at the end of the 1st month after trauma. Haptaglobin concentration (complex protein of blood serum) in effusion increases 3–15 times. Biochemical parameters of SF after trauma correlate with the similar blood parameters.

In order to determine the activity of traumatic process, the following symptoms are considered as the signs of inflammation: decreased fluid viscosity in the joint cavity, increased whole protein concentration in it; and decreased glucose content of effusion. In order to diagnose joint inflammations, additionally the level of lysosome enzymes (acid phosphatase, α- and β-N-acetyl glucose aminidase, etc.), glycolysis enzymes (glycolysis is the glucose conversion to lactic acid under anaerobic conditions with the lacking oxygen), and the cycle of three-carbon acids (lactadehydrogenase, malatdehydrogenase, and phosphpohexoisomerase) whose activity corresponds to the inflammation degree was studied.

In clinics, most often the data about effusion composition is limited due to a laboriousness of biochemical analysis and restricted laboratory capacities. Commonly, the problems of pathochemical (pathology-related) symptoms of joint synovitis remain unresolved. A complex comparison of cytological, bio- and immunochemical parameters of disease is helpful in diagnostics.

Chronic arthritis is developed from acute traumatic arthritis by a mechanism that is still not fully understood. The following causes of chronization are theoretically permissible: inflammation-maintaining factor availability and decrease in reparative (recovering) capacities of the organism. This point of view is confirmed by clinical observations. Despite operation trauma of the joint in the resection of menisci, removal of chondromatous bodies, tendon reconstruction, etc., inflammation stops and tissue regeneration is normalized. In addition to traumatic defects, synovitis can be induced by imperfect tissue reparation (hypertrophy of fat bodies and villi, commissural joint disorder, etc.) that provides conditions for a continuous traumatization of joint elements in motion. Excessive mechanical extension of the joint capsule and as a result functional insufficiency of SM is one more factor affecting the development of chronic posttraumatic synovitis.

The fluid volume in the joint can vary from normal values to 80–100 ml. Pathochemical manifestations of chronic posttraumatic synovitis are qualitatively identical to the values in the acute and subacute phases of traumatic arthritis. The protein amount in the synovial exudate increases at the cost of globulin fractions. Activity of hyaluronidase, protease, and glycolysis enzymes (hexokinase, lactatdegydrogenase, phosphohexoisomerase, etc.) enhances and the exudate viscosity decreases. In the 1980s, it was found in the CITO biochemistry laboratory that chronic posttraumatic synovitis of the knee joint was induced by the catalytically active enzyme, namely, superoxide dismutase that, as the authors [5] believed, was the most sensitive diagnostic marker in cell destruction tests. In differential diagnostics of chronic synovitis and osteoarthrosis deformans the symptoms of the latter differ by that the effusion viscosity exceeds normal values and the amount of hyaluronic acid is either normal or exceeds normal values.

Prolonged synovitis causes degenerative modifications in the joint. Proteolytic enzymes liberated from degrading cells of SM, SF, and cartilage, pathologic metabolites (intermediate products of metabolism in living cells), and metabolic disorders in the joint enhance the destruction of the intercellular cartilage substance and create premises for abnormalities of physiological remodeling of the cartilage in chronic inflammation.

3.2. Joint Diseases

Inflammatory and degenerative joint diseases along with rheumatism and rheumatic heart disease make up a group of rheumatic diseases. Etiology (causes) and pathogenesis (development mechanism) of diseases manifested as joint syndrome (a regular combination of the symptoms due to common pathogenesis) are not fully understood despite the relationship revealed between certain synovitis-inducing factors (infections, genetic peculiarities of the organism, inherited factors) and synovitis onset. Achievements in modern genetics and immunology allow immunogenetic factors in the pathogenesis of rheumatic diseases to be determined. The division of joint diseases into two groups – immune and nonimmune – helps systematize diseases at the primary stage for further purposeful investigation of joint pathology and treatment. However, clear criteria allowing consideration of some kinds of synovitis as immune or nonimmune are not found. Therefore, the diagnostics is questionable when the disease has the symptoms of both groups which can manifest at different stages and has dual diagnostic features.

The cellular composition of the joint fluid is the easiest early diagnostic test to determine a pathology mechanism. The synoviocytograms typical of some diseases are presented in Table 3.3 [8].

Table 3.3.Cellular composition in synovitis of different etiologies

Disease	Cellular composition, %					Specific distinctions
	lymphocytes	monocytes	neutrophils	macrophages	plasmocytes	
Acute traumatic arthritis	1–28	6–10	61–90	0	0–1	–
Synovitis in degenerative-dystrophic process	11–74	8–12	4–78	0–6	0–4	Gigantic multinuclear cells
Rheumatoid arthritis	20–37	7–25	55–75	0–1	0	Rhagocytes
Bekhterev's disease	0–6	0–8	50–87	0–1	0	Rhagocytes
Chronic ulna bursitis	70	20	10	0	0	–
Malignant osteoblastoclastoma of condyle of femur	2	9	69	0	1	Accumulations of malignant cells
Podagric arthritis	24	11	65	0	0	Crystals of hyperuricemic sodium found in the fresh specimen

Analysis of the synoviocytograms provides data on the availability, mechanisms, and activity of inflammation in joints as well as displays indirect symptoms of immune disorders. Nonimmune inflammatory variations manifest in acute synovitis, e.g., in traumatic arthritis which is indicated by a high amount of neutrophils (more than 61%), so-called *inflammation cells* as well as single plasmocytes. A plasmocyte or a plasma cell is a cell of lymphoid tissue producing immunoglobulins. The quantity of cell elements in degenerative-dystrophic diseases is ranged widely because this group of disorders is presented by the SF specimens taken during both acute and remission periods. Regular variations in the synovia cellular composition are observed in osteoarthrosis depending on inflammation acuteness. In the absence of exacerbations the SF cellular composition corresponds to normal one, i.e., SF variations are reversible. Inflammation-induced SF variations manifest in increasing neutrophils and decreasing lymphocytes. The appearance of macrophages, plasmocytes, and individual large nuclear cells indicate activation of the cellular chain of immune system in exacerbations. Occurrence in SF of the cells involved in immune reactions of the joint in exacerbations, and reversibility of inflammation-induced SF variations in remissions allow us to classify osteoarthrosis as a nonimmune disease. Variations in the synovia cellular composition in rheumatoid arthritis and Bekhterev's disease resemble acute inflammation of joints; however, the presence of specific cells in the specimens (rhagocytes containing accumulations of immune complexes) points to the immune mechanism of joint pathology. Malignant cells detected in the synovia make it possible to identify a neoplastic process in the joint cavity. Long thin and sharp crystals of urates (salts of uric acid) in undrained aspirates confirm podagric nonimmune joint inflammation.

Biochemical analysis of the SF specimens at all diseases stages (Table 3.4) displays distinctions in the ratio of protein fractions in acute and chronic nonimmune inflammations in diseases of immune genesis.

Table 3.4. Biochemical parameters of SF specimens in diseases

Parameter	Normal SF	Bekhterev's disease	Rheumatoid arthritis	Degenerative-dystrophic process	Acute synovitis
Whole protein, g/l including:	10	35	53	32	36
albumins, %	63	55	51	60	60
α_1-globulins, %	7	7	8	9	8
α_2-globulins, %	7	13	15	8	11
β-globulins, %	9	10	7	10	10
γ-globulins, %	14	15	19	13	11
Fibrin	–	+	+	–	–
C-reactive protein	–	+	+	–	+
Rheumatoid factor	–	–	+	–	–
Mucin clot	dense	loose	loose	dense	loose
Hyaluronic acid , g/l	2.45	2.25	2.10	2.30	1.85

In synovitis of any genesis the whole protein increases in SF mainly at the cost of α_1- and α_2-globulins, and C-reactive protein appears. Finding rheumatoid factor in the synovia of the rheumatoid arthritis patients confirms the immune and seropositive variant of the disease. The seropositive variant means the availability of positive antigen-antibody reaction recorded on the basis of one of the enzymes accompanying the immune complex formation (agglutination, complement binding, etc.). As noted, the more active inflammation in the joint the higher the density of the mucin clot. At the same time, a relation arises between hyaluronic acid concentration in the effusion and acuteness of inflammation in the joint.

However, the aforesaid tests are often insufficient for more comprehensive study of nosological forms (*nosology* is a science about diseases and their classification) and variants of diseases. Typical SF changes in some inflammatory and noninflammatory diseases will be considered in more detail in the next paragraphs.

3.2.1. Immune Rheumatic Diseases

Immune disorders of joints are systemic (referring to the functional system) immune inflammatory diseases of connective tissues of the joint of unknown etiology that are followed, as mentioned in 2.3.2, by formation of autologous antibodies against protein structures of the proper organism.

Origination of autoimmune diseases is related [2] to persistence (prolonged symptom-free existence) in SM of infectious agents such as L-forms of bacteria, atypical mycoplasmas (general name for inflammation-inducing microorganisms of the Mycoplasmaceae family), latent viruses (i.e., viruses demonstrating a period of latent activity) and their trigger role. In engineering, *a trigger* means a switching device that is in one of two states of stable equilibrium and by signal is switched from one state to another stepwisely. In medicine, *a trigger* is a launching causative factor of infectious or some other nature that initiates a disease. Because of molecular mimicry (structure similarity) of individual antigens of an infectious agent and molecular structures of SM and cartilage, the cellular and humoral response with hyperproduction of antibodies and pathological immune complexes is activated. This results in disruption of immune tolerance to the connective tissues and development of uncontrolled self-maintained immunopathological chronic inflammation of SM. The damaging effect of the infectious agent is related to its interference in the genome and metabolism of SM and SF cells, which gives rise to the synthesis of abnormal hyaluroproteins by synoviocytes [9].

Patient's genetic propensity is of crucial importance in the development of immune diseases. This is supported by autoimmune diseases inherited by the vertical in patients' families and the antigens of histological compatibility found in the families of the patients with autoimmune diseases (HLA DR4, Dw4 and DQ7 in rheumatoid arthritis and HLA-B27 in Bekhterev's disease) [10]. Antigens of histocompatibility are immobilized on the cell surfaces including lymphocytes, and can act as receptors for infectious agents. Genetic abnormalities found in the molecular structure of collagen and antibodies against it, congenital deficiency of cellular membranes and abnormalities of the ground substance of the connective tissue in the rheumatoid arthritis patients indicate the primary (genetic) nature of a collagen disorder [11].

Development of immune joint diseases is stimulated by chronic focal (mainly nasopharingeal) streptococcal infection in a human organism, allergies, joint traumas, overcooling, and hormonal changes.

Juvenile rheumatoid arthritis (JRA) manifests in children and is a typical immune inflammation of the joint. In diagnosing JRA, a decisive role belongs to the investigation of functional morphology of SM, cartilage, and SF. In children, SF is the most easily accessible component of the synovial medium [12]. The authors of [13] report the findings of the investigation into the ultrastructure (the structure invisible by a light microscope) of SF components in different forms and stages of the pathology.

It is found that with JRA in progress cytosis is observed, namely, an increased amount of cellular elements (from 7.1±0.7 to 26.0±3.4×10^9 /l) with polymorphic nuclear leucocytes (up to 92%) and increased concentration of whole protein (up to 43 g/l) in the synovial effusion. With decreasing joint inflammation an increased amount of the cellular elements due to lymphocytes is observed in 50% of patients. A large amount of polymorphic nuclear leucocytes in SF causes its purulent appearance (cloudy bright-yellow fluid). However, bacteriological analysis of SF though so changed does not reveal any microorganisms in it.

The ratio of the cells in SF in different forms of JRA (articular, systemic, or seropositive) and at different inflammation intensities is reliably equal. Rhagocytes in the effusion depend on the activity of JRA. At degrees I and II their amount reaches 9.4±1.3%, at III it increases up to 18.8±2.9%, whereas in the seropositive patients it may rise up to 6%. More than 80% of polymorphic nuclear leucocytes and 15% of rhagocytes as well as whole protein concentration 40 g/l and more correspond to the maximal intensity of joint inflammation. Electron microscopy examination of the SF cells shows neutrophil changes caused by their degranulation, appearance of lipid inclusions in the cypoplasm and fine cellular processes. Plasmocytes and rhagocytes are characterized by the hypersegmentation of nuclei, increasing number and accumulations of lysosomes and lipid drops as well as vacuoles with heterogeneous content in the cytoplasm.

In the systemic and fast developing JRA, electron microscopy reveals collagen-producing cells and a collagen net in SF. The collagen net is thinned collagen fibers of different form 20−60 nm in diameter (the so-called interfibrillary dysplastic collagen) between which detritus (a decomposition product) is found in the form of dispersed inclusions. Also, erythrocytes are detected among collagen fibers to indicate the insufficiency of the hemosynovial barrier. Degenerative changes in the articular cartilage result in chondrocytes with the signs of destruction (increasing number and size of lysosomes, formation of fine processes on the cell surface, etc.) found in SF.

Rheumatoid arthritis in adults most often starts at an age of 35−45 years. The relation between rheumatoid arthritis and infection is proved by serologic (based of antigen-antibody reactions) and microbiological studies of patients' SF and blood serum. The relation between streptococcal infection and arthritis is proved by finding the streptococci complex with hemagglutinating macroglobulin that does not differ from rheumatoid factor in its properties [14]. The staphylococcus antigen is attributed to the increasing permeability of the hemosynovial barrier in the rheumatoid arthritis patients' SF. Mycoplasmas were found in SF and blood serum [15] in rheumatoid arthritis and a number of other rheumatoid diseases. The SF immunoglobulins proved to be strongly associated with the mycoplasma membrane and stimulate the formation of rheumatoid factor. Viral etiology of the disease is considered elsewhere [16]. Electron microscopy discloses tubular ultrastructures (tube-shaped) interpreted as viral bodies in the endothelium cells of capillaries and venules of different organs and tissues as well as in lymphocytes and fibroblasts. A high concentration of antibodies against viruses was revealed in the blood serum of the patients. However, today, the viral nature of rheumatoid arthritis is questionable. The ultra-structures are interpreted as manifestations of cell damages since it appears unsuccessful to isolate tubular ultrastructures or identify viruses by the immunofluorescent method.

Immune reactions of the immediate type in rheumatoid arthritis are based on formation of immune complexes for which aggregated γ-globulin is an antigen and rheumatoid factors (Ig M) having antibody specifics against Fc-fragment of the γ-globulin molecule is an antibody. Rheumatoid factor has the nonspecific affinity with the connective tissue. In pathogenesis, its value is not still understood [5]. At a large concentration of rheumatoid factor in the human organism large complexes appear in the blood serum that consists of one molecule of the rheumatoid factor and five molecules of immunoglobulin.

Changes in SF in this disease, as in JRA, depend on the intensity of inflammatory and destructive processes in joints. Rheumatoid synovitis is characterized by the changes in SM in the form of hyperplasia (increasing quantity) of villi, proliferation (enlargement) of lining cells, infiltrates of lymphocytes and plasma cells with formation of follicles, superficial and deep deposition of fibrin, and necrosis spots. Exacerbation of inflammation is responsible for the hemorrhage in the SM, appearance or increase of a fibrinous exudate in the joint, and proliferation of synoviocytes. The diagnosis of rheumatoid synovitis is supported by biopsy (diagnostic resection) of SM and detection of the depositions of immunoglobulins, complement, and rheumatoid factor by means of immunofluorescent microscopy. The biopsy material of the articular cartilage of the patella in rheumatoid arthritis differs from a normal one in the deposition of protein masses in the cartilage matrix, pronounced dystrophic modifications of chondrocytes and their weak proliferative activity, cartilage erosions as the result of invasion (spread) of the pathologically modified SM tissue, and cystosous cavities at the place of died chondrocytes.

In rheumatoid arthritis lysosome enzymes (hydrolases) play an important role in the pathogenesis of tissue damages. Their increased number and activity is induced by infectious agents, that is, absorption of large immune complexes by synoviocytes, polymorphic nuclear leucocytes, and macrophages is accompanied by the squeezing of lysosomes from cytoplasm and their damage with liberation of their enzymes in extracellular spaces. Lysosome enzymes catalyzing hydrolysis, i.e., hydrolases (phosphatases, collagenase, etc.) destroy collagen fibers and proteoglycans, suppress the synthesis of polysaccharides of the cartilage matrix, and cause the erosion of the articular cartilage [14].

In rheumatoid SF, the whole protein increases (up to 53 g/l) mainly at the cost of γ-globulins, fibrins, and C-reactive protein (Table 3.4). The general level of the complement decreases and the C4-component fraction increases. A decrease in hyaluronic acid is reported [5], lower SF viscosity, and increased concentration of the chondrotin-4-sulfate. Destroyed metabolism of collagen manifests itself in exacerbations of inflammation in the joint by increasing amounts of collagen metabolites (protein-bound oxyproline, or monocarbonic amino acid) in urine and blood plasma.

The cellular composition of SF is distinguished by an increased amount of leucocytes up to 10^{10} /l [17] with neutrophils (up to 7%), lymphocytes (up to 3%), and monocytes (up to 25%) as constituents (Table 3.3). In the disease, specifically modified poly- and mononuclear leucocytes and microphages (rhagocytes) are detected in SF in 9% of cases. In their cytoplasm specific immune complexes (from 3 to 10) with the rheumatoid factor Ig M are found. In many lymphocytes, the activation signs are observed characterized by the margination (the edge-located nucleic chromatin), large nuclei, moderately developed endoplasmatic net, viz the system of channels, vesicles, and *cisterns* limited by membranes, an insignificant number of lysosome and mitochondria. Fibroblasts are met in SF in the form of groups or individually lying oval cells with a large nucleus and several small nuclei, the cell membrane of some of them having lashes.

Rheumatoid factor is not detected in the blood serum in 10–30% of patients with typical rheumatoid arthritis during a long time. This kind of the disease is called *seronegative rheumatoid arthritis*. Rheumatoid factor detected in SF earlier than in the blood serum reliably indicates the seropositive variant.

Bekhterev's disease (ankylosing spondylarthritis) is a chronic inflammatory ankylosing (accompanied by the adhesion of joint surfaces) pathology of axial skeleton from the group of seronegative spondylarthritis or inflammation of intervertebral joints. In this disease the cartilaginous joints and intervertebral disks are damaged (the central form of the disease). As for synovial joints, most often in Bekhterev's disease large joints of the limbs are damaged. A mixed nature of disorders manifests in rhisomelic (relating to intervertebral disks and the roots of the limbs, e.g., shoulder and hip), peripheral, (ulnar, radiocapral, knee, and ankle joints are damaged), and *Scandinavian* (small joints of hands and arms are damaged) disease forms. Inflammation mechanisms (infiltration, i.e., invasion of macrophages and lymphocytes into joint tissues) and its etiology (detection of the histocompatibility antigen HLA-B27 in 81–97% of patients) point to immune nature of the inflammation.

The study of cellular and biochemical SF composition in diagnosing Bekhterev's disease is hindered because it can be conducted only in the peripheral form of the disease when synovitis is accompanied by accumulation of effusion in the joint cavity which can be aspirated.

A similarity has been revealed [8] of biochemical changes in SF in the knee joint synovitis in Bekhterev's disease and rheumatoid arthritis except for the rheumatoid factor being absent in spondylarthritis. The cellular composition in Bekhterev's disease is distinguished by a small amount of lymphocytes and monocytes (6–8%) and absence of rhagocytes.

Arthritis of immunopathological genesis due to infection and invasion, i.e., penetration of parasites in the joint (reactive arthritis, generalized immune-inflammatory reactions in chronic infections, post-vaccine arthritis, etc.) can be included in immune joint diseases.

Reactive arthritis is an aseptic (non purulent) inflammation of joints arising during or 1 to 2 months after an infection as the result of the cascade of immune disorders. The "reactive arthritis" term was suggested in 1969 by Finnish researchers P. Ahvonen, K. Sievers, K. Aho (1969), who were the first to describe arthritis after Yersinia infection (an intestinal infection induced by microbes of *Yersinia enterocolitica* and *Yersinia pseudotuberculosis*).

Nowadays, streptococci (rheumatic), Chlamydia, Yersinia, salmonella arthritis and arthritis occurring in viral diseases (viral hepatitis and rubella) refer to reactive arthritis [18]. In the structure of rheumatic diseases the frequency of reactive arthritis is from 8 to 41% [19]. In terms of etiology, two kinds of reactive arthritis are distinguished, that is, 1) reactive arthritis associated with the antigen B_{27} of the HLA system (induced by such causative agents as Yersinia, schigella, salmonella, and campilobacteria); 2) reactive arthritis without general genetic association with the HLA-system (rheumatic arthritis, arthritis in viral hepatitis at the background of HBS-antigenaemia, rheumatic meningitis, after acute respiratory and other viral infections). Reactive arthritis arises in people with genetic predisposition due to an excessive immune response of the organism to microbe antigens found outside joint cavity with the formation of immune complexes and their deposition in SM, which results in immune complex arthritis. Reiter's disease is believed [17] to be a particular variant of reactive arthritis. It has the complex of symptoms (syndrome) of polyarthritis, uretritis, and conjunctivitis after enterocolitic (relating to intestine inflammation) or urogenital (involving urogenital organs) Chlamydia infection.

Previously it has been believed that reactive arthritis is "sterile" since neither a living disease-inducing agent nor its antigens could be detected. Afterwards, with improvements in the methodology, antigens of microbes, chlamydia DNA, as well as proper microorganisms capable of multiplication were detected in joint tissues and SF [20]. In this connection, the "reactive arthritis" term should be used carefully [21]. However, it is widely spread up to now both in literature and in the international classifications of diseases.

Synovia displays nonspecific changes of inflammatory nature, namely, the fluid is cloudy, yellowish, low-viscous, the leucocytes vary within $(2 \div 100) \times 10^9$/l, neutrophils exceed 50%, and the mucin clot is flaky. An increase in the level of α_2- and γ-globulins, occurrence of the fibrin of seromucoid and C-reactive protein in SF arte associated with the changes in the biochemical blood test. In the blood of the patients with reactive Yersinia arthritis, high antibody titers were found by passive hemagglutination and in those with dysentery high values of antibody titers to causative agents were detected by indirect hemagglutination with standard erythrocytic diagnostics. The antibody titer is an ultimate dilution of blood serum at which antibody activity is revealed by serologic reaction. In the given case, the diagnostic antibody titer is 1:200 and higher. In chlamydia infection antibodies to Chlamydia antigens were detected in the blood serum and SF by serological reactions (complement binding and direct and indirect immunofluorescence)

In viral arthritis, viral antigens and (or) immune complexes with them are revealed in the blood and SF. In some cases viruses are localized in the joint cavity, and blood demonstrates high antiviral antibody titers.

Reactive arthritis is predisposed to total remission (inverse development) but may also recur and even become chronic and involve ever more joints.

3.2.2. Nonimmune Rheumatic Diseases

Despite isolation of the "nonimmune diseases of joints" in an individual group, synovitis forms to be considered in this paragraph have immunopathological and humoral forms though insignificantly pronounced and playing a secondary sequential role in the pathogenesis. Therefore, the *predominantly nonimmune diseases* term sounds more accurate.

Infection-induced arthritis results from invasion of bacterial agents directly into the joint cavity. Infection most probably passes from the lesions in the oral cavity, the respiratory tract, the urogenital tract and some others on blood vessels. It is called hematogenic, i.e., referring to the blood stream. More rarely infection is spread by the lymphatic system. Primary infection of the joint cavity is probable in wounding or operations and punctures. Inflammation can be induced by microorganisms of the same kind (staphylo-, strepto-, gonococci, enterobacteria, blue pus bacillus, clostridia, etc.) or associations of microorganisms.

Clear local manifestations of the disease include joint pains, swelling, hyperemia (plethora), hyperthermia (temperature elevation), and regional lymphadenitis (damage of regional lymphatic vessels), in combination with general intoxication symptoms, i.e., high body temperature, chill, etc. This allows assumption of the septic (bacterial) etiology of arthritis at the earliest stage.

The exudate amount sharply increases in the affected joint. The effusion is cloudy and flaky or puruloid of lowered viscosity, leucocytosis exceeds 5×10^{10}/l, neutrophils prevailing. The glucose concentration is lowered and that of lactic acid is increased. The microscopy of the deposit, fluid inoculations, and SM biopsy material make it possible to detect an arthritic causative agent and determine its susceptibility to antibiotics to provide a purposeful individual therapy.

Lyme disease, borreliosis (the name is related to the region around Lyme, Connecticut, USA where in 1977 an outbreak of pediatric arthritis occurred) is the combination of recurring mono- or oligoarthritis with migrating erythema [22]. Erythema is a limited hyperemia (enhanced local blood flow) and skin redness. The disease etiology was discovered much later – in 1982 when its causative agent was determined (spirochete *Borrelia burgdorferi*) carried by ixodic ticks [23]. The invasion of the causative agent into human organism induces changes in all organs and systems. Intoxication and skin rash are accompanied by lymphoadenopathy, splenomegalia, neurological disorders in the form of meningitis, encephalitis, and myelitis, as well as cardiac disorders including myopericarditis, pancarditis and conductance disturbances [24]. Spirochetes' targets are collagen skin fibers, synovial membranes of joints and tendons, and other proteoglycan-containing tissues.

Within several months to 2 years after the disease onset, arthritis is developed in 60% of patients. The joint syndrome lasts for about a week, does not cause a persistent joint deformation; however, it can recur or acquire a chronic mode (in 10% of patients). Large joints are predominantly affected (hip, knee, or shoulder). Sometimes Borrelia are found in SM of the patients with chronic arthritis. The chronic inflammation is apparently due to not only the causative agent but also immunopathological antigen-dependent reactions running in the joint tissues. Borrelia are not managed to detect in the synovial effusion [2].

Serologic methods are more accessible for lab verification in practice. The immune-enzymatic method, indirect immunofluorescence, and western immunoblotting [25] are the most widely spread methods to determine anti-borreliosis antibodies. In CIS countries, the indirect immunofluorescence reaction is widely used. The corpuscular antigen from the strain Ip-21 *Borrelia afzelii* that is prepared in the laboratory of infection transmitters in Gamalei Scientific Institute of Epidemiology and Microbiology, Russian Academy of Sciences [26] is used in this reaction. Western blotting or immunoblotting as the method for detecting antibodies on microfilters is spread in the USA and Great Britain.

Immune disorders in borreliosis are supported by the cryogenic technique of globulins and immune complexes in SF and blood. Biochemical changes in SF are nonspecific, that is, the protein level increases at the cost of α_2- and γ-globulins, and fibrin appears to be deposited on SM infiltered by plasmo- and lymphocytes. The number of leucocytes is $5\times10^2\div10^5$/ml.

Microcrystalline arthritis is developed in gout, chondrocalcinosis, and hydroxyapatite arthropathia caused by the formation of crystals of some substances in articular tissues. In gout, the breaking of either the congenital (genetically caused) or acquired (in malignant tumors, endocrine, hematological, and other diseases) mechanism of uric acid metabolism results in increasing uric acid in the blood serum (hyperuricaemia) and deposition of sodium monourate crystals predominantly in the articular tissues, skin, and kidneys. This is largely because the uric acid solubility is lower in SF than in the blood plasma. In long-term treatment of gout, the urates penetrate from SF into the cartilage, subchondral bone, articular capsule, tendons, and ligaments forming the accumulations of sodium monourate crystals in them. These latter along with blood plasma become the sources of crystals for SF, which results in a chronic mode of arthritis occurrence and erosive changes of joint tissues [2, 17]. **Chondrocalcinosis** (pseudo-gout) is a chronic disease in the form of recurrences of acute arthritis due to disorder in the inorganic pyrophosphate (salts of condensed phosphoric acids) exchange and deposition of calcium pyrophosphate in the joint cartilage. Pyrophosphate is an important intermediate metabolite in the synthesis of proteoglycans and collagen with chondrocytes. It is believed that in chondrocalcinosis, either the formation of pyrophosphate is enhanced or activity of the breaking component, namely, pyrophosphase, is lowered. As the result, crystals of calcium pyrophosphate dihydrate arise, are deposited in the joint tissues and damage them. **Hydroxyapatite arthropathia** is a chronic disease induced by hydroxyapatite crystal deposition in periarticular tissues and manifesting as periodically occurring acute periarthritis. The immunopathological mechanism of the disease is unknown. The inflammation pathogenesis is similar to other joint diseases, that is, egress of crystals from tissues into the cavities of vaginal synovial membranes and bursas results in migration of neutrophil leucocytes and phagocytosis of crystals with the emergence of inflammation-inducing lysosome enzymes and biologically active substances (mediators).

For differential diagnostics of microcrystalline arthritis the corresponding crystals are searched in a synovial effusion free of anticoagulant within 6 hours after obtaining the puncture material [27]. The clots and deposits obtained on effusion centrifugation are studied. The crystals can be revealed by the common-used light microscopy. Polarization microscopy makes it possible to more accurately determine the kind of crystals. They can be disposed in the extracellular space or inside the neutrophils phagocizing them. The detection of the crystals in leucocytes cytoplasm is of the highest diagnostic importance.

In gout, the sodium monourate crystals are detected in the joint effusion in the form of thin a needle up to 10–20 μm long that tend to form packs or bunches. The crystals do not disappear with addition of ethyldiamine tetra acetate under usage in analytical chemistry, do not destroy by the uricase enzyme, and demonstrate a strong double refraction in polarization microscopy. In chodrocalcinosis, the crystals of calcium pyrophosphate dihydrate in the form of sticks 5-10 μm long as well as rectangular and rhomboid plates up to 4 μm wide are detected in the synovial effusion. The crystals are dissolved after addition of ethylamine tetraacetate but not destroyed by uricase and in polarization microscopy they demonstrate a weakly pronounced positive double refraction. Calcium hydroxyapatite crystals are seldom revealed by a conventional light microscopy because of their small size and fast dissolution when appeared in SF. They are oval or polygonal shining formations 1–5 μm in size that consist of weakly polarizing or not refracting crystal agglomerates. Electron microscopy is advisable to detect calcium hydroxyapatite crystals.

Hyperuricemia, an increased amount of uric acid in the blood, does not necessarily points to gout, as well calcification characterized by deposits of calcium salts in the joint points to pseudo-gout. In questionable diagnostic cases, to identify gout and pseudo-gout the deposit obtained in SF centrifugation is examined by means of a polarization microscope with a red filter. Needle crystals of uric acid salts or urates characteristic of gout are shining yellow if their long axis is in parallel to the axis of microscope compensator. Calcium pyrophosphate crystals characteristic of pseudo-gout are rhomboid and shining blue. In gout and pseudo-gout crystals can be detected in neutrophils.

Osteoarthritis deformans is a chronic slowly progressing joint disease due to degenerative-dystrophic lesions of hyaline cartilage. Up to 80% of all cases of rheumatic diseases fall on this pathology.

The disease is due to excessive mechanical loads to joints above physiological norms (with excessive body weight), chronic cartilage microtraumatization in professional activities or in sport, as well as to the overloading of articular surfaces in their abnormal congruency (in dysplasia, i.e., in wrong anatomic joint development, consequences of traumas and disorders, etc.). The above causes result in the lesion of collagen fibers of hyaline cartilage and restriction of its regenerative capability.

In osteoarthritis, the changes in the SF composition and properties depend on the stage of degenerative process and its periods (remission or exacerbation of secondary synovitis in traumas and mechanical joint overloading, overcooling, etc.). Typical changes in the cellular and biochemical composition of SF in osteoarthrosis are shown in Tables 3.3 and 3.4. At the remission stage of synovitis, the volume of the joint fluid, its composition, and properties are within normal values, the effusion viscosity is normal or exceeds the norm, and the hyaluronic acid amount is normal or above the normal value. In exacerbation periods, the changes in the cellular and biochemical composition correspond to aseptic inflammation, that is, the SF volume increases, its viscosity is lowered, it might become cloudy, the whole protein amount increases, and the cellular composition varies (neutrophils increase and gigantic multinuclear cells appear).

Mechanical and inflammatory damage to synovio- and chondrocytes provokes the egress of catabolic (decomposing complex organic substances) enzymes, which causes decrease and destruction of the hyaluronate in SF and destroys the structure of other proteoglycans that regulate the motion of the articular fluid and provide normal lubrication and mechanical properties of articular cartilage.

3.2.3. Arthropathies in Nonrheumatic Diseases

Pigmented villonodular synovitis is related to benign tumor diseases of joints of unknown etiology. It is characterized by the pronounced SM hyperplasia with villi and noduli enlarged. Morphologically, gigantic multinuclear cells pigment (hemosiderine) crystal deposits are recognized in SM formations. Villi traumatization results in the accumulation of hemorrhagic effusions in the joint cavity and secondary synovitis. SF becomes brownie or hemorrhagic. Impregnation of the articular cartilage with hemosiderine causes its secondary degenerative changes.

Analysis of spectrophotometric characteristics of synovial effusions [28] makes it possible to differentiate the pigmented villonodular synovitis and synovitis of traumatic and rheumatic etiology. The technique consists in measuring optical density of effusion in the region of protein (D_{280}) and pigment (D_{460}) absorption and determining their ratio ($K = D_{280}/D_{460}$). At K below12, pigmented villonodular synovitis is diagnosed.

In this disease the cellular composition of SF is characterized by a high amount of lymphocytes (28–45%) and presence of macrophages [29], which point to activization of immune cells.

Joint SM tumors are divided into benign and malign ones. Malign tumors can be primary and secondary (metastatic). Primary tumors are characterized by monoarticular damages of SM tissue with gradual onset. In tumor growth secondary synovitis is developed in SM with accumulation of noninflammatory effusion in the articular cavity.

Primary malign tumors of SM and bursas (synovioma, sarcoma, and fibrosarcoma) are characterized by a fast growth, increasing pain syndrome, and night pains. Synovial effusion is hemorrhagic (of blood color) in color. The cellular composition of SF demonstrates the presence of tumor cells and their agglomerates.

Most often the lung, breast, urine bladder, and prostate cancers give metastases in SM. In a number of cases, symptoms of joint damages precede the clinical detection of a primary tumor.

Tumors of articular bone end are classified in the same way as SM tumors. Chondroma, osteochondroma, osteoid-osteoma, chondroblastoma (Kodman's disease, E.E. Kodman, an American surgeon), osteoblastoclastoma (gigantic-cell tumor) are referred to benign tumors. A clinical X-ray picture of the diseases from this category does not differ from others. In the case of subpeiosteal (beneath the periosteum) localization of the tumor and its growth towards epiphysis with involvement of the articular capsule, secondary synovitis is probable.

Primary malign tumors of the articular bone end (osteogenic sarcoma, para-ostal fibrosarcoma, chodrosarcoma, malign osteoblasoclastoma, etc.) are distinguished by a fast growth. Secondary synovitis arises once the tumor is transferred to SM.

Both in benign and malign tumors the effusion amount in the joint varies from normal to significant. In puncturing the joint cavity sometimes just a drop of blood is feasible to obtain, which gives one a wrong idea about traumatization of soft tissues with a needle. However, even one drop is a valuable diagnostic material wherein tumor cells can be recognized.

Paraneoplastic arthritis is reactive non-oncological condition with syndromes arising from metabolic, immune, endocrine, and other changes in the organism under the effect of primary tumor growth outside joints. The relation of malign neoplasm to paraneoplastic reactions is supported by the regression or disappearance of these latter after radical tumor removal. Neither characteristic biochemical changes or cell regeneration are detected in studying the synovial effusion.

Arthritis in hemorrhagic diatheses (hemophilia, thrombocytopenic purpura) arises from hemorrhage into peri-articular tissues and subsequent penetration of blood into joints, which results in the development of secondary joint inflammation with significant pains and disturbance of limb functions. Synovial effusion undergoes the same changes in the joint as in traumatic hemarthrosis. Repeated hemorrhages lead to SM fibrosis (fibrosis is enlargement of fibrous connective tissue), obliteration of synovial torsions, cartilage destruction, narrowing of the joint fissure, and its impaired mobility.

In hemorrhagic vasculitis (Shönlein-Genoch's disease, J.L. Shönlein, a German physiscian and E.H. Genoch, a German pediatric), arthritis often induced by hemorrhage into para-articular tissues, however, hemorrhage into joint cavities does not occur. SF changes are nonspecific and similar to acute aseptic inflammation.

3.3. Age-Related Changes

Ageing is a natural process of age-related changes in organs and systems occurring in each living organism in ontogenesis, viz transformations experienced by an organism within a life span. Three age periods of ageing are distinguished, namely, middle age (from 45 to 59 years old), elderly age (from 60 to 74 years old) and old age (75 years old and older). Those who are 90 and more years old are referred to long-livers.

In contrast to osteoarthrosis deformans, dystrophic and destructive processes in joints in ageing are not considered as diseases although in both cases the cartilage degeneration and bone deformations occur. Age-related diseases of joints are characterized by the following features:

- joint ageing is due to osteoporosis and dystrophy of articular cartilage;
- clinical occurrence of age-related degeneration is of gradual slowly progressing mode; complains to muscle tiredness and weakness prevail; joints are less mobile;
- in X-ray examination and morphological analysis, sclerosis of the subchondral plate is pronounced insignificantly; changes manifest more intensively in the most heavy-duty regions and are symmetrical; edge bone-cartilage enlargements can be absent or insignificant and appear in the old age;
- decreased cartilage thickness results in gradual symmetrical shortening of limbs by 1–2 cm.

Most cells of an adult human organism is capable of division only by a certain number of doublings, which is due to shortening of DNA occurring in each division in the end portions of chromosomes, that is, telomeres [30]. During life span the changes in the DNA molecules result in the distortion of synthesis and decomposition of the enzyme-protein system with catabolic reactions prevailing, which also contribute to structural and functional changes in the cells and their dying.

The cells under ageing in the human organism tissues are featured by the changes in the form of reduction (decreasing sizes) of organoids and cytoplasm, graininess of nuclei and mitochondria, decrease and flattening of vesicles of the Golgi complex, increase of lysosome quantity, and decrease of endoplasmatic net channels and ribosomes (intracellular particles involved in protein synthesis) on their membranes [31]. Nuclei graininess and their nonuniform coloring indicate an energetically less active and more stable state of cellular metabolism.

Age-related vascular changes impair trophic processes of all organism tissues. The walls of the vessels feeding the joint capsule get thickened, sclerosized and their lumens get narrower. In some places, the wall of capillaries adjoins the joint cavity thus providing a free invasion of toxins and antigens in the joint cavity and development of reactive SM inflammation. The collagen fiber bunches of the joint capsule are hyalinized in some locations (hyalinosis is a protein dystrophy characterized by the deposition of extracellular dense protein masses in the tissue) and comprise the deposits of calcium salts and cartilage tissue elements. In old age, the capsule layers are often not differentiated. After 75 years old the amount of hyaluronic acid sharply gets lower in the joint capsule tissues and is only identified in the SM villi. SM gets rough, atrophied and the villous layer is deprived of cellular elements to decrease the production of SF and changes in its biochemical composition, cartilage dystrophy, and impaired functioning of the joint.

The knee joint cartilage undergoes age-related changes earlier than other bone systems. They occur in the most heavy-duty regions at the upper pole of patella and medial condyles of hip and tibia bones. The cartilage surface under ageing is deprived of the surface layer, namely, the perichondrium, and gets cloudy, yellowish-gray, grainy, and rough. In an old age erosions, cracks, desquamation spots, and defects within 1.5 cm in size appear on the cartilage friction surface. Chondrocytes of isogenic groups (identical morphologically) swell and are agglomerated in 6–8 cells, with their nuclei shifted to the periphery. Separately disposed chondrocytes are enlarged and have large nucleus and plenty vacuoles. The signs observed indicate dystrophic changes in the cartilage cells.

The concentration of cellular elements in the dystrophically modified cartilage is nonuniform and in some places chondrocytes are absent. The cartilage tissue is dysfibered and necrotized at the edges of cracks, not structured, and adjacent chondrocytes are lysed. Hyaluronic acid is localized in the edge zones of the joint cartilage, around chondrocytes, and in the basal layer. At 90 years old and older, hyaluronic acid is not detected in the joint tissues; instead of it because of deceleration of the metabolism, sulfated glycosaminoglycans (predominantly keratosulfates) are accumulated with the formation of larger macromolecular compounds than hyaluronic acid. The accumulation of keratosulfates in the basal substance and basal cartilage layer is a compensatory and adaptive phenomenon that increases the density of the degenerating cartilage tissue.

The properties and functions of SF vary due to increasing permeability of the vessel walls of the joint capsule, age-related depression of the production and accumulation of hyaluronic acid, decelerating metabolism between the elements of the synovial medium. Its amount in joint cavity decreases from 3–4 to 1–2 ml and biochemical composition approaches that of blood serum, i.e., the hyaluronic acid concentration decreases progressively and the protein content rises. Enzymes in SF that belong to decomposing cellular structures of cartilage and

SM grow insignificantly, which accelerates the degeneration of joint tissues. At the initial ageing stage the cellular composition of SF does not differ from normal. Afterwards, synoviocytograms changes are of inflammatory nature, viz synoviocytes and histiocytes (connective tissue cells, a kind of macrophages) are detected with the signs of degeneration as well as died tissue cells and their parts. Moreover, the cartilage wear products are present in SF in the form of tissue particles and collagen fibers of different shape and size. Impaired viscosity as the result of the loss of high-molecular components leads to the tribological and amortization dysfunctions. Therefore, age-related changes in the composition and properties of SF due to insufficiency of other elements of synovial medium contribute into their changes.

Acknowledgments

The chapter generalizes the data on the most significant nosologies in the groups of immune and nonimmune joint diseases as well typical modifications of SF. A diversity of pathological conditions of the synovial medium of joints described in medical literature is considered by the authors mainly in terms of clinical diagnostics. Analysis of cytological and biochemical changes in synovial effusions traditionally used in orthopedics is helpful in diagnostics and quality management of joint treatment. Application of the methods of molecular biology and immunology to rheumatic pathologies has made it possible to understand the nature of many diseases and discover a genetic propensity for their development. The next level of diagnostics assumes complex assessment of joint conditions with regard to biophysical variations and functional disorders of the synovial medium. The approach aims to optimize joint treatment at all disease stages as well as individually protect cartilages.

References

[1] *International statistic classification of diseases and health-related problems. 10th revised edition.* In: World Health Organization in 2 volumes, Geneve, 1995, Vol 2.

[2] Ivashkin, VT; Sultanov, VK. *Joint diseases. Propedeutics, differential diagnosis, and treatment.* Moscow: Litterra, 2005.

[3] Voronovich, IR. *Injuries of the knee joint.* Minsk: Belarus, 1971.

[4] Pavlova, VN. *Synovial medium of joints.* Moscow: Medicine, 1980.

[5] Gerasimov, AM; Furtseva, LN. *Biochemical diagnostics in traumatology and orthopedics.* Moscow: Medicine, 1986.

[6] Redin, VA; Mazaeva, GP. *Hyaluronidase-hyaluronic acid system in traumatic arthritis of knee joint.* In: Collection of Methodic Materials CITO. Moscow: Medicine, 1972, 17–19.

[7] Playtsko, VV; Levenets, VN; Stavinskii YuA. Changes in synovial medium in deforming gonarthrosis. *Orthop. Traumatol. Prosth.* 1990, N 5, 24–28.

[8] Cherniakova, YuM. *Optimization of diagnostics and treatment of synovitis by controlling biophysical properties of the synovial fluid.* PhD Med Thesis, Minsk, 2006.

[9] Smith, C; Hammerman, D. *Evidence for a viral etiology of rheumatoid synovitis*. In: Infection and immunology in the rheumatic diseases. Ed. Dumonde, DC. Oxford: Blackwell, 1976, 213−224.

[10] Soroka, NF. Clinical rheumatology at the centennial border. *Zdravookhranenine,* 2001, N 5, 2−7.

[11] Steffen, C; Ludvig, H; Knapp, W; et al. Collagen antibodies and collagen-anicollagen immune complexes in rheumatoid arthritis, *Z. Rheumat.* 1975, Bd 34, 391−399.

[12] Dulyapin, VA. Morphological features of synovial membrane and joint cartilage in different forms and variants of rheumatic arthritis. *Doctor Sci. Med. Thesis.* Moscow, 1987.

[13] Lazarchik, IV; Vasilevskii, IV; Netukova, NI. Cytological characteristic of synovial fluid in juvenile rheumatoid arthritis. *Zdravookhranenie.* 2003, N 7, 6−10.

[14] Kopyeva, TN. *The pathology of rheumatoid arthritis.* Moscow: Medicine, 1980.

[15] Gardner, DL. *The pathology of rheumatoid arthritis.* London: Arnold, 1972.

[16] Neumark, T; Farkas, K. *Virus-like particles and some ultrastructural aspects of lymphoreticular cells in rheumatoid synovial membrane*. In: Infection and immunology in the rheumatic diseases. Ed. Dumonde, DC. Oxford: Blackwell, 1976, 225−233.

[17] *Diagnostics and treatment of internal diseases. Handbook for physicians* in 3 Vol. Ed. Komarov, FI. Vol 1. Diseases of cardio-vascular system, rheumatic diseases. Moscow: Medicine, 1991.

[18] Chirkin, AA; Okorokov, AN; Goncharik, II. *Diagnostic reference book of a physician: clinical symptoms, patient examination programs, and data interpretation.* Minsk: Belarus, 1994.

[19] Cassidy, JT; Petty, RE. *Textbook of pediatric rheumatology.* Toronto: WB Saunders Company, 2001.

[20] Alekseeva, EI; Zholobova, ES. Reactive arthritis in children. *Vopr. Sovr. Pediatr.* 2003, Vol 2, N1, 51−56.

[21] Agababova, ER. Some unclear and unsolved problems of seronegative spondyloarthropathies. *Nauchno-practicheskaya revmatologia.* 2001, N 4, 10−17.

[22] Steere, AC; Malawista, SE; Snydman, DR; et al. Lyme arthritis: an epidemic of oligo-articular arthritis in children and adults in three Connecticut communities. *Arthr. Rheum.* 1977, Vol 20, 7−17.

[23] Burgdorfer, W; Barbur, AG; Hayes, SF; Benach, JL; Grundwaldt, E; Davis, JP. Lyme disease – a tick-borne spirochetosis? *Science.* 1982, Vol 216, 1317−1319.

[24] Lobzin, YuV; Uskov, AN; Kozlov, SS. *The series: Actual infections. Lyme borreliosis (ixodic tick borreliosis).* St. Petersburg: Foliant, 2000.

[25] Centers for Disease Control and Prevention. Recommendations for test performance and interpretation from the Second NC on Serologic Diagnosis of Lyme disease. *MMWR Morb. Mortal Weekly Rep.* 1995, Vol 44, 590−591.

[26] Korenberg, EI. Ixodic tick borreliosis as a group of human diseases and main results of its research in Russia. *Zh. Infect. Pat.* 1966, Vol 3, N 4, 22−24.

[27] Joseph, J; McGrath, H. Gout or "pseudogout": how to differentiate crystal-induced arthropathies. *Geriatrics.* 1995, Vol 50, 33−39.

[28] Beloenko, ED; Slobozhanina, EI; Kozlova, NM; Mamontova, MV; Chernitskii, EA. Spectrophotometric investigation of synovial effusion in differential diagnostics of pigmented villonodular synovitis. *Orthop. Traumatol. Prosth.* 1990, N 5, 32–34.

[29] Rodionova, SS; Shvedova, GL; Gladstein, AI. Cellular composition of synovial fluid in pigmented villonodular synovitis. *Lab. Delo*. 1981, N 3, 164–167.

[30] Zelenin, AV. Gene therapy at the turn of the 3rd millennium. *Dokl. RAN.* 2001, Vol 71, N 5, 387–395.

[31] Podrushnyak, EP. *Age-related changes and diseases of human musculoskeletal system.* Kiev: Zdorov'ya. 1987.

Chapter 4

RESEARCH METHODS

Modern medical science uses a wide range of microscopic, microbiological, serologic, and other methods to study biological fluids. In arthrology they are used to assess pathological conditions of synovial medium that lead to increasing SF volume in the joint thus facilitating the fluid aspiration procedure.The development of arthroscopy has allowed SF to be obtained for analysis in any pathological condition, even if exudate is absent. However, the examination of SF to diagnose a joint pathology is not always necessary. A preliminary clinical and X-ray diagnostics of synovitis as well as visual assessment of SF aspirated from the joint is in many cases sufficient to determine a spectrum of simple tests to substantiate or rule out a probable pathological process.

The chapter discusses traditional and innovative methods for analysis of SF properties, composition, and structure. These methods allow determination of the nature of synovitis and detection of accompanying functional abnormalities of the synovial medium of the joint. In medical literature the data on the alterations in the cellular and biochemical composition of SF accompanying joint diseases are commonly cited. However, any changes in SF composition inevitably result in undesirable changes in its spatial structural order and inherent functions, which in turn lead to changes in the structure and functions of other elements of the synovial medium, which are SM and cartilage. Diagnostics of structural damages to SF is becoming increasingly helpful in current arthrology. Nowadays, in order to solve the problem, ample scientific grounds are provided. SF is considered as a condensed medium and its physicochemical structure is characterized by long-range order. A liquid-crystal phase and quasi-electret effect have been found in synovia. The circulation of SF in the joint is considered as the interaction between the viscous quasi-electret medium and biophysical field of the joint that occurs under mechanical loading. To confirm and decode the interrelation of structural and functional abnormalities of SF, methods for evaluation of condensed media are widely adopted. A complex assessment of changes in the joint synovial medium by analyzing the physicochemical structure and physical properties of SF makes it possible to conceive the nature of synovitis as not an occasional disease but a chain in joint chondrodestruction.

4.1. Microscopy

4.1.1. Basic Data on the Technique

Synovial effusion for microscopic analysis is obtained by joint aspiration (arthrocentesis) under sterile conditions. In this manipulation the use of Novocain is undesirable since it destructs SF cells. For cytological examination, it is recommended to take SF in the laboratory tube with an anticoagulant [1]. Analysis of effusion specimens is advisable during first 4–6 hours after they were taken, when the cellular and biochemical composition of SF is still unchanged.

SF microscopy techniques can be specified as follows: 1) light amplitude contrast microscopy is convenient to detect SF and bacterial cells whose image contrast is increased by enhancing amplitude differences of the light beams passing through an object; 2) luminescent (or fluorescent) microscopy of microbe cells that become capable of luminescence excited by ultraviolet radiation after treatment with special substances, namely, fluorochromes; 3) polarized microscopy is called so because an object is illuminated with polarized light; it is used to detect and study the liquid-crystal SF phase characterized by double refraction; 4) dark field microscopy is aimed at examining unstained objects (cells and decomposing tissue fragments) against the dark background of SF at the lateral lightening of the specimen; 5) ultraviolet microscopy involves the illumination of an object with ultraviolet light and its visible picture is taken by means of the luminescent screen or microphotography; it is used to detect bacteria and viruses in SF; 6) phase contrast microscopy is handy to study living unstained specimens; image contrast power is increased by transforming phase differences of the light beams passing through a specimen into amplitude ones; 7) electron microscopy makes it possible to take an enlarged picture of dried or specially treated specimens by the electronic beam.

Fresh undried specimens as well as stained specimens and dried smears and drops are studied using microscopy. In bacteriological study, the SF specimens are centrifuged and the deposits, clots, and flakes are examined. The study of the native material makes it possible to estimate the cellular element amount, detect rhagocytes and extracellular structures including endoprosthesis fragments, suspensions of drugs, crystals, cartilage fragments, etc.

Extracellular structures of SF are detected in the following manner. Before the native SF smear is totally dried, cholesterol crystals in the form of rhomboid or polygonal flakes can be seen. As the specimen is dried up, the crystals “disappear” from the field of vision. In SF microscopy in the common and polarized light, the sodium monourate crystals and calcium pyrophosphate dihydrate can be visualized. The former is characteristic of gout while the latter points to pseudo-gout. Sodium monourate crystals are found in the form of long needles or clusters 10–20 μm long. They are seen well against the black background as “white sparks” due to double refraction and may be revealed in neutrophils. Sodium pyrophosphate dihydrate crystals are shaped as obtuse-ended rhombs or rectangles. Their size ranges from 10 to 2 μm and can be even smaller. They are hard to detect even in the polarized light because of their small size and weak luminescence. In hydroxyapatite arthropathy, the calcium hydroxyapatite crystals are hard to detect by traditional light microscopy due to their small sizes and fast dissolution in SF. They are seen as polygonal shining structures 1–5 μm in size consisting of crystal agglomerates which weakly polarize or do not refract light. It is recommended to use electron microscopy to detect calcium hydroxyapatite crystals.

Cytochemical methods of microscopy assume investigation of the internal structure of cells, intracellular structures, and products of vital activity with application of special staining methods. The SF cells do not vary much in shape; therefore, special staining of the cells or the substance accumulated in them is enough for identification.

The microscopy of stained fixed SF smears is used to detect microorganisms, study their morphology, and compose synoviocytograms. Fixation is the treatment of a living object to interrupt living processes in it with retaining its fine structure. As the result of fixation, cells are attached strongly to the slide and stained better. While operating the pathogenic microorganisms, fixation is necessary for safety. At a low concentration of microorganisms, their detection in a common SF material is often impossible. The purposeful search for causative agents needs the enrichment of the specimen via centrifugation and subsequent microscopy of the deposit and its bacteriological examination.

In order to detect microorganisms in SF or causative agents of a joint disease, two and more stains are used in smear staining. The most popular Gram's staining is based on distinctions of chemical composition of the cell wall of prokaryotic microorganisms (with lack of a shaped cellular nucleus and typical chromosome system). This method was developed by a Danish microbiologist H. Gram in 1883. Gram-positive microorganisms are capable of holding the complex of stains of iodine-containing trimethylphenol type whereas gram-negative microorganisms of different chemical structure of their cell wall do not hold these stains. Gram-positive bacteria are stained bright-black (dark-blue) while gram-negative ones get red or brown depending on a stain; cell nuclei are bright-red and cytoplasm is pink. The accuracy in determining the microbe species or sensitivity by Gram's method is 75% in gram-positive infection, 50% in gram-negative infection, and less than 25% in gonococcal arthritis. Microscopy of SF allows differential diagnostics of infectious disorders and aseptic inflammation induced by damage to the synovial medium with microcrystals in microcrystalline arthropathies.

For detection of chemically resistant pathogenic microorganisms in effusions, in particular, acid-resistant ones, containing a great amount of fatty substances, the Ziehl-Neelsen staining method is used. The method was suggested by a German bacteriologist F. Ziehl and morbid anatomist F. Neelsen late in the 19th century. The fixed smear is stained with Ziehl carbolic magenta, decolorized with 5% solution of H_2SO_4 for 20–25 s and after that stained again with methylene blue [2]. Special methods called after the names of their authors, such as Neisser, Keffler, Ozheshko, and others are used to study the morphology of microorganisms, i.e., to reveal filaments and spores and their movability.

4.1.2. Evaluation of SF Structure by Microscopic Examination

Hypotheses about structural ordering and spatial arrangement of SF have been substantiated elsewhere [3, 4]. By examining dried out SF drops, researchers observed formation of textures of characteristic pattern such as dendrites, needles and individual spherical crystals against the background of homogeneous semitransparent film. Microscopic examination of synovia textures taken from joints afflicted with different diseases proved their difference, which formed grounds for creating a new method for SF testing to diagnose a rheumatic disorder [5]. The simplicity of the experiment allows researchers to compare microtextures of dried synovia specimens for primary evaluation of SF structural order. It has been used to study the influence of the electromagnetic effect on the structure of lubricating film in joint diseases [6].

Such structures as dendrites and spherulites in the dried SF drops taken from joints with different pathology levels were compared using optical microscopy (Fig. 4.1). In healthy SF (*a*) the dendritic textures are well pronounced and distributed rather uniformly over the specimen. In degenerative dystrophic disorder (*b*) there are smaller dendrites that are not seen so clearly. It may be due to unequal amounts of protein in specimens *a* and *b* (10 and 32 g/l) as one of the causes. Acute joint inflammation (*c*) is responsible for even greater disordering of SF structures, i.e., the sizes of dendrites and noncrystalline inclusions are unequal at different specimen spots. In Bekhterev's disease (*d*) and rheumatoid arthritis (*e*) the textures of the dried drops are similar. Rather fine texture fragments are distributed uniformly, which can be attributed to a large amount of protein (35 and 53 g/l), appearance of its pathological fractions, and decreasing mass of protein molecules.

The study of the effect of a constant electromagnetic field on the ordering of the SF structural components has shown the following [7, 8]. In order to simulate the magnetic therapeutic effect on the joint, a SF drop was held on the slide for 10 min in the solenoid field under intensity $H = 1.2$ kA/m. After that, the solenoid was switched off and the specimen was dried up on the slide without displacing it. Under the same other conditions, the crystalline texture fragments are seen more clearly in the SF drops dried out in the magnetic field (*f–j*) than in the initial similar specimens (*a–e*). In Fig. 4.1 *g, h* the texture of the specimens corresponding to the nonimmune diseases is shown. One can see that the texture dendrites are equal in size and similar in shape to those in the (*a, f*). This proves the idea that a therapeutic effect of magnetic field on joints consists in recovering of the damaged SF coordination structures. However, in immune inflammation, the effect of the magnetic field results in total disordering of texture elements and disappearance of dendrites (*i, j*).

Therefore, the texture of the dried drops gives us an idea about distribution of the SF protein components in the bulk of the saline solution. Analysis of the textures indicates that the higher the activity of inflammation in joint the stronger the disordering of dendritic structures in synovia specimens.

Electron microscopy is finding increasing applications in biological and medical research [9, 10]. The technique assumes the use of specimens 2–200 nm thick. For distinguishing the specimen details at a distance of 1 nm from each other in the picture produced by electron microscope, magnification of 100000–200000 is necessary. Best microscopes can produce specimen pictures on the photographic plate with such magnification, yet they cover a too small area. Commonly, the micropicture with a lower magnification is taken and afterwards, it is magnified photographically. The photographic plate resolves about 10000 lines on a length of 10 cm.

For electron microscopic examination, the SF sample is prepared as a thin homogeneous smear on the slide that is dried out at 18–20 °C in a shadowed place. After that, a layer of hard metal is applied by vacuum spraying to the specimen. The layer called "replica" is examined instead of the layer itself by an electron microscope. The picture of SF crystalline fragments is determined by the orientation, period, and perfectness of the lattice. Through varying the contrast of the picture, it is possible to study the lattice and its imperfections at atomic scale.

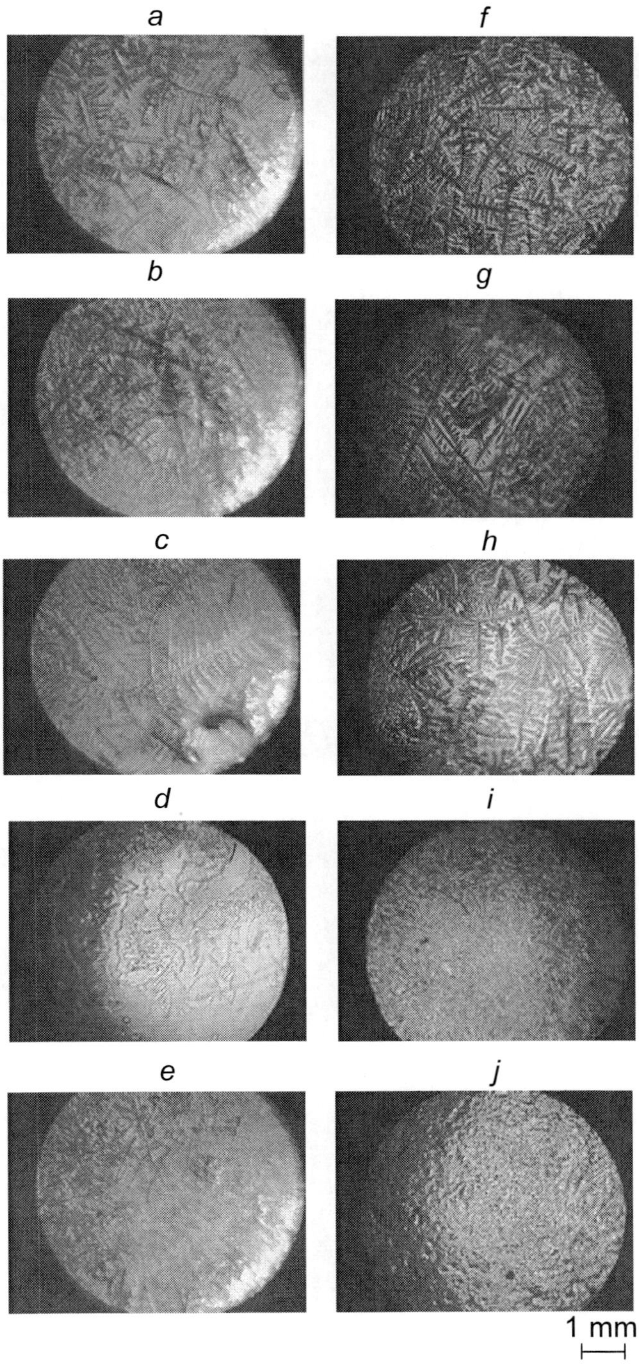

Figure 4.1. Texture of the dried SF drops taken form joints: *a, f* –conventionally healthy; *b, g* – degenerative-dystrophic; *c, h* – afflicted with acute synovitis; *d, i* – afflicted with Bekhterev's disease; *e, j* – afflicted with rheumatoid arthritis. Specimens *a-e* are dried out without application of magnetic field; *f–j* are dried in the constant magnetic field of intensity $H = 1.2$ кA/m.

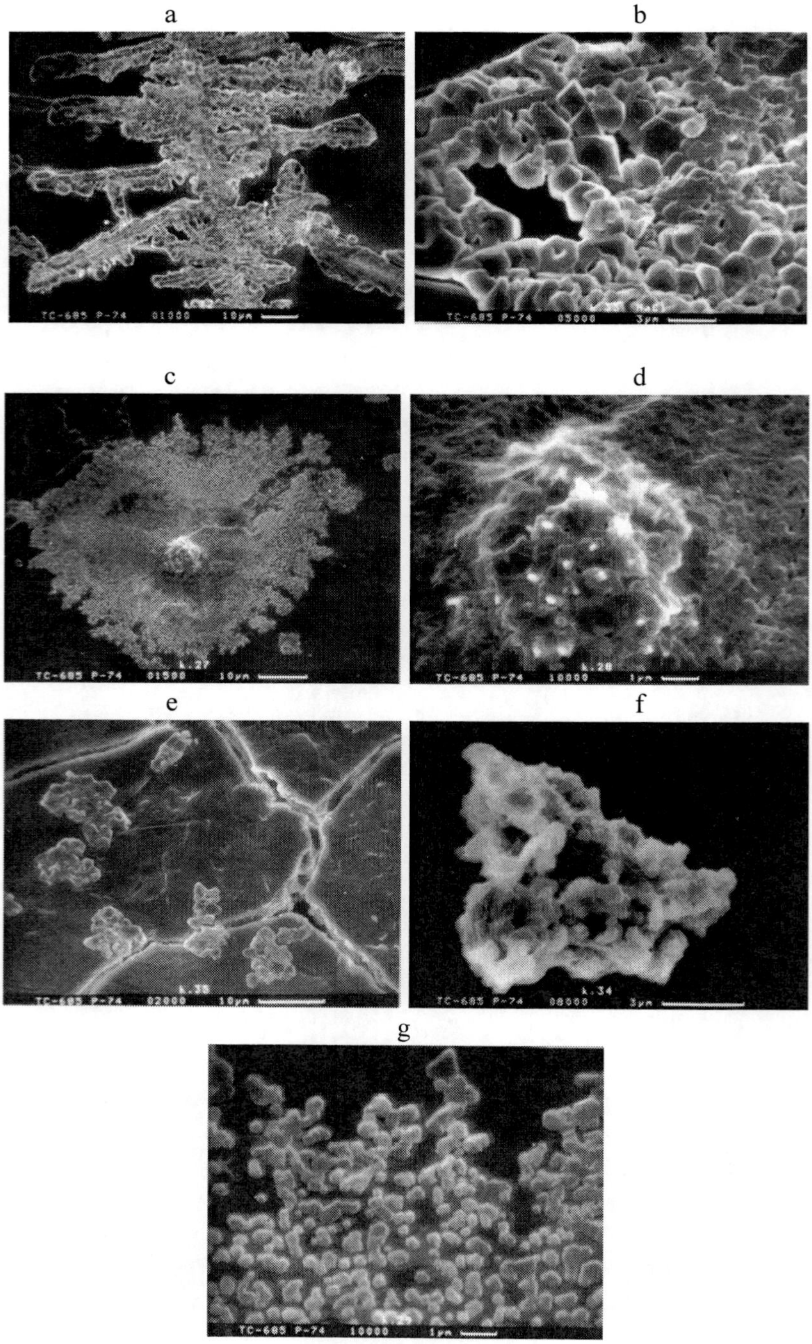

Figure 4.2. Electron microphotographs of texture typical elements of the dried SF specimen: *a* – dendrites (×1000); *b* – dendrites (×5000); *c* – microcrystal agglomerate (×1500); *d* – agglomerate center (×10000); *e* – crystalline agglomerates in the protein film (×2000); *f* – singular crystalline agglomerate (×8000); g – microcrystals (×10000).

The pictures of the typical dendrites and spherulites in the SF taken from a conditionally healthy joint are produced by a Cam Scan-4 scanning electron microscope (Fig. 4.2). The dendrites are mineral aggregates of the ordered dendritic shape up 100 mcm long with numerous finer branches (*a*). They arise in SF drying as the result of salt crystallization in the viscous protein synovium base. At magnification 50000, the salt crystals involved in dendrite formation (*b*) are clearly seen. Their agglomerates are concentrated around the long core of the dendrite and its branches. The sites of the salt crystallization can be shaped as spots within 60 µm in diameter with the saturated center and the rarefied edge zone (*c, d*) that are formed by the numerous salt microcrystals. SF fixed on the slide can form homogeneous films up to 2.5 µm thick (*e*) with involvement of the unsaline polysaccharide component of synovia. Individual irregular agglomerates 3-10 µm in size (*f*) and numerous probably saline monocrystals less than 0.5 µm (*g*) are disposed mainly in the center of the films.

4.2. Biochemical Analysis

Quantitative and qualitative evaluation of the SF biochemical composition is performed by the techniques under usage in analysis of blood serum, transsudates, and exudates. The SF specimens are studied to detect enzymes and electrolytes within four hours after its aspiration. SF can be kept within 7 days at 4 °C. Keeping synovia at −20 °C for a week allows determination of protein and alkali phosphatase and after 3 month-freezing – cholesterol and immunoglobulins [11].

One of the features of SF is its capability of forming a mucin clot upon being mixed with acetic acid. The addition of acetic acid to SF results in lowering pH of the mixture owing to which the hyaluronates bind covalently with proteins and become incapable of dissolving in water forming mucin clots. In mixing normal SF and acetic acid, a dense clot arises evaluated as “good”. The reduced polymerization of hyaluronic acid in synovitis gives rise to a less dense clot that is ranked as “loose” and “very loose”. Loose clots are characteristic of septic, gouty, rheumatoid, and tuberculosis arthritis. The test is normal in dystrophic disorders of joints.

Nowadays, unified techniques to determine protein concentration in biological fluids are unavailable. It is unfeasible to create a universal method because of a unique structure of each protein. In order to determine the whole protein concentration photometric methods have found practical application [12]. They are divided into the following groups:

1) turbidimetric (syn. nephelometric) methods based on the precipitation of proteins, e.g., the sulfosalicylic method;
2) methods based on the formation of stained substances in reagent solutions, e.g., the method using Coomassie Blue dye, the methods with stains Ponseau S, bromcreosol, bromphenol, pyrogallol, etc., and biuretic methods;
3) direct spectrophotometry based on the capability of aromatic amino acids of absorbing light with a wave length of 280 nm.

Methodically, low protein concentrations typical of SF, spinal, lachrymal, and other fluids containing protein in significantly lower concentrations than in blood are most difficult to determine.

Turbidimetry and nephelometry (**Greek** *nephele* is a cloud, Latin *turbidus* is cloudy and Greek *metreo* is measure) is determination of the concentration of suspended particles and high-molecular substances in solution based on evaluating the intensity of light dissipation passing through the solution. Nephelometry is used to determine the concentration of immunoglobulins IgG, IgA, IgM, and IgE, subclasses IgG, C3, and C4, factor B, C-reactive protein, and some other serum proteins. Concentration of the substance in question is found by calibration charts or visually, i.e., by comparing the suspension under study to the series of standard suspensions with known concentrations of the substance in question. The lower limits of the concentrations of suspended particles reach 10^{-4} % in nephelometry. Also, nephelometric or turbidimetric titration is used when the solution under study is titrated by precipitator solution. The equivalence point is found by the break on the titration curves. Due to its low precision the method is only applied to find the components for which other satisfactory methods, first of all photometric, are absent.

Presently, in order to determine the concentration of whole protein under laboratory condition n the sulfosalicylic method is unified. The method performed by photoelectrocalorimeter at a wave length of 590–650 nm was suggested by an English physicist and chemist D. Kingsberry et al. in 1926. It is based on the photoelectric registration of variations in light diffusion of a liquid specimen due to protein solution getting turbid in the presence of sulfosalicylic acid. Its undisputable advantages are simplicity of analysis and accessibility of reagents.

Methods based on application of stains including Coomassie Blue G-250, biurethane reagent, and pyrogallol solutions have found limited applications in clinical diagnostic laboratories. An English expert in organic chemistry M. Bradford reported the possibility of determining protein concentration by Coomassie G-250 in 1976. The reagent is capable of being sorbed on proteins producing absorption maximum at a wave length of 595 nm. The reagent susceptibility is rather high and manifests at a protein concentration of 1–2 mg/ml. Modern spectrophotometers can register protein concentrations from 10 μkg/ml to 10 mg/ml using the Bradford method. In the Bradford reaction the ratio of reagent and specimen volumes 50:1 is used. The Lowry method is also high-sensitive for determining low protein concentrations. It was suggested by an English pharmacologist O. Lowry in the 1950s and was realized at the wave length 750 nm. The method is not widespread in laboratory practice in medicine because of its technological complexity. In 1986, a Japanese physicist and chemist N. Watanabe et al. proposed pyrogallol for determining the protein concentration in biological fluids. The method is based on binding pyrogallol molybdate with protein in the acidous environment. Maximal absorption of the reaction products corresponds to 600 nm.

The biuretic method includes the photoelectrocolorimetric evaluation of the solution staining intensity upon protein reaction with copper sulfate at the wave length 540–560 nm. Although this method is believed to belong to the most reliable ones in determination of protein concentration in biological fluids, it is not universal. Unfortunately, it has limited applications when dealing with small protein concentrations in SF, urine, and spinal fluid.

Adsorptive spectrophotometry is a physicochemical method for studying solutions and solid substances based on the analysis of adsorption spectra in ultraviolet (200–400 nm), visible (400–760 nm), and infrared (>760 nm) spectrum regions. Spectrophotometry studies the dependence of the intensity of light absorbed by an object on wave length. Spectrophotometry was helpful in detecting in preliminarily deposited SF proteins increased concentrations of mediators of immune inflammation (interleukins 1b and 6, circulating immune complexes, stable metabolites of nitrogen oxide) with employing the Griess reagent (the mixture of synthetic compounds was suggested by a German chemist J.P. Griess in the 1850s). Thus the chondrodestructive effect of SF in osteoarthritis was justified. Mediators are chemical substances whose molecules are capable of reacting with specific receptors of the cellular membrane and varying its permeability for certain ions thus generating an active electric signal or action potential. The mediator concentration in the aforesaid SF appeared to be reliably higher than in blood serum [13]. Analysis of spectrophotometric characteristics of synovial effusions makes it possible [14] to differentiate pigmented villonodular synovitis (PVNS) and synovitis of traumatic and rheumatic etiologies. The technique consists in measuring optical density in the region of absorption of proteins (D_{280}) and pigments (D_{460}) and determining their ratio ($K = D_{280}/D_{460}$). At $K < 12$ PVNS is diagnosed.

In order to unify the analysis conditions, calibrators are prepared in advance. They are standard aqueous solutions of albumin of a known concentration and on their base calibration charts are constructed or plots of protein optical density (*I*) of samples versus protein content (*C*). Unfortunately, protein concentrations in the same biological fluids found by the above-mentioned method are reliably different. In some standard samples with identical protein content, the concentrations found by different methods differ twice and even more depending on the ratio between albumin and globulin amounts in proteins (A/G-coefficient). The protein concentration in solution can only be reliably determined when A/G-coefficient of the sample in question corresponds to A/G-coefficient of standard solution. If the albumin-globulin spectrum of solution differs from the A/G-coefficient of calibration solution, either higher or lower than actual protein concentrations are disclosed. The effect of protein spectrum of the fluid in question on analytical error depends greatly on the method employed. The phenomenon can be explained via amino acid composition of proteins. Albumin and globulins differ considerably in amino acids, namely, glutamine, serine, tryptophan, phenylalanine, and cysteine [15].

In the 1990s, mathematical analysis was used (B.Yu. Altshuller, S.S. Rakov, and G.A. Tkachev) to determine the influence of *A/G*-coefficient on the whole protein concentration error when applying the Bradford, Lauri, pyrogallol, sulfosalicylic, and biuretic methods. It is seen (Fig. 4.3 *a, b*) that the photo transducer signal at the "final point" is governed by not only protein concentration but also the ratio of protein fractions in the fluids under study, namely, albumin and serum.

The experimental dependences are approximated by the following functions:

- sulfosalicylic method: $C(A/G) = 1.85 - [5.43 : (A/G + 4.42)]$;
- Lauri method: $C(A/G) = 0.82 + [0.79 : (A/G + 1.12)]$;
- Bradford method: $C(A/G) = 1.22 - [1.72 : (A/G + 4.73)]$;
- pyrogallol method: $C(A/G) = 1.04 - [0.06 : (A/G + 0.20)]$,

where C(A/G) is the protein concentration to be found; (A/G) is albumin/globulin ratio of the sample of the biological fluid under study. The functions serve objective quantitative criteria for the method reliability as a way for revealing certain proteins in a fluid. Thus, the reagents of the Lauri method have a close affinity to globulins. In other three methods, globulins available yield, on the contrary, underestimated results. Only the biuretic reagent stains identically the proteins of different structures.

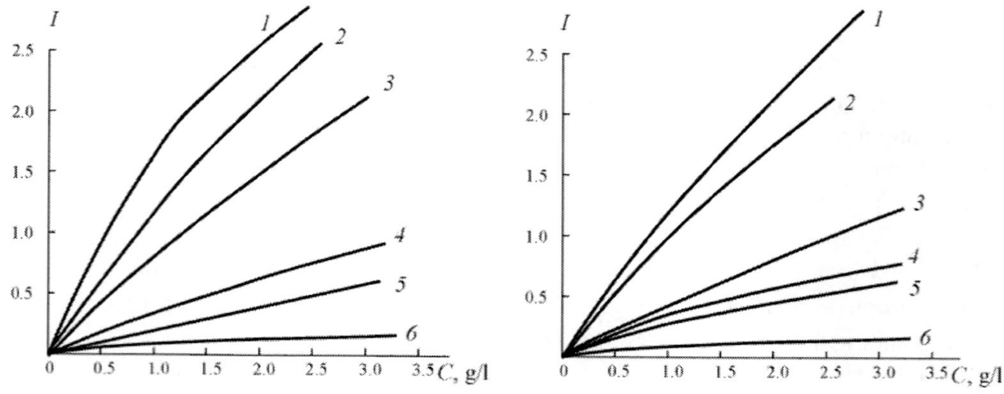

Figure 4.3. Calibration charts to determine protein concentration in biological fluids by different methods employing calibrators (by the data of B. Altshuller, S. Rakov, and G. Tkachev): *a* – aqueous solution of human globulin; *b* – serum, A/G = 2.14. The curves correspond to the methods: *1* and *3* – sulfosalicylic at wave lengths 340 and 600 nm, *2* – Bradford; *4* – pyrogallol; *5* – Lauri; *6* – biuretic.

SF protein fractions differ in structure and functions. The division of the protein mixture into fractions is based on different protein molecule movability in the fluid under the effect of the electric field. Commonly 5–6 standard fractions are separated by electrophoresis: albumins and 4–5 fractions of globulins (α_1-, α_2-, β-, and γ-globulins and sometimes β_1 and β_2-globulins are separated individually).

The albumin fraction is homogeneous and its normal share is 40–60% of the whole protein amount.

Globulin fractions are dissimilar in composition. The α_1-globulin fraction includes the acute-phase proteins, viz α_1-antitripsin (the main component of the fraction) that is the inhibitor of numerous proteolytic enzymes such as tripsin, chimotripsin, plasmin, etc. and alpha-acidous glycoprotein (orosomucoid). It has a wide spectrum of functions and favors fibrillogenesis (formation of fibers in the intercellular space of connective tissue) in the zone of joint inflammation. Also, α_1-globulins include α_1-lipoproteins (involved in lipid transportation), protothrombin and transport proteins or thyroxin-binding globulin and transcortin (involved in binding and transporting cortisol and thyroxin).

The α_2-globulin fraction mainly includes the acute-phase proteins, namely, α_2-macroglobulin, haptoplasmin, ceruloplasmin, etc. Its main component is α_2-macroglobulin involved in the development of infectious and inflammatory reactions. Haptoglobin is a glycoprotein that forms a complex with hemoglobin libererated from erythrocytes in intravascular hemolysis. Ceruloplasmin binds copper ions in a specific way and is an oxydase (an enzyme catalyzing oxidative-reducing reactions) of ascorbic acid, adrenalin, and dioxyphenylnealanin; it is also capable of inactivating free radicals.

The β-globulin fraction contains transferrin (iron-carrying protein), hemopexin (binds hemes or iron-containing compounds found in proteins and preventing from their excretion by kidneys and iron loss), complement components involved in immunity reactions, beta-lipoproteins (responsible for cholesterol and phospholipid transportation), and some immunoglobulins.

The γ-globulin fraction consists of immunoglobulins that refer to antibodies providing the humoral immunity. Immunoglobulins (Ig) are globular proteins found in human blood serum and SF. Immunoglobulins form the group of the chemically similar compounds having carbohydrates as constituents. All immunoglobulins are apparently antibodies against some antigens. 5 classes of human immunoglobulins are known: G, M, A, D, and E. The immunoglobulins G (IgG) are the most fully understood. Their molecules are built of two identical light (molecular mass 22000) and two identical heavy (molecular mass 55000–70000) polypeptide chains connected by disulfide bonds. An immunoglobulin molecule cleaved by proteolytic enzymes (e.g. papain) is divided into three parts, namely, two identical fragments Fab, each of which retains the capability of binding with an antigen, and a fragment Fc that helps immunoglobulins pass through biological membranes. All three fragments are connected by short flexible links located in the middle of the heavy chain. Owing to flexibility, the immunoglobulin molecules are associated optimally with the antigens of different spatial structures. The areas of the molecule responsible for binding to the antigen (active centre) are formed by N-ended (carry the NH_2 amino group at the end) links of heavy and light chains. The sequence of amino acids in these chains is specific of each IgG while it is almost the same in other sections of the chains. Immunoglobulins are divided into the following classes depending on heavy chain structure (Table 4.1).

Table 4.1. Immunoglobulins of a healthy man

Immunoglobulin class	Molecular mass	Carbohydrate amount, %	Amount in serum, mg %
IgG	140 000	2	800–1680
IgM	900 000	10	50–190
IgA	170 000 and more	7	140–420
IgD	180 000	12	3–40
IgE	196 000	10	0.01–0.14

Most antibodies are found among IgG, therefore, gamma-globulin medication to be used for treatment purposes consist mainly of IgG. IgM are the most "ancient" immunoglobulins – in terms of evolution, i.e., they are synthesized at the first stages of immune reaction. Their molecules consist of 5 monomer subunits each of which resembles IgG molecule. IgA is characterized by its capability of invading in the secretions produced by glandular cells (saliva, colostrum, and intestinal juice) where they are met in the polymer form. The antibodies involved in allergic reactions are IgE.

In joint disorders, the ratio of protein fractions varies (dysproteinemia) in SF and blood serum at normal whole protein (Table 4.2). Dysproteinemia occurs oftener than variations in whole protein amounts and while being observed in dynamics can characterize a disease stage, its duration, and efficiency of the treatment.

Table 4.2. Dysproteinemia of SF and blood serum in joint disorders

Protein fractions	**Increased values**	**Decreased values**
albumin	Nonspecific	• tumors of SM • hemorrhages, hemorrhage of the joints • collagenosis • severe (purulent) inflammations of joints
α_1-globulins	• acute, subacute, and chronic inflammatory processes in joints • trauma and surgical invasions in joints • joint tumors	• inherited deficit of alpha-1-antitripsin, deficit of alpha-1-lipoprotein
α_2-globulins	• acute, subacute and chronic inflammations • diffusive diseases of connective tissue • joint tumors	• joint trauma • hemarthrosis (blood hemolysis of the joint cavity, 3−4th day after trauma)
β-globulins	• myeloma or leucosis with predominant bone damage	• congenital hypobetalipoproteinemia, deficit of IgA
γ-globulins	• parasite invasions • autoimmune diseases	• immune-deficit conditions (HIV)

C-reactive protein (CRP) is one of the main markers of acute-phase inflammations. It is synthesized mainly in the hepatic cells or hepatocytes. Its synthesis is provoked by antigens, immune complexes, bacteria, and trauma (within 4−6 hours after lesion). In joint inflammation, its concentration in SF and blood increases 10−100 times. There is a direct correlation between CRP level variations and dynamics of clinical manifestations of a disease; therefore, CRP is the most specific and sensitive indicator of inflammation and necrosis of joint tissues. The determination of CRP concentration is widely used for monitoring and control of treatment adequacy of rheumatologic, chronic, inflammatory, and oncological diseases and complications in traumatology and orthopedics [16].

Immunoturbidimetry, nephelometry, and radial immune diffusion are classical methods for determination of CRP concentration [17].

Increased concentrations of CRP occurring in SF in pathologies fall within 5–500 mg/l and correspond to the concentration range determined by the above-said methods. The reagent sets are introduced in laboratory practice that allow CRP concentrations considered as "normal", "minute", or just "background" to be distinguished whereas CRP concentrations lower than 5 mg/l indicate the absence of inflammation response, that is, exact CRP concentration is taken as clinically insignificant. The basic CRP concentration is about 0.5 mg/l that is found in essentially healthy people and in patients without acute inflammation or exacerbations. In order to determine the basic CRP level, high-sensitive CRP (hs-CRP) immunoturbidimetry with preliminary latex enhancement is applied. Immobilization of antibodies to CRP on the latex particles enhances the sensitivity of quantitative determination of the protein approximately 10-fold. The results of hs-CRP determination in fresh and frozen samples of biological fluids do not differ essentially.

Immunodiffusion is the most widely spread method for determining CRP based on precipitation reaction or precipitation of solved antigen interacting with antibody. The essence of radial immune diffusion is as follows. Wells are cut in the thin layer of the gel (agar) containing antibodies (monospecific antiserum) of a given concentration. There antigens are placed (a test antigen of known concentration and a biological fluid) that diffuse in the gel. Around the wells the so-called precipitin rings arise, that is, nontransparent bands (precipitates) on the boundary of the antigen-antigen superposition whose diameter is proportional to antigen concentration. The results are used to build the calibration graph that expresses the dependence of precipitate diameters on antigen concentration in the solutions in question (Fig. 4.4). The method of double radial immunodiffusion is distinguished by that in the thin layer of the conventional gel the wells are cut for an antigen and antibodies. The antigen and the antibodies placed in different wells diffuse towards each other forming precipitin lines at a distance from the wells. The antigen concentration is found by the distance from the antigen-containing well to the precipitin line. The principle of radial diffusion forms the grounds for the method applied to study toxic genesis of bacterial cultures and choose clones of high toxicity from bacterial population.

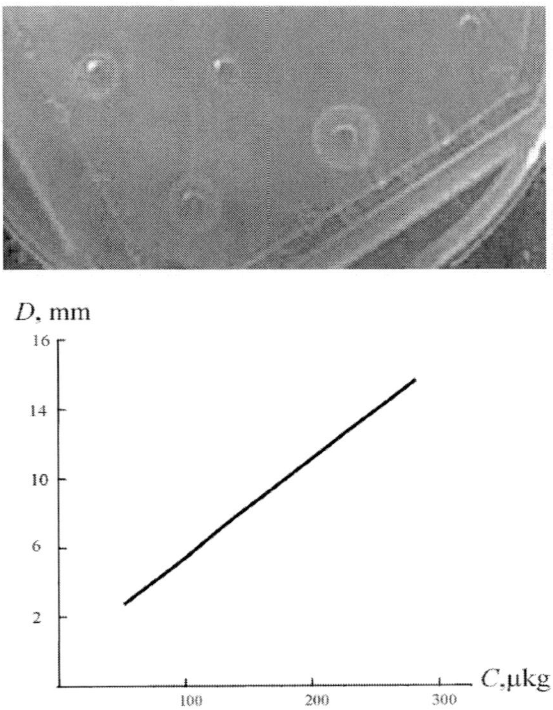

Figure 4.4. Radial immunodiffusion: *a* – precipitin rings in the gel with antiserum; *b* – calibration graph (*D* is precipitin ring diameter, *C* is antigen concentration).

Increased CRP concentration in SF depends on the nature of joint inflammation. In viral infections, tumor metastasis, subacute chronic and some systemic rheumatic diseases CRP concentrations increase sometimes up to 10–30 mg/l. In bacterial infections, exacerbation of some inflammations (e.g., rheumatoid arthritis), and tissue injures (surgical operations) CRP can increase up to 40–100 mg/l (and sometimes up to 200 mg/l). Severe infections, burnings, and sepsis are accompanied by the highest CRP level up to 300 mg/l and higher.

Rheumatoid factor is antibodies to the IgG Fc fragment that are revealed in the serum and SF in rheumatoid arthritis and is evaluated by laser nephelometry and immune-enzyme methods. Counting rheumatoid factor of IgM class is of clinical value. The rheumatoid factor is found in the serum (synthesized by B-lymphocytes CD5+) and in SF, the titer being higher in the latter case. This is due to its local reproduction with the plasmatic cells of the damaged joint.

Agglutination methods including the Waaler-Rose (E. Waaler, the contemporary Novergain bacteriologist and immunologist and N.M. Rose, the American bacteriologist) agglutination reaction with sheep erythrocytes and latex-test are also sensitive to rheumatoid factor IgM. To provide a more accurate diagnostics, the combination of two methods is recommended for determining rheumatoid factor (Waaler-Rose and latex-test) since the patient's blood serum can contain several different rheumatoid factors one of which is agglutinated by only erythrocytes and others only by the latex particles [18]. In agglutination, a negative charge on the latex particle surface that prevents their spontaneous agglutination is of significance. The charge should be diminished in order to form cross links between the particles that result in agglutination. For this purpose, IgM antibodies are used whose molecules contain many active chains, which favor the bond formation between particles and help overcome their mutual repulsion caused by a unipolar charge available. The ion strength of the solution where the agglutination occurs is chosen so that to diminish the charge on the particle surface. For this the molecules having an uncompensated charge, in particular, of albumin, are added to the incubation environment. With neutral pH, a high concentration of electrolytes also favors a decrease in the negative charge of latex particles. Increasing viscosity of environment because of polymer solutions (dextran) facilitates cooperation of the charged particles.

Hard-phase enzyme linked sorbent assay ELISA is the most sensitive method to find rheumatoid factor *in vitro.* It is based on the double binding of the immunoglobulin in question with an antigen (Fc-fragment of IgG) fixed in the wells of the immunological plate. Once the reaction between SF and the fixed antigen is finished, the plate is washed. Unbound components of the sample under study are removed and the antigen-antibody complexes remain on the well walls. To detect them, the second immunological reaction is performed where the bound specific immunoglobulin serves an antigen and an enzyme-labeled (commonly peroxidase) immunoglobulin (e.g. rabbit's one) is an antibody to it. Once the second immunological reaction stops, the wells of the plate are washed and then the third stage or enzyme reaction catalyzed by the enzymatic part of the immunoglobulin molecule follows. A colorless substance or chromogen (ortho-phenylene diamine or tetramethylbenzidinin) is a substrate of the reaction during which it forms a stained substance. The intensity of the staining in the well depends on the number of immunoglobulins in a sample. Upon finishing the enzymatic reaction the wells undergo photometering. Afterwards, based on the values of optical density of the control samples, the results are mathematically processed. The higher the optical density of the substance in the well in question the more specific antibodies are present in the sample and, consequently, the higher the titer of the SF to be analyzed. In the absence of the antibodies in SF the wells stay unstained.

Cholesterol is determined in biological fluids with use of chemical, enzymatic, electrochemical, and chromatographic methods [19].

The Ilca method (S. Ilca, the contemporary Italian clinician) is adopted as a direct chemical unified method for determining cholesterol based on dehydroxyling cholesterol with the Liberman-Burkhard reagent (the mixture of concentrated H_2SO_4, CH_3COOH, and acetic anhydride in a proportion 1:1:5). The ratio of reagent and sample volumes is 21:1. Cholesterol gives a green color in the presence of the mixture of acids and acetic anhydride (see 2.7.1). Photometering is preformed at a wave length of 625 nm. The method is simple, accessible and cost effective. Its disadvantage is its unspecific mode when numerous components of the biological fluid, proteins denatured by acids as well as medical drugs including those injected into the joint cavity can interact as the result of dehydration in the endogenous thermal reaction. Due to these effects, the cholesterol appears to be increased by 2–12%

The Zlatkis-Zak (A. Zlatkis and B. Zak are contemporary American biochemists) chemical reaction is widespread in laboratory practice. It is based on oxidation of free cholesterol or cholesterol ethers found in a biological fluid with salts $FeCl_3$ in the presence of H_2SO_4 and CH_3COOH. Photometering of the unsaturated products stained in red-violet is performed at a wave length of 560 nm.

Enzymatic determination of cholesterol is employed in three stages. The first one is enzyme hydrolysis of cholesterol ethers with cholinesterase (hydrolysis-catalyzing enzyme) resulting in cholesterol and fat acid mixture. The second stage is cholesterol oxidation with the air dissolved in this mixture in the presence of cholesterol oxidase (the enzyme that catalyzes reduction-oxidation of cells). The third stage is finding the products of reaction or oxygen loss. Traditionally, the H_2O_2 amount is found in reaction with phenol and 4-aminoantipyrin in the presence of peroxidase (it catalyzes oxidation in cells by means of hydrogen peroxide) by measuring light absorption at 500 nm.

Electrochemical measurement of cholesterol is based on registration of decreasing partial pressure O_2 or increasing concentration of H_2O_2 during oxidation. In order to find O_2 the Clark (proposed by L. Clark, an American biochemist) electrode consisting of a platinum electrode polarized at -0.6 V and chlorine-silver one. H_2O_2 is found amperometrically by the output of the reduction reaction on the platinum electrode or indirectly by the concentration of $K_3[Fe(CN)_6]$ from $K_4[Fe(CN)_6]$.

Liquid chromatography allows lipids, cholesterol, and its ethers to be extracted from biological fluids. Silicogels with chemically grafted groups C_{18}, sometimes C_4 or C_8 are used as adsorbents. Adsorbent C_{18} makes it possible to separate cholesterol and its ethers within 30 min with a high quality. The whole cholesterol is determined by the absorption in the ultra-violet spectrum region (a wave length is lower than 210 nm) or refractometrically. Liquid chromatography has a high resolution; thus only 5–20 μl of a biological fluid is enough for analysis. The SF lipid fraction is examined by thin-layer chromatography (see 2.7.1).

Glucose level is the parameter that characterizes a pathological condition of SF. Its reduction is believed to be a more specific yet less sensitive indicator of inflammation in the joint than the protein structure. Its normal concentration in SF is within 0.1 mmol/l whereas in rheumatoid arthritis, glucose may increase up to 0.5–3.5 mmol/l. In order to determine the glucose content, one of the three unified methods is employed, namely, ferricyanide, or Hagedorn-Jensen, orthotuloidine (colorimetric), and glucose oxidase (enzymatic) [20]. The Hagedorn-Jensen method is named after Danish scientists H.Ch. Hagedorn and B.N. Jensen. It is based on glucose ability of being involved in reduction-oxidation. Oxidized glucose reduces the iron of red blood salt in the alkaline medium and transforms it into the yellow one. Unreduced red blood salt is determined iodometrically, and by the amount of the reduced red blood salt the sugar is found in SF.

The sugar is determined by color reaction with orthotuloidine in acid in heating. The complex compound stains the solution in green. The solution intensity is recorded photoelctrocolorimetrically and is in direct proportion to glucose concentration.

The glucose oxidase method consists in glucose oxidation with air oxygen in the presence of glucose oxidase with formation of H_2O_2. The latter forms a stained compound whose staining intensity is proportional to glucose concentration.

Recently, the interest has been growing to lactic acid level determination in SF whose increase is believed to be the marker of bacterial arthritis. Express diagnostics of this disease is based on the control of lactic acid levels in SF.

Numerous pathochemical modifications in SF in joint pathologies do not allow us to characterize the whole spectrum of diagnostic biochemical methods within the scope of this book. We have considered those to be in the greatest demand in clinical arthrology and orthopedics. More detailed data on testing metabolic disorders in joints are described in manuals on biochemical analysis of blood serum.

4.3. Microbiological Analysis

Medical microbiology used to study SF in rheumatology is helpful in diagnosing infectious arthritis induced by pathogenic microorganisms and arthritis of immunopathological genesis caused by modified reactions of immunity.

Pyoseptic lesions of joints are mainly induced by traumas and unskilled operative interventions when microorganisms invade in joint cavities. Upon regular surgical interventions purulent complications occur comparatively rarely [21]. An infectious agent can invade into the joint not only if its integrity is broken but also via lymph or blood. Infection is spread by lymphatic tracts from neighboring regions, e.g., from infected bones (an osteomyelitis focus) or from soft tissues (abscess and phlegmone). SM is damaged by hematogeneous metastases from the purulent focus earlier and more often than other elements of the synovial medium and is the main localization of inflammation. Hence, SF becomes the nutrient medium for microorganisms. The articular cartilage deprived of vessels is involved in the inflammatory process due to microbe invasion in the cartilage micropores together with SF. Mono- and polyarthritis can result from staphylococci, streptococci, gonococci, brucellosis, typhoid, meningococci, tuberculosis, viral (influenza, arboviruses, hepatitis viruses, HIV-infection, mononucleosis, and rubella), spirochete (Lime disease, rat bite disease, secondary syphilis), mycotic, and chlamydia infections.

Parameters of anatomic composition, blood supply and surrounding tissue structure are main factors that govern the current of a wounded joint infection. Large muscles of the hip joint, large volume and complex torsions of the internal capsule of the knee joint, multicomponent composition of all joints and bone structures of lower limbs lead to the development and more severe manifestation of purulent processes. Small dimensions of the elbow joint compared to other large human joints and small volume of periarticular tissues cause a lower intensity of the inflammation in infections.

Diagnostics of most infectious arthritis is based mainly on the methods for the detection of agents in the joint effusion and SM biopsy material. In infectious and para-infectious arthritis, the agents are searched in biological fluids (blood, urine, feces, sputum, smears from fauces, and urethra smears) and extra-articular tissues (enlarged lymphatic nodes, marrow, spots of skin rash).

Microbiological analysis includes the orienting test or bacterioscopy of the material (see 4.1), bacteriological (culture) examination, immunobiological (serologic and allergologic) analysis, as well as experimental (biological) examination of the biomaterial.

4.3.1. Examination of Synovia for Cultures

Examination for cultures is the main test of microbiological analysis that unites the set of methods for determining micoroorganisms by isolating a pure culture using nutrient media and identifying it. The pure culture of a microorganism (strain) is a colony of cells born from one cell.

To isolate pure cultures of microorganisms, the SF sediment inoculation by infected loop or spatula of the dense medium in the Petri cap is traditionally used (J.R. Petri, the German bacteriologist). More rarely in clinical laboratories the biological or chemical methods are employed to isolate the agent of a disease. They need the availability of laboratory animals sensitive to certain microorganisms, supplementary chemical equipment, and specialists in microbiology.

As the result of the inoculation of medium and incubation (growing of young cells) the colonies of microorganisms appear in a thermostat at 37 °C within two days (Fig. 4.5). They can differ from each other in appearance, color and cell distribution over the cap area. Gram's stained smears are prepared from different colonies and examined by a microscope. The residues of the colonies are inoculated on medium for reproduction of microorganism cultures by placing them in the thermostat.

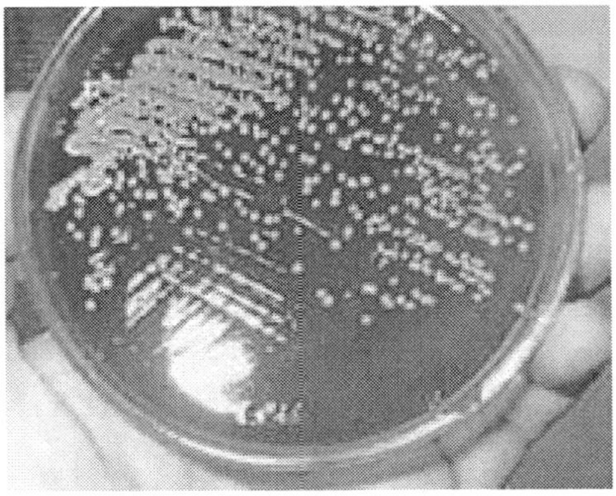

Figure 4.5. The growth of the colonies of microorganisms on the nutrient medium in the Petri cap.

The purity of the culture obtained is assessed by morphological and tinctorial (affinity of the cellular wall to certain stains) properties of microbial cells. The species of the microorganism is defined based on its features using the set of five criteria. It includes:

1. Morphological criteria:

a) the shape of cells;

b) tinctorial properties by Gram stain or by target differential diagnostic methods;

c) movability of cells.

2. Culture-related criteria:

a) dynamics of cell growth on special nutrients;

b) appearance of colonies.

3. Biochemical criteria consisting in revealing the enzymes that:

a) decompose protein and amino acids, namely, proteinases, peptidases (identified by dissolution reaction of fresh serum, gelatin, and casein) decarboxylases (identified by arising amines in electrophoresis), desaminases (by isolated ammonia), triptophanases (by revealing indol), desulfurases (hydrogen sulfide formation), etc.;

b) decompose sugars or carbohydrases (inoculation of Hiss medium (Ph.H. Hiss, the American bacteriologist) comprising mono-, di, and polysaccharides and detection of acid and gas), amylases (inoculation of starch medium and subsequent testing with iodine);

c) decompose erythrocytes or hemolysines (determination of hemolysis, i.e., blood erythrocyte decomposition in inoculation of blood agar);

d) decompose lipids and lipoids, i.e., lecitinases (in inoculation of yolk the opacity arises in the places of colony growth);

e) oxidation-reduction enzymes, i.e., oxidases (blue staining of the colonies under the effect of paraphynelene diamine), peroxidases (reduction of methylenum blue), and catalases (testing with H_2O_2).

4. Serologic criteria assess the microorganism interaction with special diagnostic sera.

5. Biological criteria:

a) assess the degree of pathogenesis (virulence) of the microorganism in animals;

b) determination of the microorganism susceptibility to a specific bacteriophage;

c) determination of microorganism susceptibility to antibiotics.

Cultural investigation of SF yields positive results in 90−100% of non-gonococci joint infections. The information value of bacteriological tests decreases drastically in the case of preceding antibiotic therapy. In a number of cases, an additional study of SF is required to detect mycobacteria, fungi, and atypical agents. In microbiological investigation of SF it is advisable to use experimental condition and media that allow both aerobic and anaerobic bacteria to be detected. The long-standing comparative evaluation of the efficiency of various techniques permits us to consider the cultural method as the most precise in microbiology.

4.3.2. Some Other Methods of Microbiological Analysis

Culture examination of SF is supplemented by serological and allergologic analysis as well as bacteriological investigation of the synovial materials.

Immunodiagnostics of SF assumes immunology methods to be employed to recognize structural lesions and functional disorders of synovia at the genetic level. Above all, it is a serologic investigation, i.e., examination of the SF antigen–antibody indicator reactions that can be registered on the ground of one of the phenomena accompanying the formation of immune complex such as precipitation, agglutination, and complement binding.

As shown in 2.3.3, agglutination (sticking and sedimentation from the homogeneous suspension of erythrocytes and other antigen-carrying cells under the effect of agglutinin antibodies) that is traditionally used to determine the blood group allows one to determine a SF group. In the following subsection 4.3.3 the examples are given to demonstrate the use of SF agglutination to determine the kind of proteins and identify infectious agents in joints.

Precipitation is a phenomenon of sedimentation of a dissolved antigen in its interaction with the antibody due to insolubility of their complex in isotonic fluids. Isotonic solutions being similar to blood serum in composition, pH, and other properties are called physiological solutions and used to register immunological reactions with SF involved. As shown in 4.3.3., precipitation is used to form and sediment insoluble complexes of soluble SF antigen (precipitinogen) – specific antibody (precipitin) in the diagnostics of articular infections.

The complement is the system of serum proteins contained in SF that is activated by the antigen-antibody complex with the formation of biologically active substances responsible for irreversible disturbances of cellular membranes. The complement as one of the factors of natural immunity is widely used in diagnostic immunological reactions with participation of SF. The reactions include the attachment of complement to antigen-antibody complex on the surface of cellular membrane that lead to the lysis of bacteria, erythrocytes, and other cells treated by respective antibodies; involvement in the antigen-antibody reaction that do not lead to cell lysis; and enzymatic catalysis of biological phenomena related to the "recognition" at the molecular level. Below the examples are cited how complement materials are used in SF analysis for the diagnostics of some infectious joint diseases.

Allergologic analysis, i.e., the study of SF reactions to antigens of exoallergen classes penetrating into the joint cavity from the environment and autologous allergens arising from the autologous tissues of the joint under certain conditions (trauma, burning, and infection) is rarely employed in arthrology. In allergy due to pathological immunity modifications [22], the synovial medium responds to a specific antigen via excessive reaction that damages the autologous cells and tissues of the joint. The damage occurs as edema and inflammation of tissues, spasm, and relaxation of unstriped muscles, microcirculatory and hemodynamic injures. As a rule, the reaction develops at the secondary rather than primary contact of the synovial medium with an allergen. The allergen reaction occurs as immediate or delayed type hypersensitivity. Unfortunately, allergology, the domain of medicine that studies the causes, mechanisms of development, manifestation, diagnostics, prophylaxis, and treatment of allergic reactions and diseases, is not widely employed to diagnose joint disorders [22, 23, 24].

Experimental biological investigation of SF has two directions. The first direction aims to set the immunological memory, i.e., the capability of joint immunity to respond to the secondary invasion of an antigen after their first interaction. The immunological memory is the most intrinsic property of immune response. There are two kinds of immunological memory.

Positive immunological memory is an accelerated and enhanced specific response to the secondary encounters with the same antigen. In primary immune response (Fig. 4.6, *a*) after antigen invasion in the joint tissues or SF the antibodies appear in SF within several days (latent period t_1). Afterwards, the number of antibodies increases up to maximum with follow-up decrease. In secondary response of the joint synovial medium to the same antigen dose (*b*), the latent period t_2 is reduced and the curve of the kinetic dependence of antibodies in SF becomes higher and steeper and lowers down more slowly. Positive immunological memory of the synovial medium to antigens is the basis of allergic diseases of joints.

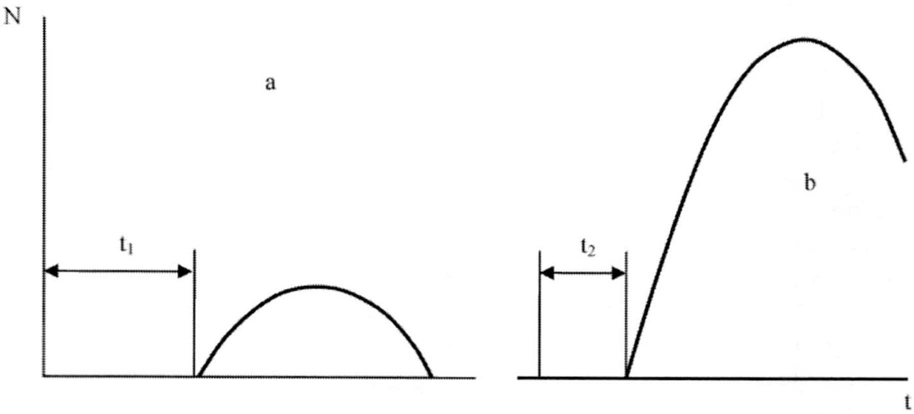

Figure 4.6. Kinetic dependences of the number (*N*) of antibodies in SF in primary (*a*) and secondary (*б*) immune responses.

Negative immunological memory is the innate and acquired immune tolerance that manifests in a weakened response to both primary and secondary antigen invasion. Disturbances of negative immunological memory to autologous antigens of the synovial medium provide the grounds for pathogenesis of certain autoimmune joint diseases. Activation of the negative immunological memory is the most promising method for overcoming tissue incompatibility (histoincompatibility) in osteoplasty and arthroplasty [25]. Immunological memory of joints in response to different antigens is different. It can be short-term (days or weeks), long-term (months and years), and life-long. Immunological memory is a kind of biological memory that differs principally from neurological (brain) memory in its performance and data storage level and volume. Long living T- and B-lymphocytes arising in primary immune response and circulating in SF as specific precursors of antigen-reactive lymphocytes are main carriers of immunological memory in joints. In secondary response, these cells are reproduced ensuring the clone increase (a number of generations following each other) antibody-forming or antigen-reactive lymphocytes of the same specificity. Immune complexes, cytophilic and blocking antibodies have a certain effect onto immunological memory. Immunological memory can be transferred from an immune donor to a non-immune recipient by invading living lymphocytes carrying a “transfer factor” or immune RNA into the joints. The problem is discussed in more detail in 5.3.3.

The second direction in microbiological analysis of SF presumes the study of infectious diseases of synovial joints in experiments involving animals, such as mice, dogs, monkeys, and cavies. To cultivate viruses and intracellular microorganisms, the chicken embryos and cell cultures under development are used. They are grown outside the organism on special media of human and animal tissue cells and retain inherent metabolism and susceptibility to certain viruses. Laboratory animals are subjected to viral infections when the viruses do not cause the cytopathic effect on the cell cultures and are not reproduced in chicken embryos as well as when pathogenesis and immunity of viral infections is studied. Experimental biology which provides the basis for many fundamental propositions in arthrology deals with animal vivisection. In all times, these experiments are believed unethical if they do harm to them. In all developed countries the laws are adopted concerning the strict control over animal tests. The tests over human beings are even more intricate. In Russian medicine the founder of the home scientific immunology school, Nobel Prize winner (1908) I.I. Mechnikov has attracted the attention to this problem as of utmost seriousness [26]. Currently, the problem of physicians' responsibility for the aftereffects of their work has become of even greater urgency in connection with the boom in genetic engineering. Its methods differ from manipulations with microbes since the propagation of "constructed" organisms can have serious consequences for humanity. In 1982, in Strasbourg the recommendations on application of genetic engineering methods to people were approved. In 2001, English parliament approved the law that allows the cloning of human cells with regulations of donors' rights and their obligatory consent to investigations.

Below an example is considered of the results of the biological study of horse's SF [27]. Age-related dynamics of phosphatase activity in horse's blood serum (the enzyme that maintains the level of phosphates in the organism) and ceruloplasmin (the protein that binds and carries copper in the organism, the main antioxidant) is similar to the dynamics of these enzymes in the synovia. So it was concluded that the age-related variation in substance activity responsible for the regulation of general biological reactions of inflammations, immunogenesis, adaptation, and compensation corresponded to the decreasing efficiency of metabolism both in the organism as a whole and in the joint with SF involved.

4.3.3. Causative Agents of Joint Infections

In arthritis, staphylococci are detected the most often, mainly, *Staphylococcus aureus* (Greek *staphyle* is grape, Lat. *coccus* is coccus and *aureum* is golden). Bacterioscopy of the Gram stained smears detects gram-positive (violet) round microorganisms up to 1 μm in size, arranged as conglomerates, pairs, or short chains.

In bacteriological investigations, the synovial effusion is inoculated in the Petri caps with 3–5% of blood agar or yolk-saline agar, after which it is placed in the thermostat for 18–24 hours at 37 °C. Within 24 hour-period, the staphylococci form mean-sized convex turbid colonies of fine-grainy structure with the hemolysis zone on the blood agar or turbid zone on the yolk-saline agar. To obtain a pure culture, staphylococci are inoculated from the colonies for 3 days on the medium called "the slanting agar". It is produced by filling a sterile tube with the liquid agar by 1/3 which is thickened in the sloped tube; afterwards the free surface of the thickened agar becomes elliptically shaped and located at an angle to the tube axis. Plasma coagulation activity of microorganisms is detected in the tubes with citrate plasma, i.e., the blood plasma containing the citric acid salt. The test is considered positive if the plasma is coagulated within two hours of being held in the thermostat.

Afterwards, staphylococci are phagotyped to determine the affiliation of the isolates to a set of isolates. Phagotyping is executed by four groups of phages included in the international set of twenty three phages. Serotyping or staphylococci reaction with antibodies – is done using the set of typical adsorption sera. The pathogeneous golden staphylococcus is distinguished from the conditionally pathogeneous ones by formation of golden, capability of hemolyzing blood, coagulating plasma, isolating hyaluronidase, lecitovitellase, DNA-ase, oxidizing manit in aerobic conditions and fermenting it in the absence of oxygen, and producing α-toxin that leads to skin necrosis of laboratory animals [28].

Streptococci or gram-positive microorganisms in the form of cocci arranged in smears as short chains, their groups, or individually lying cells also refer to arthritis causative agents. For detecting streptococci, the biomaterial is inoculated on the laminar sugar or blood agar plates and cultivated in the thermostat. Within a day the growth of streptococci is observed in the form of fine flat colonies of grainy structure with the hemolysis zone (*Streptococcus pyogenes*) and a green edge of methemglobin (a hemoglobin derivative) around them (*Streptococcus viridans*) or free of it (*Streptococcus anhaemolyticus*). In the sugar broth the streptococci display the bottom and wall growth in the form of flakes or grains. To identify β-hemolytic streptococci of group A their high resistance to antibacterial chemical compound bacitracin is determined.

To determine the virulence of streptococci, their capability of producing toxin, i.e., fibrinolysin (streptokinase) is studied. For this purpose, the streptococcus culture (0.5 ml) and 25% solution of $CaCl_2$ are added in the laboratory tube to the human blood diluted in a 1:3 proportion. The mixture is placed in the water bath for 1–2 hours at 42 °C. The streptococci releasing fibrinolysin dissolve the fibrin clot in the laboratory tube. Most often the arthritis progress coincides with elimination (absorption) of a causative agent that initiates the development of acute rheumatoid fever and rheumatic arthritis in a genetically predisposed organism.

If it is impossible to detect a causative agent in SF, the serological examination of patients is performed, i.e., the streptococcus antigen is found by the binding reaction of the complement in SF and the antibody titer to streptococcus toxins (O-streptolysin) is determined. Anti-streptococcal immune serum required to bind the complement is obtained by immunization of rabbits by the group-A streptococcus. Maximal serum dilution that inhibits the hemolysis less than by "+" is taken as the antigen titer. The determination of O-antistreptolysin in SF is based on its capability of neutralizing hemolytic activity of O-streptolysin. For this, multiple dilutions of patient's SF are prepared adding the standard O-streptolysin. The mixtures are incubated in the thermostat for 15 min at 37 °C, afterwards, 0.2 ml of suspension of rabbit's erythrocytes is introduced in all laboratory tubes and incubation lasts for about an hour after which the reaction results are evaluated.

Blue pus infection in joints is initiated by the blue pus bacillus *Pseudomonas aeruginosa,* the gram-negative bacillus (1.5–3.0)×(0.5–0.8) μm in size having 1–2 filaments located in the smear individually, in pairs or chains and stained pink. To grow this causative agent, just one organic compound, namely, citric acid salt (citrate) as a source of carbon and energy is enough in the medium. The blue pus bacillus is cultivated on the media as convex pigmented colonies with uneven edges, metallic shine, and jasmine smell. The bacteria produce fluorescein and pyocyanin (blue) pigments. Some isolates synthesize pyorubin (a red-brown pigment), erythrogen (red), melanogen (black), and about 20% of the colonies are pigment-free. Biochemically, the microorganism is inactive, i.e., it only oxidizes glucose. The oxidation is executed in two laboratory tubes containing a beef-extract broth, glucose, and bromthymol blue. One of the tubes is filled with Vaseline oil. The blue pus bacillus changes the mixture color in the oil-free tube. High proteolytic activity (capability of cleaving proteins) of the blue pus bacillus manifests in dilution of the gelatin and coagulated blood serum, casein hydrolysis, amino acid cleavage, and enzyme production, namely, catalase and oxidase.

Brucellosis arthropathy is caused by microorganisms of *Brucella* species (*B. melitensis, B. abortus, and B. suis*). To diagnose it, SF, blood, and more rarely urine, puncture material of bone marrow and lymphatic nodes are inoculated using special laboratory facilities. The microorganism is immobile gram-positive bacilli or cocci sized up to 1.5 μm. Brucellas grow slowly during 25 to 30 days. Their growth in the hepatic or ascitic broth makes it turbid with mucous sediment arising. In the Petri caps with the hepatic agar the bacteria form fine, smooth, white turbid colonies with pearly hue. The brucella culture does not ferments carbons, does not coagulate milk, and does not dilute gelatin. Brucellas are differentiated by hydrogen sulfide liberation (*B. abortus* and *B. suis*), susceptibility to the bacteriological effect of aniline rosein (*B. melitensis* and *B. abortus*) and thionine (*B. melitensis* and *B. suis*) stains , as well as by the need in carbonic acid for the growth of *B. abortus*.

Serological methods for brucellosis diagnostics are most accessible among other microbiological methods for confirming brucellosis. They include the Wright reaction (A.E. Wright, the English bacteriologist and infectiologist); agglutination of brucellas killed by heat in brucellosis-infected patient's SF and blood serum; the Huddleson reaction (J.F. Huddleson, the American bacteriologist), namely, agglutination of the bacteria of the stained specimen (for diagnostics *in vitro*) with different-volume patient's serum drops performed on the slide; binding of the complement; indirect hemoagglutination; immunofluorescence, etc. In a number of cases, intracutaneus allergic Burnet testing is applied (E. Burnet, the French microbiologist) with a brucellosis antigen, namely, melitin.

Tuberculosis microbacteria (*Mycobacterium tuberculosis*) when observed by a microscope look like straight or slightly curved structurally homogeneous or grainy bacilli sized (2−8)×0.3 μm and disposed individually, in pairs or small agglomerates. Owing to mycolic acid and lipids found in large amounts in the cell wall, microbacteria are resistant to the effects of alcohol, acids, and alkaline. In Ziehl-Neelsen staining of smears (the method was suggested by a German bacteriologist F. Ziehl and pathological anatomist F. Neelsen) to detect alcohol- and acid-resistant bacteria as well as fuchsin-philic intracellular inclusions characteristic of viral infections), the microbacteria become bright-red. Gram staining takes 2 to 3 hours due to poor susceptibility of the microbacteria to aniline stains. In express diagnostics of tuberculosis, luminescent microscopy is used for which the specimen is stained by auramin, decolorized by hydrochloride alcohol and stained by acid fuchsin. The microbacteria shine golden green against a dark background. The agent culture can be detected at a concentration of 20−100 microbe bodies in 1 ml of the biological material.

In tuberculous arthritis, the culture investigation of SM specimens is the most informative since the causative agent is detected in 80−94% of cases. For cultivation, the Löwenstein-Jensen protein-yolk medium is used (A. Löwenstein, the Austrian pathologist and bacteriologist and K. Jensen, the Danish bacteriologist) with malachite green, glycerin broth or liquid saline media with asparagine and glycerin. Within a 3−4 day incubation at 37−38 °C, the colony growth is observed in the form of wart or cauliflower on the solid medium. In the glycerin broth, the mycobacterium growth is seen in the form of brittle wrinkled yellowish film within 10−14 days. The tuberculosis mycobacteria produce enzymes such as catalase and peroxidase and nicotinic acid.

An intracutaneus allergic Mantoux test with tuberculin (a material obtained from tuberculous mycobacteria cultures) is used to diagnose tuberculosis. It is named after French physician Ch. Mantoux who created the method in 1908. To verify the borreliosis etiology of arthritis, a wide spectrum of direct and indirect microbiological tests is used. Microorganisms

Borrelia burgdorferi are anaerobic gram-negative curled movable bacteria sized (20–30)×(0.2–0.3) μm. The spirochete cytoplasm is arranged as a spiral around a curled axial thread. Romanovsky-Gimze staining (gray violet staining) or Burry (black and white "negative" specimens) is used. A Russian physician D.L. Romanovsky proposed the staining method, a German chemist and bacteriologist G. Gimza created a stain, and R. Burri proposed to use black ink as a stain. Living microorganisms are observed by phase contrast or dark-field microscopy. A low diagnostic value of SF microscopy in borreliosis limits its wide employment.

Borrelia are extremely demanding to cultivation conditions. Long-standing empirical experiments have resulted in the medium termed BSK-II (modified medium proposed by American microbiologists A.G. Barbour, H.G. Stoenner, and R.T. Kelly) that is applicable to isolate and cultivate borreliosis causative agents.

Borrelium can be isolated from the biopsy material taken from migrating erythema in about 60% of cases. In chronic atrophic acrodermatitis (when inflammatory nodes or swollen bluish red spots arise on the extension surface of joints) the percentage of the positive results is 80–90%. The percentage of the positive results is lower in blood (1–3%), cerebrospinal liquor (15–20%) or SF (20–25%) inoculations.

Standard (indirect) serologic methods (immunofluorescent, immunoenzymatic, immune blotting) are most commonly used to diagnose borreliosis (see 3.2.2).

Indirect immunofluorescence reaction has been developed and proposed for clinical diagnostics of borreliosis prior to others. This laboratory test is widely used in medical institutions being the most cost-effective, accessible, and not requiring any special lab facilities [23]. Specific antibodies arising in the reaction are registered in the form of complexes (antigen + specific antibody + serum against human globulins marked by fluorescin) that are fixed on the corpuscular antigen (Ip-21 *Borrelia afzelii*) and shine in ultraviolet beams. Blood serum, SF and liquor can be the objects of investigation. The sensitivity of the serologic reaction (the ratio of object brightness to cell number) is within 40–50% with a reliability of 96–98%.

Recently, the polymerase chain reaction (PCR) is used to diagnose borreliosis. This high-sensitive method allows detection of singular DNA or RNA molecules in the biological specimen under testing. In PCR, genome loci of borrelia (locus is a gene location in the cell) are used as targets. The structure of the genome of *Borrelia burgdorferi sensu stricto* B31 isolate of American origin is completely disclosed and serves a reference isolate for the whole *Borrelia burgdorferi* group. However, the genetic structure of similar gene loci in different borrelia differs essentially. Therefore, the PCR method to diagnose borreliosis is not unified and remains inaccessible for practical medicine. Nevertheless, its employment in clinical diagnostics of borreliosis is advisable, since it, primarily, allows detection of DNA borrelia in different biological materials (the tick as a carrier of microorganisms, skin specimen, blood, urine, cerebrospinal liquor, SF, etc.); second, its high sensitivity makes it possible to detect a patient's infection 7–14 days after the moment of tick bite, i.e., within an incubation period. Control investigation after a month treatment is the optimal term during which DNA and RNA borrelia are removed totally from the organism in the case of adequate treatment.

The involvement of chlamydiae (*Chlamydia trachomatis*) into infectious processes in joints (see 3.2.1) has recently been revealed. Chlamydiae are assigned to obligate parasites, i.e., those surviving only inside the host cells. They can have the coccus, ovoid (vesicular) or rod-shaped form sized from 200 to 800 nm. In urogenital infections and Reiter disease (syndromes of polyarthritis, ureteritis, and conjunctivitis) the microorganisms are detected in smears and scrapes from the mucous membranes upon Romanovsky-Gimza staining. Here one can see violet intracellular inclusions, namely, Prowazek-Halberstädter bodies (S. Prowazek, a Czech microbiologist and L. Halberstädter, a German physician) against the blue background. For antigen detection, the smears are treated with monoclone (marked with fluorochromes) antibodies against the cellular membrane protein using the indirect immunofluorescence. Chlamydiae are detected by infecting chicken embryos and human cell cultures with the biological material. The antigens of microbes, DNA, chlamydiae as well as proper microorganisms capable of reproduction are isolated from the joint tissues and SF [29]. Specific antibodies such as IgA, IgG, and IgM are detected in the biological fluids by binding the complement, indirect agglutinations, and immune-enzymatic analysis.

Gonococcus arthritis is initiated by the *Neisseria gonorrhoeae* microorganism, the gram-negative diplococci arranged in pairs as agglomerates inside leucocytes and outside cells. In hematogeneous infection this microbe can cause the development of purulent arthritis. Smears from the cellular membranes and specimens of synovial effusion are stained with methylene blue and by Gram. Bacterioscopy and inoculation allow one to detect gonococci in the synovial effusion only in 1/4–2/3 of all cases. Certain difficulties in detecting and identifying gonococci arise even at the stage of taking and transporting the material since the causative agent is extremely sensitive to drying. In a number of cases the procedure is successful if the SF obtained within first 7–10 days after the disease onset is placed immediately after aspiration in the Petri cap on the nonselective medium, e.g., chocolate agar and held in the desiccator in the presence of 10% carbonic acid. 24 hours after incubation at 37 °C the convex mucous colonies grow that resemble dew drops. Bordet-Gengou (J. Bordet, the Nobel prize winner (1919), O. Gengou, the French microbiologist) serological reaction is of diagnostic value within 2–4 weeks after the gonorrhea onset as well as intracutaneus testing with a gonovaccine.

Anaerobic infection of joints is a wound infection accompanied by heavy intoxication, edema, and necrosis of soft tissues. It is caused by spore-forming microorganisms of *Clostridium* kind (*C. perfringens*, *C. novyi*, *C. septicum*, C. *histolyticum*, *C. tetani*). The symptoms of anaerobic infection are so specific that a correct diagnosis can be easily set by the clinical picture. In difficult cases the specimens taken from the wounds and joints are analyzed. In the smears large gram-positive bacilli arranged individually or as chains are detected.

For express diagnostics of anaerobic infections, passive hemagglutination of an antibody erythrocyte specimen with an exotoxin antigen-containing biological material is performed. Exotoxin is a toxic protein substance produced by a toxigenic bacterium accumulated in the medium in cultivation. Other diagnostic methods include immune enzymatic analysis and precipitation reaction. Clostridia are isolated in the biological material on the agar media in Petri caps in aerostats, on the Kitt-Tarocci liquid medium (in the late 18th century a German veterinary physician Th. Kitt and Italian physiologist G. Tarocci proposed a liquid medium for cultivating anaerobic microorganisms consisting of concentrated beef-extract broth), in defatted milk under butter, and in the columns of the beef-extract agar.

To detect the pure culture *C. perfringens* the material is inoculated in the Wilson-Blair agar medium (E.B. Wilson, the American cytologist and embryologist and E. M. Blaier, the American microbiologist) containing glucose, potassium sulfite, and ferric chloride. After 3 hours, the clostridium microcolonies get black and glucose fermentation results in gas occurrence and rapture in the medium layer. In *C. perfringens* inoculation in milk under butter milk turns with casein clots within 6 hours.

Among arthritis-inducing viruses the causative agents of chickenpox, measles, epidemic parotitis, and viral hepatitis prevail [24]. They can cause a reactive joint inflammation and once invaded into SM and SF cause immune inflammation. In practical rheumatology the serologic diagnostic tests of viral hepatitis are the most widely spread. They allow detection in the blood serum and SF of an increased level of specific antibodies and their at least fourfold titer increase in dynamics (the virus titer is the number of infectious plaque-forming hemagglutinating or other units of viral activity found in a volume unit of a virus-containing fluid). For the cultivation of viruses the cell cultures, chicken embryos, and more rarely laboratory animals are used. A pathological effect of the viruses on the cell cultures manifests in the variation of their shapes, i.e., after initial proliferation (reproduction) they are rounded, and the layer is wrinkled and destroyed. If the cytopathic effect of viruses is not revealed then hemosorption is applied when erythrocytes are applied to the virus-infected cell culture and the infection is detected by the rate with which the virus hemagglutinins cause the accumulation of erythrocytes on the cells.

The microbiological study of SF does not exclude a probable detection of the infectious agents not described above. Theoretically, any microorganism can cause joint inflammation. Detailed microbiological and serological, if necessary, analyses of patient's SF and blood are the main point in the diagnostics and selection of the effective therapy of arthritis.

4.4. Rheological Methods

Rheology (Greek *rheos* – flow) is a physical science dealing with the flow and deformation of media, in particular, fluids. The subject of rheology is irreversible residual deformations of media developed in time. The rheology term was suggested in 1929 by an American chemist Eu. Bingham. Biorheology studies the flow of biological fluids, namely, blood, SF, cerebrospinal fluid, etc. Biorheology is the part of biomechanics of fluids where the theoretical views of the mechanics of liquid media are used to describe the motion of fluids in biological processes [30].

4.4.1. The Main Concepts

Viscosity (internal friction) is the property of gases and fluids that characterizes their resistance to the action of external forces causing the flow. Viscosity of fluids mainly depends on the intermolecular interaction restricting the movability of molecules. Viscosity leads to dissipation and transition of fluid flow-inducing external forces to heat. A fluid without viscosity, or ideal fluid, is an abstraction.

The law of viscous flow was discovered in 1687 by an English mathematician and physicist I. Newton. Newton's formula

$$F = \eta \frac{dv}{dz} S,$$

where F is the force of internal friction arising between the fluid layers in their shearing relative each other; η is the coefficient of fluid dynamic viscosity; dv/dz is a velocity gradient showing how the velocity varies on unit length in the direction z; S is the area of fluid contact layers. The force of internal friction F impedes the movement of fluid layers moving very fast and accelerates the layers that move more slowly. The coefficient of kinematic viscosity is v=η/ρ, where ρ is fluid density.

The fluids termed Newtonian follow the law of viscous flow. Their coefficient of viscosity η only depends on the fluid nature and temperature. The coefficient η of non-Newtonian fluids also depends on the fluid velocity gradient dv/dz, therefore, for them

$$F \approx \left(\frac{dv}{dz}\right)^n,$$

where n characterizes the mechanical properties of fluid under given conditions of flowing.

Synovial fluid is non-Newtonian since it has the structure of protein-polysaccharide complexes bound to water molecules and the features of long-range order. Its main component, namely, blood serum, is essentially a Newtonian fluid. SF found in healthy joints is a gel, i.e., the system of liquid dispersed medium with protein particles forming a spatial structure (network) distributed in it. Its normal viscosity is 5–7 arbitrary units [31] (arbitrary unit is water viscosity, see in more detail 4.5.2). In joint diseases the SF viscosity decreases down to 2–3 standard units and the serum viscosity is 1.2 standard units [32]. The SF viscosity, as any fluid, rises with decreasing temperature, thus, at a temperature drop from 37 down to 17 °C the SF viscosity grows by 10%.

The mode of SF flow is laminar, i.e., the fluid moves by layers without mixing. In a pathological joint and viscosity loss the flow rate of the SF lubricating layer might increase so that the laminar flow will change to turbulent at which intensive mixing of the fluid layers occurs. The SF flow in joints is most often characterized by volume rate $Q=V/t$, where V is fluid volume and t is time. As the fluid is incompressible, equal volumes of SF pass through all gaps in a joint per unit time, i.e., $Q=VS$=const, where S is the cross section area of a gap. The linear rate is a path covered by a SF particle per unit time $v=L/t$.

For a stationary fluid flow on the pipe the Poiseuille law is valid

$$Q = \frac{\pi R^4}{8\eta} \cdot \frac{\Delta p}{\iota},$$

where R and ι are tube radius and length, $\Delta p=p_1-p_2$ is the pressure difference at input (p_1) and output (p_2) of a tube. The regularity was revealed empirically by a French physicist and physician J. Poiseuille. From this law describing reliably the laminar flow of SF it follows that the drop of fluid pressure in the joint depends on the volume flow rate, yet even to a higher degree on the gap between the mated cartilages wetted by SF. The linear rate of the SF flow is higher in narrow gaps.

In 1806, a French physicist P. Laplase discovered one of the main laws of capillary phenomena called by his name:

$$p_\sigma = \sigma\left(\frac{1}{R_1} + \frac{1}{R_2}\right),$$

where p_σ is capillary pressure, i.e., the difference of the pressures at both sides of the curved interface of two fluids or a fluid and a gas; σ is surface tension equaling the work for the formation of an area unit of the surface; R_1 and R_2 are curvature radii of two mutually normal sections of the interface. Analysis of the Laplase formula highlights the following conclusions:

1) capillary pressure in the gap of the joint friction pair increases with increasing surface tension of SF;

2) an increase in the capillary pressure of SF in the gap of the friction pair evidently causes an increase in stresses in cartilages;

3) since the capillary pressure is in reverse proportion to the curvature radius of the interface, the SF pressure is higher in narrow gaps.

The Laplase law was discovered during the study of capillary gaps formed by the rigid solids. In this case there is a direct relationship between pressure and fluid flow rate. A lower increase in the SF volume flow rate corresponds to increasing pressure in the joint gaps formed by elastic cartilages (Fig. 4.7).

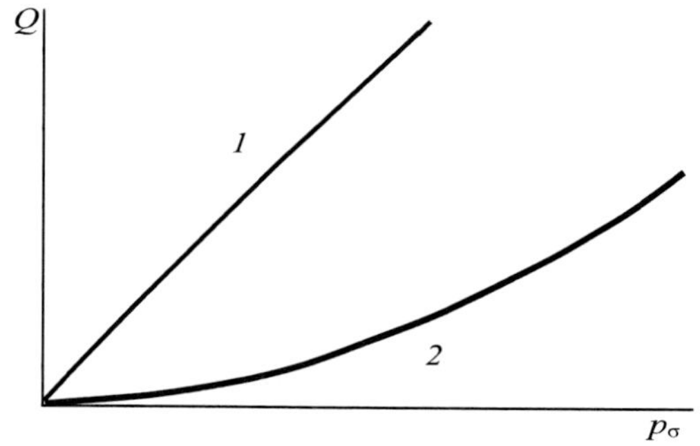

Figure 4.7. Volume fluid flow rate Q vs. pressure p_σ in a capillary formed by: *1* – rigid, *2* – elastic walls.

The total SF volume found in a joint can be divided into an active part circulating along the gap between the cartilages and deposited one uninvolved in circulation though can be involved under certain conditions. The loss of the circulating fluid volume due to filtration of low-molecular SF fraction in the cartilage pores is compensated by the deposited SF.

4.4.2. Viscosimetry of Synovial Fluid

Viscosimetry is the set of methods for measuring viscosity. The viscometer is an instrument to measure the viscosity of fluids and gases. The viscosity of SF is measured by capillary and rotation viscometers as well as those that realize the method of a falling sphere.

Capillary viscometers are based on the Poiseuille law by action principle. The designs of capillary viscosimeters under usage in medicine are shown in Fig. 4.8.

The Ostwald viscometer was developed by W. Ostwald, the German physicist and chemist, Nobel prize winner (1909). The viscosity measurement technique by the instruments shown in Fig. 4.8, *a* and *b*, consists in the recording of the time required for SF to flow via capillary *2* under the action of gravity force at a known pressure difference. It is specified by the shape and dimensions of measuring bath *1*. The volume of the transported fluid is registered by the marks on the bath. Ostwald viscometers are designed for measuring the viscosity of media within the limits from 10^{-5} to 10^{4} Pa·s, i.e., from gases to consistent greases. The SF viscosity (2–7)·10^{-3} Pa·s falls within this range.

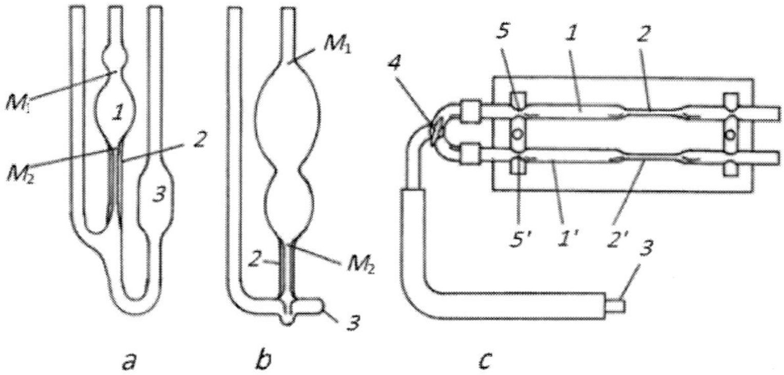

Figure 4.8. Capillary Ostwald viscometer (a) and its variant (b) and Hess one (*c*) [33]. 1 and 1′ – measuring tubes; 2 and 2′, 5 and 5′ – capillaries; 3 – receiving tube; *4* – tap, M_1 and M_2 – marks of the tube boundaries.

Clinics widely use the Hess viscometer with two capillaries developed by the Russian chemist G.I. Hess to measure the viscosity of biological fluids. Producing vacuum in tip 3, measuring tubes are filled by turns up to zero marks through a branch equipped with tap *4* and technological capillaries *2* and *2'*: *1* with distilled water and *1'* with SF. Afterwards, by means of the same vacuum system both fluids move simultaneously through capillaries 5 and 5′ to the left until SF reaches the mark and water reaches the other mark in its tube. Filling of tubes 1 and 1′ will be different because of different viscosities of water and SF. Without regard for SF as a non-Newtonian fluid we can approximately take that $Q_1/Q_2=\eta_2/\eta_1$, where indices *1* и *2* correspond to water and SF, respectively. With homogeneous fluid flows $V=Q/t$, then $V_1/V_2=\eta_2/\eta_1$, where V_1 is tube *1* volume from zero to the mark recorded in measurement; V_2 is tube 1′ volume between the zero and specified marks. The value of η_2/η_1 is called relative SF viscosity and measured in standard units. For measurement convenience, tubes 1 and 1′ have different diameters to provide approximately equal levels in the tubes despite different volumes of the escaped water and SF.

Rotational viscometers are instruments whose main unit is a pair of co-axial cylinders one of which (a rotor) rotates while another one is stationary. The fluid in question is placed in the gap between the cylinders. The gap is sufficiently small to provide equal conditions for the deformation of the liquid sample to be studied. This is the main point why rotational viscometry is advantageous over the capillary since a nonuniform distribution of the flow rates and surface tension of the fluid on the channel radius is inevitable in a capillary. Viscosity is found by measuring:

- angular velocity ω of the rotor rotation which produces the specified moment of force through the fluid layer on the stationary cylinder;
- moment of force acting on the stationary cylinder at a specified angular velocity of rotor.

In Newtonian fluids M/ω=const. While calculating η corrections are introduced primarily, to edge effects, i.e., the variation of the parameter under registration on the spots adjacent to the cylinder edges.

Falling sphere viscometers (the Stokes method) are a tube filled with the fluid in question in which a sphere is emerged and the velocity of its uniform falling is recorded. The sphere is surrounded by the laminar flow of the fluid in its uniform motion at a low velocity. The fluid viscosity is measured by the Stokes' formula:

$$\eta = \hat{E}\left(\rho - \rho_0\right)/v,$$

where v is the sphere's setting velocity, ρ and ρ_0 are densities of the sphere material and the fluid, and K is an instrument constant. The law governing the resistance force of a viscous fluid at a slow progressive movement of a solid in it was derived in 1851 by an English physicist J. Stokes.

A sphere falling in a fluid is affected by 1) the gravitational force directed normally down; 2) upthrust Archimedes force directed normally upwards; and 3) the Stokes force also directed normally upwards. Under the action of these forces the sphere acquired acceleration and its velocity rises up to a limiting value. Then acceleration becomes equaling zero and the sphere moves uniformly. The viscometer records the velocity. In finding viscosity the corrections are introduced to the inertia effect (the sphere acceleration before staring uniform movement is taken into account) and the effect of the tube walls on the velocity of sphere drop. The method is convenient to measure the viscosity of the fluids under excessive pressures. Such conditions are provided in the lubricating interlayer under synovial joint loading.

The aforesaid methods allow the viscosity of SF and other biological fluids to be measured at an error of about 1%. By observing uniformity of the measurements at the methodical level and improving the accuracy of the viscometer records, it is possible to reduce the error down to 0.1%. Viscometers are commonly calibrated by measuring the viscosity of standard fluids whose viscosity is known in advance. In viscometry, distilled water is the most accurate reference with a viscosity of 1.002 mPa·s at 20 °C.

4.4.3. Rheology of Synovia in Joints

Synovial fluid flow in joints is a necessary condition for their functioning. One of urgent problems in current arthrology is to prevent the joints from development of essential alterations in joint tissues by ensuring optimal movement of SF in the joint cavity. Disturbances of optimal regimes is caused by SF deficits, closure of the channels of its flow to the joint cavity, and variations in SF rheological characteristics.

The deficit of SF formation and secretion occurring in arthrosis induces deteriorated lubrication, increased coefficient of friction in joints, appearance of tissue degeneration spots on the cartilage surfaces, broken congruency and continuous microtraumatization of cartilages in joint movement [34].

Channels for SF motion in the joint are governed by morphology. For instance, SF runs in the knee joint along the submeniscus channels in the horizontal direction and along vertical channels near the patella in the frontal direction forming the united functional system of SF movement. The direction of the flow and functioning of the channels depend on phase and angle of flexing and extending movements in joints. The SF motion along the channels performs certain biomechanical functions. First and foremost, this is an effect of the synovial pad to reduce the concentration of contact pressure on the cartilage friction surface. Second, local concentration of SF at some sites of the friction surface causes the compulsory diffusion of the nutrient SF components in the cartilage tissue of these sites. Traumas and degenerative-dystrophic disorders of joints often result in the occurrence of commissure in the channels for SF motion ("the commissure" of the joints). The commissure of the knee joint is most often localized in the channels for SF motion, namely, above and beneath the rear horns of both menisci, in the superior exterior lateral torsion and in the anterior chamber of the knee joint [35]. Disturbance of optimal hydrodynamic parameters of SF motion in joints induces pathological disorders in tissues and accelerated cartilage wear.

Rheological characteristics of SF in a healthy joint are temperature-dependent. During motion and increased loads to the joint the temperature in its cavity elevates by about 3 °C. This leads to the following adaptive variations in the synovial medium of joints [36]:

- with temperature elevation the viscosity decreases and SF lubricity improves;
- in long-term operation of the joint the low-molecular part of SF is squeezed out from the cartilage tissue micropores and comes to the friction surfaces;
- a hydrodynamic effect of the lubricating interlayer of SF is enhanced under the action of these factors.

Owing to adaptation, the normal conditions of joint lubrication is recovered, friction decreases, and functional congruency of movably mated cartilages and joint mobility are ensured.

The viscosity of SF taken from a conventionally healthy joint (a donor is healthy somatically and no abnormalities detected in diagnostic arthroscopy) measured by the rotational viscometer decreases exponentially depending on shear rate (Fig. 4.9).

In terms of fluid mechanics, SF can be presented as a disperse system consisting of the set of protein aggregates suspended in the saline solution and moving as the whole. The model assumes that:

- aggregate sizes govern system fluidity;
- the aggregates are refined under the action of shear stresses;
- the system fluidity depends on aggregate deformation rate.

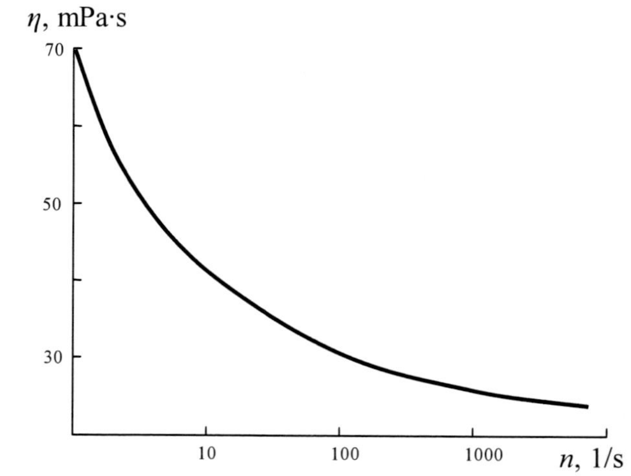

Figure 4.9. SF viscosity versus shear rate [36].

The viscosity of SF taken from conventionally healthy joints varies essentially at variations in pH, salt concentration, and degree of polymerization of hyaluronic acid that binds electrolytes and low-molecular proteins in gelatinous structures. It is noted [37] that hyaluronic acid serves a "synovial filter" relative to proteins of large (<160000) molecular mass. The amount of these proteins (fibrinogen, coagulability factors, globulins α_2 and β_2) is lower in SF than in blood serum.

Rheological abnormalities of SF flow in the joint cavity arise in joint diseases that are responsible for decreasing viscosity of SF. In aseptic joint inflammation, SF is diluted due to depolymerization and decreased concentration of hyaluronic acid. Its layer is less elastic and incapable of ensuring lubrication, absorption of impact loads in the joint, and cartilage protection. In its motion within the joint it leaks from micropores of the cartilage tissues and a gap between the cartilages. Pathological immune complexes and destructive enzymes are accumulated in low-viscous SF. This enhances the progress in degenerative processes, limitation of joint functional capacities, and gradual destruction of the cartilage [34].

The lowest concentration of hyaluronic acid is characteristic of the joints afflicted with infectious arthritis and rheumatoid arthritis. Consequently, the SF viscosity is the lowest in such joints. In traumatic synovitis, osteoarthritis, and systemic lupus erythematosus a decrease in hyaluronic acid in SF is less evident [38]. The viscosity of SF decreases in gouty and psoriatic arthritis, Reiter disease, and ankylosing spondylarthritis. Table 4.3 presents the quantitative assessment of viscosity and accompanying characteristics of SF in joint diseases [39].

Assessment of the functional mobility of SF within joints has become one of the diagnostic characteristics in traumatology and orthopedics in identification of degenerative-dystrophic disorders of joints. Thus, the drainage function of the channels for SF motion is determined by contrast microscopy [40] and the dysfunctions of the joint can be diagnosed by the channel narrowing or disappearance at an early stage of a disease.

The high-efficient yet not fully understood method of controlling SF rheological parameters uses the effect of the electric and magnetic fields. Electro- and magnetorheological effects are displayed in enhanced non-Newtonian flow and increasing SF yield point in shear due to enhancement of structure formation in a pathologically modified SF. The main physicochemical regularities of the processes are specified in 5.2.1.

Table 4.3. Assessment of SF variation in joint disorders

Nosological form	Viscosity	Color	Transparency	Mucin clot	Cells
Normal condition	High	Pale-yellow	Transp.	Good	–
Post-traumatic arthritis	High	Pale-yellow and bloody	Transp.	Bad	–
Secondary synovitis	Low	Amber-yellow	Turbid	Bad	–
Rheumatoid arthritis	Low	Yellow and green	Turbid	Bad	Rhagocytes
Rheumatism	Low	Yellow	Turbid	Good	–
Bekhterev's disease	Low	Yellow	Turbid	Good	Rhagocytes
Psoriatic arthritis	Low	Yellow and Green	Turbid	Good	–
Systemic lupus erythematosus	High	Yellow	Turbid	Good	LE
Gouty arthritis	Low	Yellow	Turbid	Bad	–
Chondrocalcinosis	Low	Yellow	Turbid	Good	–
Septic arthritis	Low	Bloody	Turbid	Bad	–
Pigmented arthritis	High	Brown	Turbid	Good	–

4.5. WETTING

Synovia performs its functions in contact with joint tissues. It invades in the capillary gap between the cartilage surfaces. Under joint loading, a low-molecular part of SF is filtered in the cartilage tissue micropores and provides one of the main functions of synovia, i.e., metabolism in the synovial medium of the joint. The high-molecular component of SF is adsorbed on the cartilage surface owing to which the lubricating layer is not squeezed out from the gap in the friction pair even under considerable loads thus protecting the cartilage from mechanical damages and providing lubrication. These interrelated and complex processes as far as physicochemical and biological processes are concerned, are due to a surface phenomenon termed wetting. Wetting is a phenomenon occurring in a fluid contacting a solid or another fluid. It is displayed in a fluid spread on the interface surface, its invasion in capillary channels, and occurrence of menisci in them.

Estimation of wetting parameters is based on the following ideas The position of a fluid drop on the solid surface is governed by the surface tension of fluid σ_f and solid σ_s at the boundary with air and on the fluid–solid contact surface σ_{fs} (Fig. 4.10). Under equilibrium conditions (i.e., in the absence of capillary effect, diffusion, chemical interaction, etc.) it corresponds to the Young equation:

$$\cos\theta_0 = (\sigma_s - \sigma_{fs})/\sigma_f,$$

where Θ_0 is a so-called equilibrium contact angle reckoned from the surface under wetting to the wetting fluid. The equation was derived by an English physician and physicist Th. Young in 1804.

The contact angle is the measure of wetting. Its value depends on the ratio of energies of adhesion, i.e., fluid adhesion to a solid, and cohesion, i.e., intermolecular attraction in a fluid. It is $0° < \Theta < 90°$ for the water-wetted (hydrophilic) solid surfaces (e.g., a cartilage). Unwettable (hydrophobic) surfaces are characterized by $\Theta > 90°$.

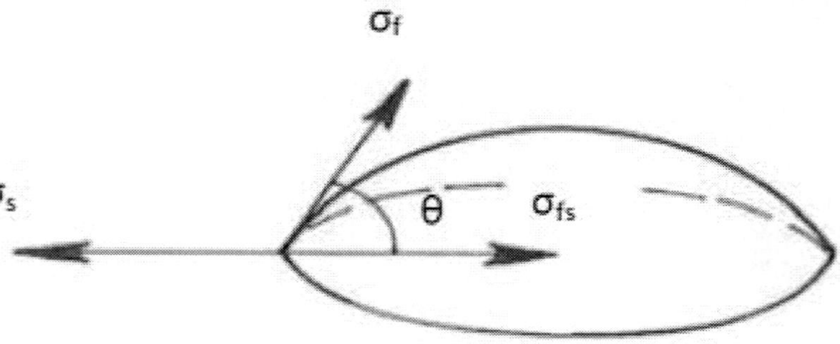

Figure 4.10. A drop on the solid surface.

Wetting depends on the quality of solid surface. Surface roughness is the set of its microasperities. Its microrelief is a chaotic or ordered alternation of protrusions and hollows different in shape and size. It is characterized by six height and spacing parameters regulated by State Standard 2789-73. Under other conditions being the same, the wetting indicators of solids depend on these parameters, the ratio of drop size and microasperity spacing, drop motion under inleakage or flow around, microasperity direction, etc. It is believed [41] that the surface roughness of hydrophilic solids improves wetting and that of hydrophobic solids impairs wetting. The rubbing surface of the hyaline cartilage has the ordered roughness in the form of microgrooves oriented in a certain way [42]. As reported elsewhere [43], such microrelief regularity favors the spread of SF along the grooves and, as known, friction in the joint is minimal if the directions of microgrooves and sliding coincide.

Cartilaginous tissue has the system of micropores in which SF is filtered. The cartilage friction surface is nonuniform, i.e., its part φ_s is a solid phase and the remaining part φ_p is pores so that $\varphi_s + \varphi_p = 1$. The equilibrium contact angle of wetting of porous bodies depends on φ_p [44]. The case occurs in SF contacting an artificial cartilage based on microporous ultra high-molecular polyethylene [45]. Under the effect of surface tension forces, the SF layer contacting the micropore walls in the cartilage is curved and produces an additional pressure in relation to external pressure caused by joint loading. SF penetrates into the pores of cartilage tissue and performs the metabolic function as the result of these pressures in total.

Temperature variations which fall within the range of human physiological temperatures do not have a significant effect on the wetting of cartilage and structural materials (used in manufacture of endoprostheses, namely, titanium, alloys Co-Cr-Mo, silicate and zirconium ceramic, ultra high-molecular polyethylene) with synovial.

Electrocapillary phenomena are variations in the surface tension at the fluid-solid interface caused by the difference in electric potential at the interface. The phenomenon was discovered in 1876 by a French physicist, Nobel Prize winner (1908) G. Lippmann. A potential jump occurs due to spatial division of charge carriers in the double electric layer. The latter is formed by two sets of electric charges concentrated in the surface layers of a solid and a fluid. The charges in these layers are opposite in sign but of the same surface density. The SF particles of a certain sign are adsorbed to and fixed motionlessly on the cartilage surface carrying a bioelectric potential of the opposite sign. The rest particles form a stationary so-called diffusive part of the double electric layer. The charge density and SF flow rate that governs the wetting depend on the distance x to the cartilage surface, i.e., on the electric potential distribution F(x) in the diffusive part (Fig. 4.11). In the plane standing at a distance δ from the cartilage surface the SF flow rate is zero. This plane is called a sliding plane. The potential in the sliding plane F(x) = ζ.

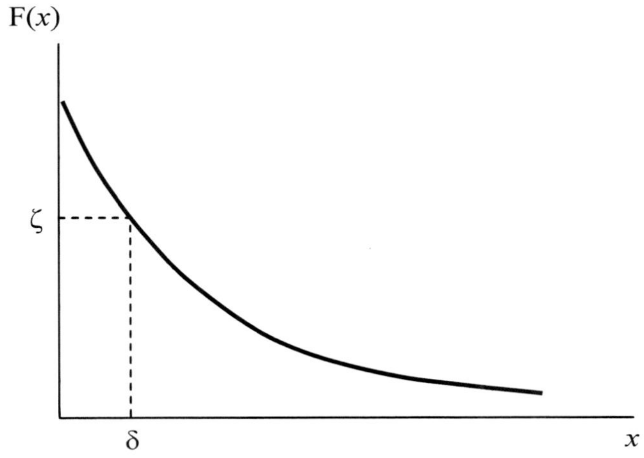

Figure 4.11. Potential distribution F(x) in double electric layer vs. distance to solid surface.

A parameter ζ (ζ-potential) is the main characteristic of electrocapillary phenomena and an indirect characteristic of wetting in the cartilage-SF system. Variations in ζ depending on pathological conditions of SF allows us to judge about the structure of the lubricating layer and degree of cartilage tissue lesion.

The contact angle is measured in the following way. A SF drop is applied with a pipette or a syringe onto a flat sample under study (cartilage, metallic, ceramic or polymer plate) that is placed on the horizontal surface of a measuring microscope. The optical axis is oriented in parallel to the sample axis. The drop is placed into a microscope's field of view and the overlap of the viewfinder lines are aligned to the contact point of three phases, namely, liquid, solid, and air. The viewfinder lines are set by turning, i.e., the first one is set in parallel to the sample surface and the second – at a tangent to the drop contour. The contact angle φ is registered by the microscope's angle measuring device.

Unfortunately, the ζ-potential of SF contacting a solid substrate is not used in laboratory clinical analysis. This is due to methodological and technological difficulties in measurement and necessity to use the expertise of specialists in biophysics, physics of condensed media and electrochemistry to interpret the results obtained.

4.6. TRIBOMETRY

Tribometry is a division of tribology dealing with methods of friction and wear testing as well as measurement techniques of the parameters of frictional interaction of solids. One of its objectives is to valuate the lubricity as a property of a lubricant to reduce wear and frictional force. SF serves a lubricant that reduces joint friction, cartilage wear, and lesions of their friction surfaces. Below, SF tribometry methods are considered.

4.6.1. Methodology of Tribometry

Current views on the biomechanics of synovial joints have shaped as the result of experimental studies of friction in joints obtained mainly by means of conventional friction machines with rotational or reciprocating motion [46] as well as pendulum friction devices which are more adequate in terms of simulation of biophysical interactions in joints. Conventional methods make it possible to study tribological characteristics of cartilage under friction against any solid counterbody and evaluate the lubricity of any lubricants at different parameters of dynamic contact which varies in shape and overlapping area.

The geometry of friction surfaces is the main characteristic of triboengineering test machines that governs contact loads.

The following types of tribometers can be distinguished using this criterion. Tribometers having a specified easily controllable geometric contact area are the most widely spread ones. The diagrams of the sample-counterbody contact in the machines of this type are shown in Fig. 4.12. Figures *a* and *b* show plate to plate schemes with reciprocal and rotating motion and figures *c* and *d* demonstrate a rotating shaft – sliding bearing (one or two) scheme. The diagram *d* is traditionally called a shaft–conformable block. In these friction diagrams the nominal pressure onto the support projection can reach 80–100 MPa.

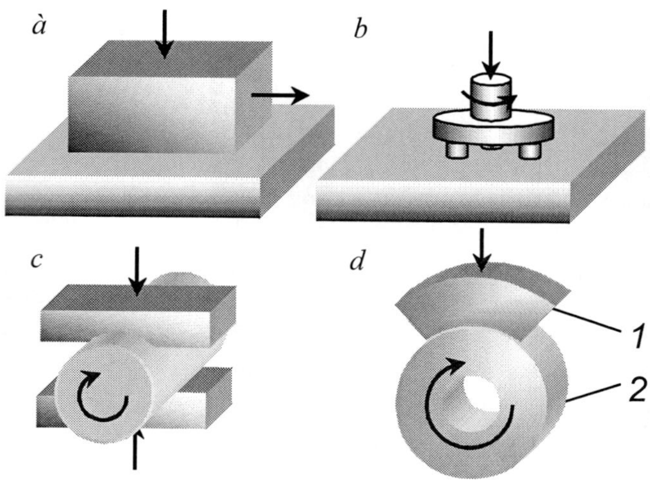

Figure 4.12. Diagrams of friction units of tribometers with a specified geometric contact area. 1 – specimen, 2 – counterbody.

Other contact schemes of samples in test machines are conditionally called “linear contact” and “point contact”.

The linear contact of friction surfaces (Fig.4.13) is provided in cylinder–on–plate (*a*), cylinder–on–cylinder element (*b*), and flexible cylindrical wire–on–cylinder (*c*) schemes. In these cases the contact occurs on the friction surface of an insignificant width that depends on elastic deformations of specimen and counterbody. During the specimen wear, the contact area will increase and can be determined by wear traces on the stationary counterbody. Maximum pressure at the contact of working elements can reach 1000−1500 MPa.

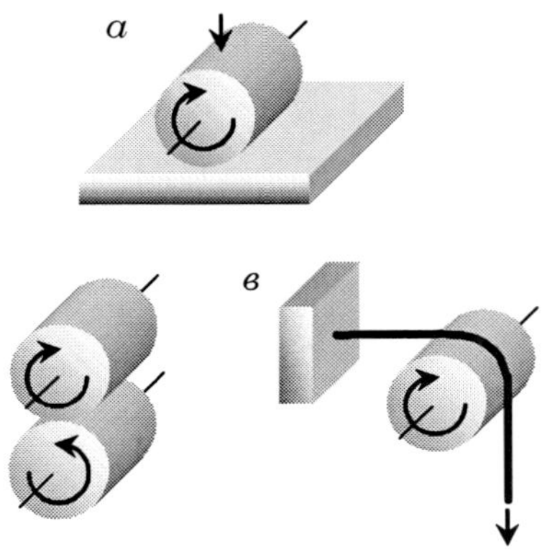

Figure 4.13. Diagrams of friction assemblies of the tribometers implementing the linear contact.

The point contact occurs (Fig. 4.14) during the contact of specimen and counterbody in the form of a pair of cylinders with mutually perpendicular axes (*a*), cone and cylinder - one or several (*c*), sphere and plate (*d*), and sphere with three spheres (*e*).

This contact can be encountered in rolling bearings. Maximum pressure in the contact of friction pairs can reach 5000 MPa.

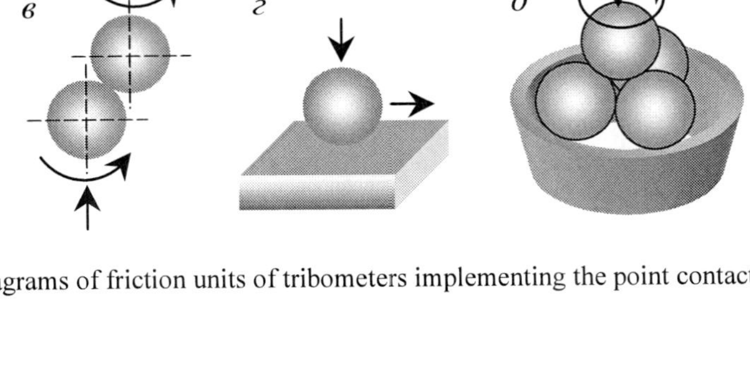

Figure 4.14. Diagrams of friction units of tribometers implementing the point contact of friction surfaces.

SF functions as a lubricant whose efficiency is determined in tribotesting by the following criteria:

- friction losses found by the values of friction torque, frictional force, or coefficient of friction;
- either the load under which the critical state of the friction pair occurs (seizure or scoring) or an ultimately permissible frictional force and temperature.

The higher the load under which one of the above-mentioned critical states occur the better protection of the friction surface against damages is ensured by the lubricating layer. A critical temperature characterizes the resistance of a lubricant to breakdown under constant loads and sliding velocities. In comparative tests the quality of the lubricant is assessed by the temperature of the lubricating layer.

The wear of specimens and breakdown of their friction surfaces occurs once the lubricating layer is broken down and a direct contact of the friction surface microasperities arises. In partial breakdown of the lubricating layer the parts are worn gradually and in complete breakdown the catastrophic wear, seizure, and scoring take place. For simulation of damages of the first kind the tests are carried out under comparatively low loads, velocities, and temperatures. The second kind of damages is simulated by testing under stepwise increase of the loading parameters mentioned above.

4.6.2. General-Purpose Tribometers

Commercially manufactured machines and instruments to study friction of solids allow evaluation of the lubricity of liquid media.

An Almen-Viland machine comprises a steel spindle 6.35 mm in diameter rotating at a frequency of 600 min^{-1} (0.2 m/s) to which two bearings made of soft steel or bronze are pressed under loading (Fig. 4.12, *c*). A hydraulic or mechanical device is used to provide loading by increasing it by 500 N every 30 seconds up to ultimate 20 kN. The spindle rotation is actuated by a drive called a motor-weighing and by its stator rotation angle a friction torque is determined. A sharp increase in the friction torque is characterized by seizure which can cause the failure of a safety pin. The quality of the lubricant is evaluated by critical friction torque.

A *rotating ring – conformable block* instrument comprises a specimen in the form of bushing *1*, mating counterbody ring *2* which is immersed in lubricant *3* found in chamber *4* (Fig. 4.15). The ring is mounted to the spindle of synchronic electric motor *5* which is also located in the chamber. Bushing *1* is pressed to the roller with lever *6*. The force acting on the lever is produced by adjustable spring *7*. Spring adjustment system *8* is found outside the chamber.

Chamber *4* is filled with gas with valve *9* and the pressure is checked with manometer *10*. Gauge *11* serves to continuously record the specimen wear. The friction torque is found by the current consumed by the motor. The temperature of the block, ring, and lubricant is measured with thermocouple *12*. In testing, friction units can be observed through a transparent cover of the chamber.

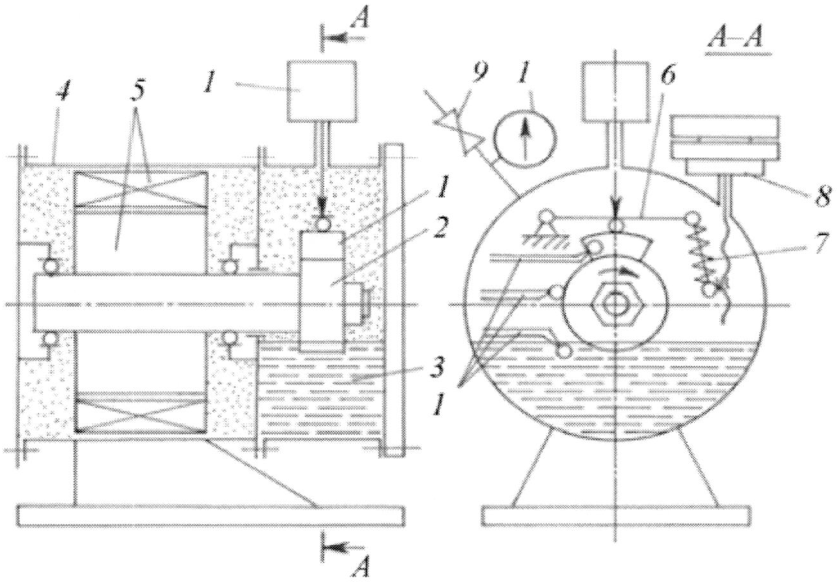

Figure 4.15. Rotating ring – conformable block assembly.

A reciprocal friction machine is provided with a friction unit presented in Fig. 4.12 *a*. Its diagram is shown in Fig. 4.16. Slider *1* is actuated with a crank mechanism and moves to the left and to the right. Counterbody *2* is mounted to steel platform *3* isolated from the slider with plate *4* made of asbestos cement. Heating device *5*, installed between the platform and the plate allows heating of the counterbody that carries the layer of the material in question up to a specified temperature. Specimen *6* is fixed in the cage of measuring unit *7* to provide a continuous specimen–counterbody contact area within a motion cycle. The specimens are loaded with lever *8*.

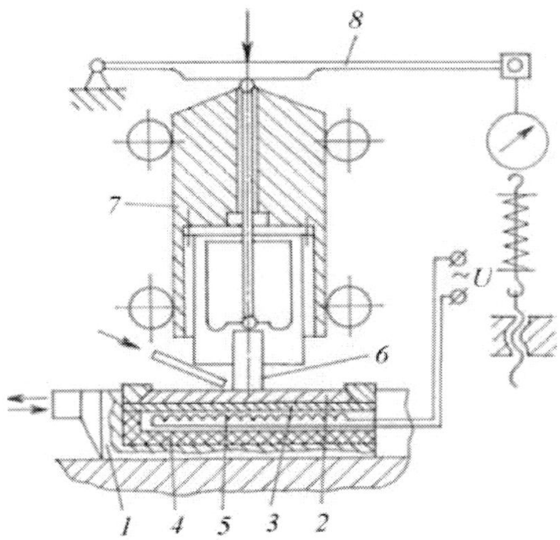

Figure 4.16. Reciprocal friction machine.

The frequency of counterbody movements can be regulated within 260 per min. The contact area is 0.8 cm^2. A micrometric dosing apparatus supplies a lubricant to the counterbody by a few drops per minute.

During the tests, the frictional force and its variation on counterbody length, temperature of the counterbody in the vicinity of its contact with the specimen, and frequency of its motion are recorded. Before testing, the specimen is run-in under stepwise loading. The load increases from 300 N in a stepwise manner by 160 N. Transition from one load stage to another takes place after the temperature stabilization in the contact zone. Critical seizure load and temperature at which it occurs are the criteria for estimating antiscoring properties of lubricants.

A Falex test machine comprises a friction assembly as shown in Fig. 4.12 *c*. It consists of a steel spindle 6.35 mm in diameter and hardness ~ HB. The spindle rotates at a constant frequency of 290 min^{-1} (0.1 m/s). The contact of the friction surfaces of block and spindle forms a linear contact. A lubricant in question is tested. The temperature of the lubricant can vary from room value to 200 °C with a heating system. Stepwise loading within18 kN is used. The breakdown of a pin that connects the working spindle with the drive spindle is the criterion for ultimate efficiency of the lubricant at a determined loading stage.

A Timken machine has a friction assembly consisting of a rotating ring 49.2 mm in diameter with two flat specimens pressed to it (Fig. 4.13, *a*). The sliding velocity is within 18 m/s and maximum load is within 570 MPa. The specimen temperature is regulated with a heater up to 270 °C. During the tests the friction force is registered. A special electronic system provided with a display is used to measure a linear wear at an accuracy of up to 2.5 μm.

A SAE machine corresponds to Fig. 4.13 *b*. Its friction assembly consists of two cylindrical rollers secured to spindles located one beneath another. The rollers rotate at different velocities and the ratio of their velocities is 14.6:1. The lubricant in question is placed in a bath wherein the lower roller is in part immersed. The upper roller is lubricated only in contact with the lower roller. A load between 0 and 1800 N is imparted to the lower roller with a lever. The pressure to roller contact can reach 2000 MPa. The tests are carried out by increasing load up to a value at which seizure occurs that can be detected visually on the friction surface of the upper roller. A disadvantage of the machine is the absence of systems to measure friction torque and wear of rollers as well subjective assessment of the onset of seizure by damages of the friction surface.

The contact scheme of the specimens as used in the SAE machine is implemented in friction machines MI-1, SMTs-2, and 2070 SMT-1 developed and manufactured in Russia.

A ChMT-1 four-ball machine corresponds to the scheme shown in Fig. 4.14 *e*. A spindle with a chuck for driving an upper ball rotates at a frequency of 1420−1450 min^{-1}. Standard balls 12.7 mm in diameter (Russian State Standard 3722-81) with accuracy not lower than degree II made of ball bearing chromium steel are used in testing. Three lower stationary balls are fixed in the cup with a lubricant under testing. An electric heater heats the lubricant and is switched off automatically once an ultimate friction torque occurs between the balls. A method for determining the lubricity of liquids is a standardized procedure (Russian State Standard 9490-75). According to the standard, two kinds of tests are carried out: short-term tests under stepwise increase of axial load and long-term (60 min) ones under constant load. In the course of short-term tests the test duration is 10±0.2 s under each specified load. Each test under a specified load is carried out using a new portion of lubricant and new balls. After that the diameter of the wear spot is measured on each of the three lower balls and its average value is found. The tests are iterated twice under each load.

Short-term tests are intended for determination of ultimate lubricity of lubricant and its antiscoring ability. The evaluation criteria are critical load under which a wear spot diameter rises sharply on lower balls (by more than 0.1 mm); welding load that causes automatic stoppage of machine (friction torque $M \geq 1200$ N·m) or welding of the balls; scoring index – a dimensionless value found by the ball wear measurement results within the loading range from initial to welding loads by the technique outlined in Russian State Standard 9490-75. In the course of the long-term tests the wear index is determined that characterizes the effect of lubricant on the ball wear under constant loads lower than critical. An average diameter of the contact spot of the lower balls after one-hour testing is taken as the wear index.

A Falex Roxana four-ball machine is based on the same principle. A rotating ball 12.7 mm in diameter contacts three stationary balls of the same diameter made of the same material (Fig. 4.14, *e*). There are three stages of upper ball rotation – 600, 1200, and 1800 min^{-1}. The load from1 to 500 N is applied through a lever to the upper ball. The test duration is constant under each load (10 s). The temperature of the specimens and test lubricant can be regulated with a heater within 300 °C. The wear of the lower balls and friction force are registered at different loading stages.

KT-2 and MACT-1 machines are designed for determining thermal resistance of lubricants in friction and make possible tests to be conducted using six schemes (Fig. 4.17): *a* – rotating ball – three stationary balls 8 mm in diameter; *b* – rotating ball 12.7 mm in diameter – spherical flange on the ring face; *c* – rotating ball 12.7 mm in diameter – three specimens with flat faces; *d* – rotating ball – elements of three cylindrical rings; *e* – rotating conical specimen – elements of three cylindrical rings; *f* – rotating conical specimen – conical flange on the ring face.

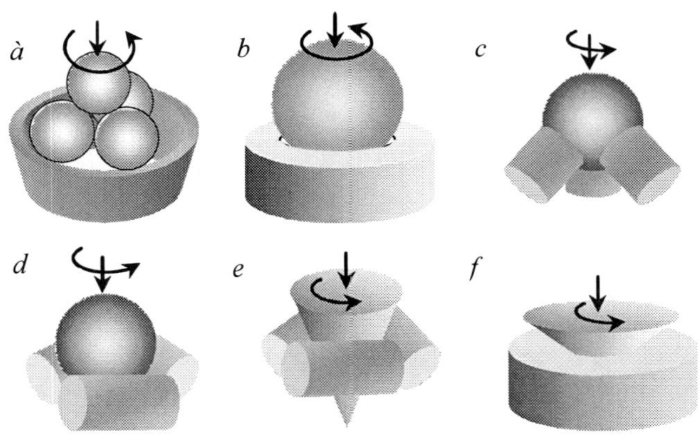

Figure 4.17. Test schemes on KT-2 and MACT-1 machines when finding thermal resistance of lubricants.

The vertical spindle of these machines rotating at a frequency of 1 min^{-1} has a chuck to hold an upper specimen (ball or cone). The upper specimen contacts stationary specimens fixed in the cap containing the test lubricant. The vertical pressing force can be 10–150 N.

The temperature of the friction assembly and lubricant layer varies within 20–300 °C and held at a specified level with an electric heater at an error ±3 °C.

The tests are carried out at constant sliding velocity, axial load and stepwise temperature elevation. The test duration is 60 s at constant temperature. The test at each new temperature is carried out using a new portion of lubricant and new specimens. The tests by schemes *b* and *f* are carried out at all temperatures with the same specimens but the lubricant is periodically replaced. During the one-minute tests the temperature in the lubricant volume and friction torque between specimens are measured. The test technique is standardized (Russian State Standard 23.221-84).

A universal friction machine (UFM-1) makes it possible to conduct tests on the areas using three schemes: rotating disc - flat cylinder face (Fig. 4.18, *a*), contact of two bushing faces (Fig. 4.18, *b*), and spindle - bushing (Fig. 4.18, *c*). The last of the three schemes provides both sliding and reciprocal wobbling motion.

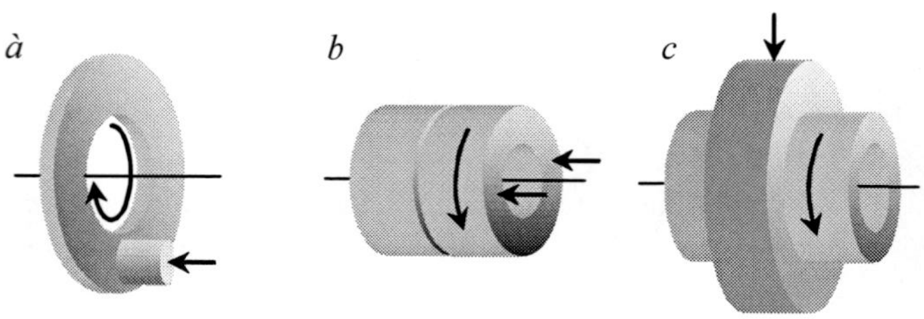

Figure 4.18. Schemes of specimen contacts performed on UFM-1 machine.

Specimens are loaded through a pneumatic system and a spindle rotation frequency is smoothly regulated. The machine is provided with devices to measure torque and heat the specimens and test lubricant within a range of 20–220 °C. The specimen wear is determined by weighing.

A standard friction machine (SFM-1) is designed for conducting tribotests using the ring-on-ring (Fig. 4.13, *b*), block-on-ring (Fig. 4.12, *d*), and shaft-bush (Fig. 4.18 *c*) geometries. The ring-in-ring scheme is used to test lubricants in sliding when one of the rings stays stationary, rolls, and rolls with slippage. Specimens are loaded through a helical loading device. During the tests rotation frequency, torque, and number of operating cycles are recorded. The specimen wear is determined by weighing and micrometering.

The tests are carried out under stepwise loading up to the breakdown of lubricating layer (seizure) or under prolonged loading at constant velocity and load to determine the wear rate of specimens in comparative tests of lubricating materials.

A SRV vibration tribometer has been developed by the Optimol-Olwerke Company. The instrument is designed to test materials at oscillating movement of the upper specimen relative to the stationary lower one using the schemes shown in Figs 4.12, 4.13, and 4.14. The specimens are placed in a chamber isolated from atmosphere, which makes it possible to conduct tests in a controllable gaseous medium. It has a device to heat the chamber up to 120 °C. A load to the specimens can vary within 120 N depending on the shape of the upper specimen the pressure on the movable contact can be from 1 to 5000 MPa. Oscillation frequency is 50 Hz and oscillation amplitude can vary from 50 to 1200 μm. In the course of testing the friction force variation is recorded. The wear is determined after testing by measuring friction traces on tghe3 specimens.

A pin-on-disk machine for face friction is designed to test lubricants by the indenter-to disk scheme (Fig. 4.12, *b*) at a sliding velocity of 0.1 m/s and under specific loads 0.2–10 MPa (Fig. 4.19).

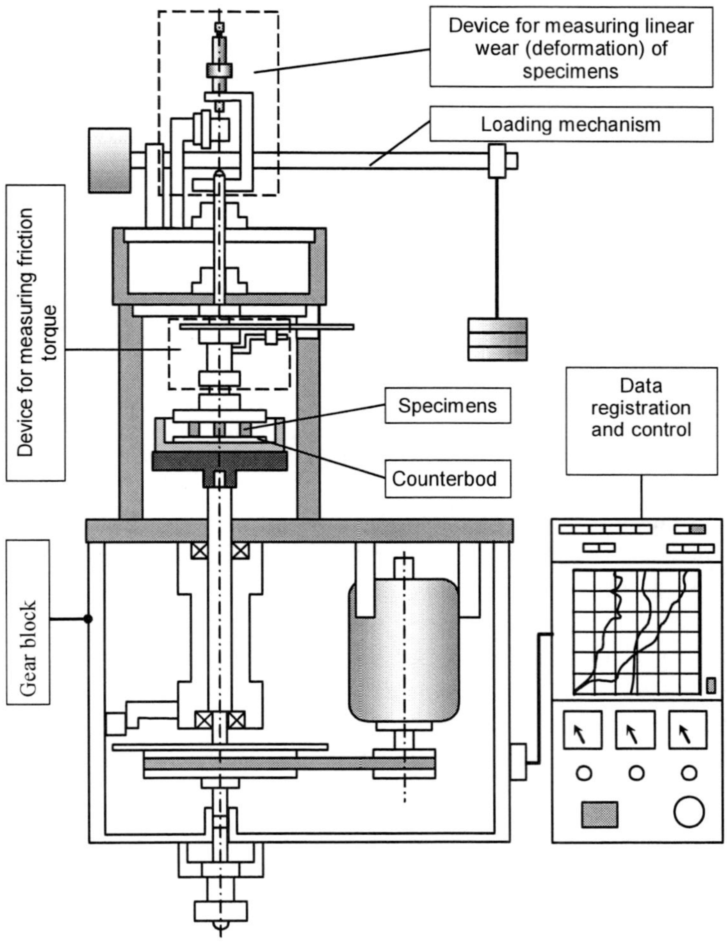

Figure 4.19. Diagram of the pin-on-disk machine for face friction.

Cartilage tissues can be used as specimens and SF or its substitutes can be used as media. The instrument is provided with an original system for determining a torque. It is equipped with inductive gauges and makes the influence of angular and vertical motions of a drive on the measurement accuracy impossible The block of data registration provides automatic recording of friction force, deformation of cartilage specimens, and sliding velocities.

A sloping tester for measuring small coefficients of friction in sliding and rolling (Fig. 3.20) has been developed in Russia [47].

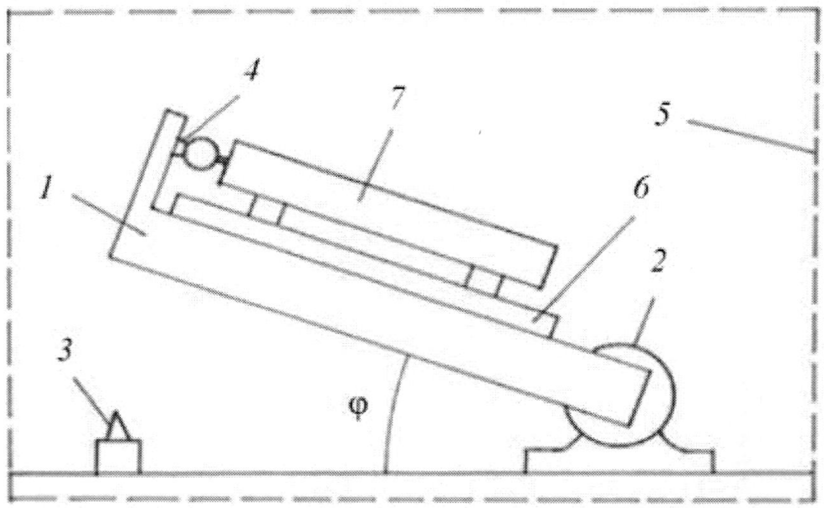

Figure 4.20. Sloping tester for measuring small coefficients of friction.

The tester consists of platform *1* equipped with drive *2* (motor with reducer) to provide rotation around horizontal axis, time measuring device, automatic recorder of start moment, and stoppage means *4*. The tester is placed into thermal chamber 5 to perform studies at regulated temperatures. A high-precision mechanism for determining coefficient of friction comprises a time measuring device to record the period of time between the moments of the onset of platform slope angle changes and the start of specimen movement on it. Substrate 6 is attached to platform *1* on which carrier *7* with three specimens *8* is set. The specimens can be cut from the tissues of synovial joints. Substrate 6 is made of glass, quartz, or Johansson plates are used. Drive 2 brings platform 1 into rotation at angular velocity ω. Measurement of angle φ between the horizontal and platform 1 plane, once the specimens start moving on it, is reduced to measuring the period of time at the moment of start τ between the start of platform turning and start of specimen movement $\varphi = \omega\ \tau$.

At the moment of initiation of platform rotation the time measuring device is switched on with start recorder *3*. As the specimens move, the circuit of feeding of the time measuring device is automatically broken with stoppage device *4*. The stopwatch (electric seconds counter) records the time at an accuracy of 10^{-2}, and the angular velocity of platform rotation with the reducer can be decreased down to $\omega = 10^{-3}$ rad/s, therefore, the setup makes it possible to measure small φ with high accuracy and determine small coefficients of friction:

$$\mu = tg(\omega\tau)$$

Different modifications of the devices [48, 49] differ by the accuracy measurement of angle φ and coefficient of friction.

4.6.3. Pendulum Tribometers

General-purpose tribometers inadequately simulate friction processes that occur in natural joints since a counterbody differs greatly from the cartilage in these test schemes. This, in turn, does not fully take account of the evaluation of SF lubricity in joints.

Beginning from the 1930s, pendulum friction machines are believed to be the best means for simulating friction in joints. First, cyclic pendulum motions are similar to cyclic motion of human and animal joints. Second, kinetics of pendulum damping allows us to judge about lubrication mechanisms in the pendulum support [50]. Third, measurement errors made during pendulum tribometer operation are minimal since the instrument has only one (under study) friction pair [51]. Pendulum tribometers are divided into three types: gravitation pendulum, frictiometers, and arthrotripsometers. The frictiometer, a pendulum with a spring load, and the arthrotripsometer, a pendulum with a motor [52], are not used in medical practice. Therefore, the main attention is given to the first type of pendulums. The gravitation pendulum or Stenton pendulum (after the name of British physicist T. Stenton) contains a friction unit in the its support. Kinetic dependences of pendulum amplitude carrying the data on friction mechanisms in the support are recorded. Fundamental findings concerning friction and lubrication of fluids have been obtained using this method [53, 54]. The method of sloping pendulum turned out to be very sensitive when studying lubrication. Its oscillation plane from the vertical line is achieved through the pendulum contact with the counterbody sloped surface on which lubricants are placed [54].

As mentioned in 1.3, the kinetics of pendulum oscillation damping might have either linear or exponential character depending on the thickness of lubricating layer. The linear dependence is characteristic of Coulomb friction (dry friction of smooth surfaces) and of friction under boundary lubrication. The exponential dependence is characteristic of viscous friction at which viscoplastic properties of rubbing materials are displayed. The exponent index equals the ratio R_0/R_m of radii of pendulum prism rounding (R_0) and the distance from the hanging point to the center of pendulum mass (R_m) [55].

The basic model of pendulum tribometer designed for studying friction in joints is described in work [56]. The setup comprises the elements for joint fixation, pendulum mechanism, and oscillation recorder. The lubricity of SF and its substitutes is judged by the time of oscillation damping or by slope angle of the time dependence of oscillation amplitude. As a rule, mechanical oscillations of pendulum are transformed into analogous electric signal and by its amplitude the lubricity of a fluid in question is assessed [52]. Unfortunately, the method is insufficiently accurate and impedes the automation of the study process. This shortcoming is eliminated by means of an optical device. The cross section of the light beam is measured with a wedge-shaped diaphragm set on the pendulum normally to the beam. The photo element current to which the beam is directed varies proportionally to beam section.

This principle of oscillation amplitude recording is used in an integral counting pendulum tribometer [57, 58]. It comprises the blocks for recording analogous electric signal and its transformation with a logic element into the pack of impulses that comes to the microprocessor. The latter determines variations of oscillation amplitudes in time and the coefficient of friction in the pendulum support. The instrument is adapted to study friction in natural dissected joints [59].

Human and animal joints operate in the natural biophysical field of a living organism. To simulate it, the pendulum support unit is equipped with an inductor connected to an external electric source [60]. Study of SF lubricity with this device has made it possible to set that healthy SF is susceptible to the effect of electromagnetic field [61], which is discussed in more detail in 4.6.4.

Pendulum devices that allow friction to be studied directly in the joints of living organisms are referred to a specific kind of tribometers [50, 62]. This group includes the apparatuses with controllable operation regime intended for training joints during rehabilitation period [63, 64].

4.6.4. Tribology of Synovia and Drugs

The lubricity of SF and drugs injected into the joint cavity has been assessed with a pendulum tribometer whose support simulates a joint endoprosthesis and is provided with an electromagnetic coil that simulates the biophysical filed in the joint [60].

The pendulum support is made of the ultra-high molecular weight polyethylene certified for orthopedic applications. It is shaped as a round plate on which a semi-spherical groove is diametrically applied d = 5 mm. A pendulum-carrying triangle prism made of stainless steel contacts the support dynamically. The supporting edge of the prism is rounded to a radius r = 2.5 mm and is conjugated with a groove. The pendulum mass is 2 kg and the sliding velocity on the support is 1 m/s. The lubricants were placed in the groove and the coefficient of friction in the pendulum support was recorded depending on the duration of the action on the lubricating layer of the electromagnetic field under voltage N = 1.2 kA/m. This SF test technique was first proposed in work [61].

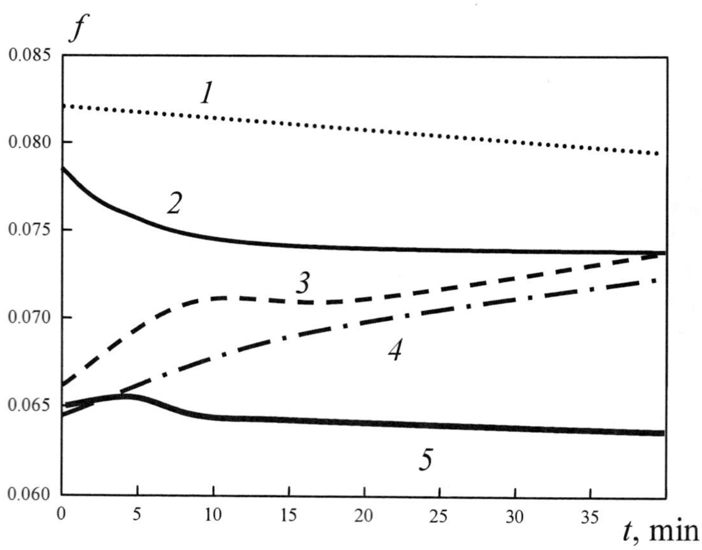

Figure 4.21. Coefficient of friction (f) versus duration (t) of exposure to electromagnetic field of the pendulum tribometer support under lubrication with SF taken from: *1* – acute synovitis joint; *2* – degenerative-dystrophic joint; *3* – Bekhterev's disease joint; *4* – rheumatoid arthritis joint; *5* – joint devoid of pathology.

Figure 4.21 presents the plots of coefficient of friction f in the pendulum support versus duration of field exposure of the lubricating layers of SF taken from knee joints with different pathologies. The studied SF samples give the following row according to the initial coefficient of friction f_0 that are found in the absence of the field: conventionally healthy and rheumatoid arthritis (0.065) < Bekhterev's disease (0.067) < degenerative-dystrophic process (0.078) < acute inflammation of non-immune genesis. Under the action of the field initial f either does not vary or may increase or decrease with time depending on SF kind. To explain the mechanisms by which electromagnetic field influences SF lubricity, the findings of synovia structure investigation by microscopy (4.1.2) and electret-thermal analysis (4.7.2) were used.

The spatial structure of hyaluronic acid (HUA) associates and proteins as well as liquid-crystal fractions of cholesterol is initially ordered and balanced in the synovia sample taken from a conventionally healthy joint (curve *5*). Apparently, this is the reason why the field does not have a significant effect on the structure and lubricity of healthy SF under the studied friction conditions. The findings of works [61, 65] indicate a possible decrease in f with increasing field voltage and duration of its effect on the lubricating layer of healthy SF.

Joint inflammations of non-immune nature (curves *1* and *2*) lead to variations in the ratio of HUA and proteins in the synovia complex compounds. The amount of HUA decreases and its molecules become shorter while the amount of protein essentially increases (up to 36 g/l) but its molecular structure remains unchanged. Part of protein macromolecules is associated into the HUA-protein complexes and the dissociated excessive macromolecules and molecules of cholesterol derivatives form permolecular structures. They are apparently susceptible to the field exposure, which causes an insignificant (within 0.002−0.004) decrease in the coefficient of friction. The physicochemical mechanism of the triboeffect needs to be further understood.

Inflammations of immune genesis are also accompanied by decreasing concentration of HUA in SF and increasing whole protein [66]. However, in these diseases, pathological conformations prevail among protein macromolecules of synovia. They together with HUA form the structures atypical of a healthy synovia. It can be conceived that agglomerates of the pathologically modified proteins form a lubricating film wherein the concentration of cholesterol ethers as well as normal HUA-protein associates is small and does not provide an expedient lubricity. The lubricity of SF of the aforesaid structure is much lower than that of a healthy synovia, deteriorates with the duration to field exposure, and results in increasing friction in the pair under investigation (curves *3* and *4*).

The reported results indicate, first, that SF tribometry is a high-informative means to assess a functional insufficiency of the synovial medium of joints [8] and, second, confirm the ideas that the electromagnetic field while affecting the SF lubricity in the absence of immune pathology normalizes the synovial medium of joints [7].

Presently, intra-articular injections of drugs are considered as the most efficient methods of treatment in orthopedics. The choice of a drug depends on the treatment objective. For instance, in treatment of synovitis antibacterial and anti-inflammatory corticosteroid-based drugs are used. In order to diminish the progressive destruction of the cartilage in degenerative-dystrophic disorders the protective SF substitutes are used that perform the functions of a lubricant similarly to natural SF (see 5.3.2). The achievements of modern pharmacology allow drugs for orthopedic treatment to be chosen individually [67]. The drugs injected into the joint cavity have a curative effect on the synovial medium and if mixed with

SF alter its biomechanical properties. The drugs of the same pharmacological group with a similar action mechanism can have a different effect on the friction in joints. However, presently, the drugs are not evaluated from the tribological point of view [68, 69]. The data of this kind are unavailable in the literature on laboratory medical analyses [70]. Nevertheless, a possible combination of two medicinal factors, namely, anti-inflammatory and tribological, makes it possible to provide the tribometering of the drugs to be injected. The experiment was first performed with a pendulum tribometer equipped with an electromagnetic field source [71].

The drugs tested are shown in Table 4.4.

Table 4.4. Drugs chosen for testing

Drug	Composition	Manufacturer	Therapeutic effect
Hydrocortisone	Hydrocortisone acetate 125 mg, lidocaine hydrochloride 25 mg	Gedeon Richter A.O. (Hungary)	Anti-inflammatory
Kenalog-40	Triamcynolonacetonide 40 mg, benzyl alcohol 9.9 mg	Bristol-Myers Squibb SpA (Italy)	Anti-inflammatory
Diprospan	Betamethasone dipropyonate 6.43 ммg, betamethasone sodium phosphate 2.63 mg	Schering-Plough (Germany)	Anti-inflammatory
Lincomycin hydrochloride	30 % solution of lincomycin hydrochloride	Borisov drug factory (Belarus)	Anti-bacterial
Synvisc	Hylan A and B (8.0 mg in 1 ml)	Biomatrix, Inc. (США)	SF substitute
Hyalart	Hyaluronic acid, 0.9 % solution of sodium chloride 2 ml	Bayer AG. (Germany)	SF substitute
Diasynol	1.5 % solution of sodium carboxymethylcellulose 1 % solution of Tekon-20, 0.9% solution of sodium chloride	Belbiopharm state concern on production and sales of pharmaceutical and microbiological products (Belarus)	SF substitute

The plots of the coefficient of friction in the pendulum support lubricated with the drugs in question versus the duration of the action of electromagnetic field are shown in Fig. 4.22.

Visual evaluation of wetting and colloid stability of lubricating fluids placed in the groove of the support plate indicates essential distinctions in their physicochemical characteristics. Synvisc is a viscous jelly-like substance that poorly spreads over the support in friction. Even after unloading the drug is spread uniformly on the groove surface. Hyalart has a more liquid consistency and wets uniformly the friction surface of the hydrophobic support thus providing favorable conditions for pendulum prism slippery. This agrees with the opinion [72] that the clinical curative effect of Sinvisc is due to its viscoelastic properties that prevent the cartilage from peak mechanical loads with further improvement in the functioning of an injured joint owing to SF production rather than better slip conditions in the joint.

Steroid drugs (Kenalog-40, Diprospan, hydrocortisone) having a pronounced anti-inflammatory effect deteriorate the friction significantly when introduced into the support. Lamination of the suspensions of these drugs occurs once they are taken out of ampoules. These steroid drugs form the following series according to increasing time needed to form a crystalline sediment in drop drying: hydrocortisone < Kenalog < Diprospan. Hydrocortisone and Kenalog demonstrate the highest *f*, rapid phase lamination, fallout of the crystalline sediment on the friction surface and forcing out of the liquid phase from the groove at prism oscillations. After that, the lubricating layer in the tribometer support consists mostly of the crystalline phase that acts as an abrasive. Therefore, Kenalog and hydrocortisone are characterized by significant deviations of current *f* from the average values (within 0.04). These are due to impossibility to provide a constant ratio of the crystalline and liquid phases in the lubricating layer found in the friction zone decease of their rapid lamination. Diprospan is a suspension of finer particles whose precipitation rate is much lower than that of the outlined drugs, which causes its satisfactory lubricity.

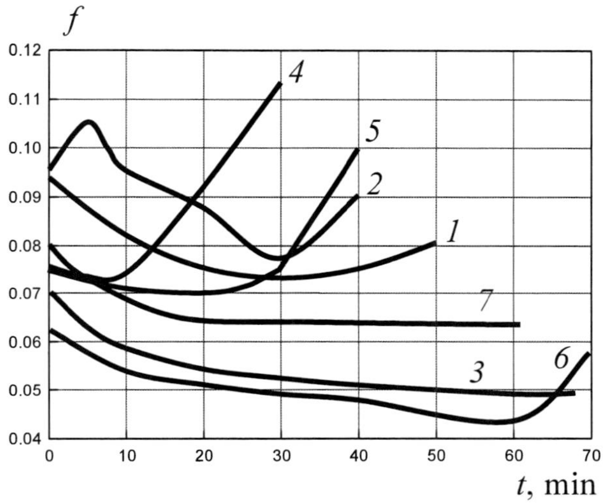

Figure 4.22. Coefficient of friction (*f*) vs. exposure time (*t*) lubricating drug layers to the field in the support of pendulum tribometer: *1* – hydrocortisone; *2* – Kenalog-40; *3* – Diprospan; *4* – lincomycin hydrochloride; *5* – Synvisc; *6* – Hyalart; *7* – Diasynol.

Lincomycin hydrochloride used for treatment of bacteria-induced inflammations is a saline solution which easily crystallizes during friction in air. One can assume that when mixed with SF this drug does not exert an abrasive effect on the cartilage since it does not contain water-insoluble components and easily invades through the synovial membrane into the bloodstream.

Comparison of initial f_0 characteristic of these drugs and SF (Fig. 4.21) highlights the following conclusions. The lubrication of the tribometer support with Diprospan, Lincomycin, and Synvisc corresponds to chronic synovitis ($f_0 \sim 0.07–0.08$). The coefficients of friction characteristic of Kenalog and hydrocortisone are higher than those of the SF modified maximally in acute synovitis ($f_0 > 0.08$). Only Hyalart has the same coefficient of friction as healthy SF ($f_0 \sim 0.06$).

Under the action of the electromagnetic field the lubricity of drugs varies essentially. Hyalart not only favors the normalization of tribological processes once it is injected into the joint but also noticeably improves them under the action of the field (Fig. 4.22, curve *6*). The similar regularity is characteristic of healthy SF (Fig. 4.21, curve *5*). As for steroid anti-inflammatory drugs, Diprospan demonstrates the highest susceptibility to the field (3). It also has the lowest in this group initial f_0 that noticeably drops under field exposure. Statistical processing of the test results of Hyalart and Diprospan confirms the effect of the field on decreasing f in Hyalart and Diprospan with a reliability of 95.5%.

Therefore, despite the same pharmacological group, each of the studied drugs displays individual tribological behavior. The method of pendulum tribometer provided with an electromagnetic field source to test the drugs turns out to be efficient for express evaluation of the drugs to be injected in joints [73]. Other conditions being equal, the choice of the drug that provides the least coefficient of friction seems to be expedient.

A diagram in the form of superposed tribological series of the drugs and SF (Fig. 4.23) reported elsewhere [6] is convenient to make primary estimates of drug lubricity in a pathologically altered joint. The ordinates of the hatched areas correspond to the confidence intervals at a risk of error 0.05. The size of these regions on the x-axis has been chosen arbitrarily.

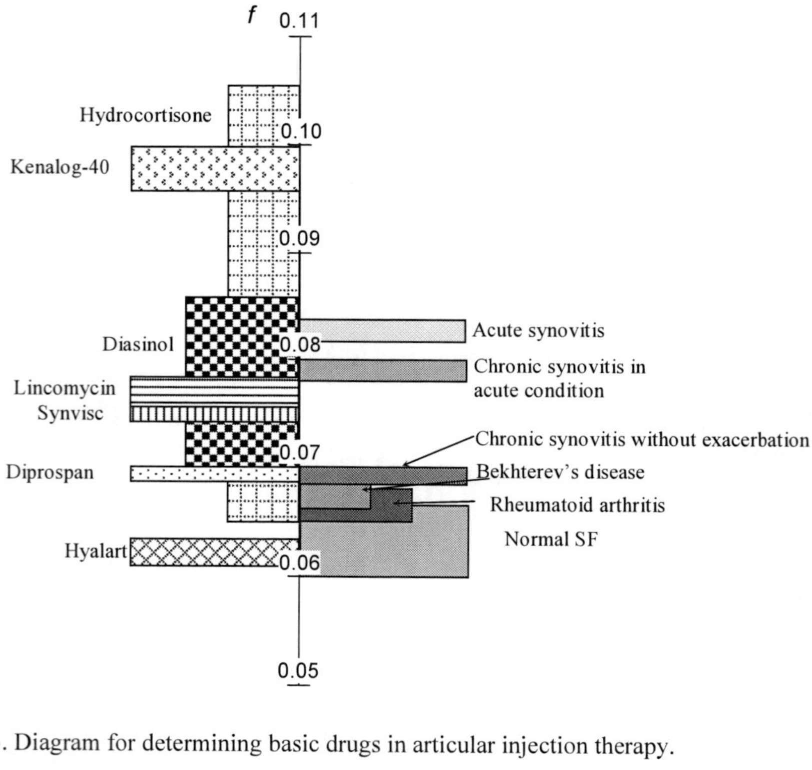

Figure 4.23. Diagram for determining basic drugs in articular injection therapy.

It is preferable to choose a drug whose coefficient of friction f_0 measured before exposure to the field is equal or lower than f_0 of the pathologic synovia. Therefore, it is recommended to use steroid anti-inflammatory drugs demonstrating broad variations in f because of the suspension delamination if an alternative medication is absent. The abrasive effect of delaminating drugs can be weakened by observing a mild orthopedic regime (immobilization, restricted load to the joint, etc.) during which the crystalline phase completely dissolves and the drug starts to exert a therapeutic effect. If f_0 of the drug C > f_0 of SF, it is worthwhile to estimate the dynamics of reduction in the coefficient of friction of the drug when an electromagnetic field acts on the lubricating layer. If the minimal coefficient of friction reaches f_0 of patient's SF the injection of this drug is recommended in combination with magnetic therapy. The test allows assessment of possibilities of structural recovery of pathologically altered SF by way of magnetic therapy. Once biomechanical resources of synovia are exhausted, which is seen in increasing f and insensitivity to electromagnetic effects, local articular therapy of joint with SF substitutes is desirable.

4.7. Electret-Thermal Analysis

Synovia performs its functions in the joint owing to its specific biochemical composition (proteins, polysaccharides, hyaluronates, liquid-crystal compounds of cholesterol, etc.) and hierarchically ordered spatial arrangement of its viscous colloid system. In joint disorders the cellular and biochemical parameters of SF vary, which is used for orthopedic diagnostics (see 4.2 and 4.4). However, they allow indirect estimation of deviations of the SF structure from the normal condition under which a satisfactory functioning of joints is ensured. In order to properly assess functional resources of SF, the data are required on the volume structure of the components of its complex compounds including bound water, ions and liquid-crystalline formations; intensity and density of the chemical bonds between them; and the hierarchic structure of larger molecular aggregates in SF that demonstrate the signs of long-range order. In principle, these parameters can be determined when performing complex investigation of synovia with application of fluid analyzers, i.e., optical (absorption, luminescent, polarization, etc.), electrochemical (potentiometric, voltammetric, coulometering, etc.), thermal (thermochemical, thermogravimetrical, distillation, etc.), chromatographic, magnetic, radioisotope, mass-spectrometric [74] methods, as well as X-ray diffraction analysis, electronography and neutronography. Unfortunately, these studies cannot be conducted in clinical conditions.

Electret-thermal analysis (ETA) has emerged in the physics of dielectrics to determine the mechanisms and parameters of electric polarization of solids [75]. It is used to study electrets [76], that is, dielectrics that maintain energy for a long time, sources of direct electric field and electric analogs of permanent magnets. By means of ETA, the effect similar to the electret one has been revealed in biological tissues and their components, namely, collagen, polysaccharides, myoglobin and hemoglobin of the frozen human blood [75, 77]. In the 21st century ETA is used to analyze biological fluids [78]. In heating, the currents, as mentioned in 2.6, display an effect that is similar to electret (quasi-electret effect), that is, in thermal destruction of chemical bonds between the fragments of biological fluid structure they move in the external electric field like free charge carriers (electrons and protons) that release in electret heating.

4.7.1. ETA Technique

The ETA technique or thermostimulated depolarization consists in recording the thermostimulated currents (TSC) generated in heating of a dielectric sample that is placed between a pair of electrodes (one of which is grounded) and contacts them. The specimen heating leads to relaxation of the charges "frozen" in the electret. Free charge carriers move within the specimen to the electrodes under the action of the electret field and a current arises in the external circuit that connects the electrodes. The temperature dependence of current is presented by a TSC spectrum that carries information on the mechanisms responsible for the appearance of the electret effect.

The diagram of a device for measuring TSC of biological fluids suggested in work [78] is shown in Fig. 4.24. Fluid drop *1* is placed in hollow *2* in the lower electrode. Dielectric gasket 3 (annealed Teflon film with zero proper TSC) brought in contact with the specimen and is covered with other electrode *4*. This measuring cell is compressed with a calibrated force and placed in dismountable electromagnetic screen *5*. The lower electrode and the screen are grounded. The cell is heated at a constant rate. The thermostimulated current signal arising in the cell is delivered with transducer-amplifier *6* to personal computer *7* with special software. The TSC spectrum is recorded.

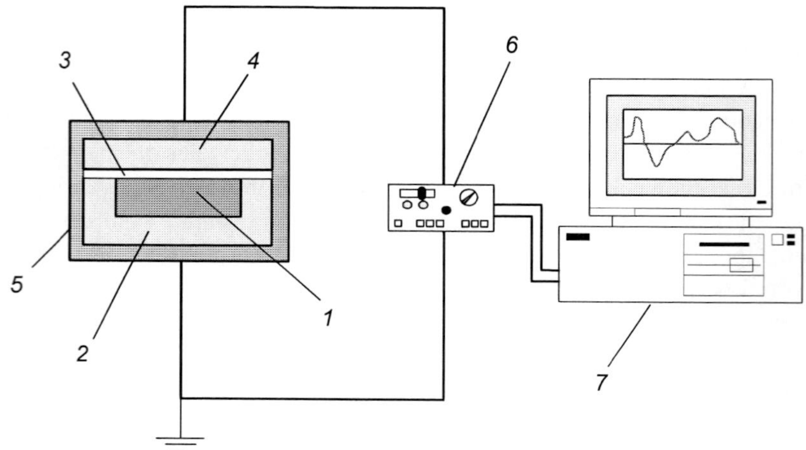

Figure 4.24. Diagram of recording of TSC of biological fluids: 1- sample, 2 and 4 – lower and upper electrodes, 3 – dielectric film; 5 – electromagnetic screen, 6 – amplifier; 7 – PC with special software.

This schematic has been improved [79] in order to reduce "the noise" of the heating system in the measuring cell and provide digital filtration of signals by statistical methods.

Recording of TSC in liquid-phase samples encounters methodic problems due to fluid spreading over the electrode surface. Uncontrollable spreading is responsible for instability of measurements and short circuit of the electrodes that can occur sometimes even when using dielectric films whose area is larger than that of the electrodes. With availability of high-resistance films in the cell, the current signals are of 10^{-12}A order. To record them, electromagnetic screens capable of absorbing external fields and electronic amplifiers of small currents are required, which make the devices far more complicated and expensive.

A new approach to the solution of these problems is in placement of a dielectric element between the pair of electrodes to avoid uncontrollable spreading of a liquid sample. In addition, it cannot produce the proper electric signal in the measuring cell. Dispersed silicon dioxide SiO_2 with particles sized 10–90 μm can be used in this case [80]. SiO_2 is a dielectric with a high (~1700 °C) melting temperature. Within a temperature range to be used in the investigation of biological fluids (up to 200 °C), TSC in silicon dioxide is essentially zero and does not distort the current signal from biological fluid. The latter, when applied to the monolayer of dioxide particles, wets the powder particles and does not leak out from the area occupied by the monolayer. When compressing the cell, a monolayer of solid particles arises in the gap between the electrodes, the space between which is filled with the fluid contacting both electrodes. The absence of a high-resistance dielectric film in the cell causes TSC of 10^{-4}–10^{-5}A order. Recording of such large currents is possible without any electric amplifiers and bulky screening systems. This allows improvement of resolution of the current recording and reproducibility of the measurement results.

The technique proposed makes it possible to study the physicochemical structure of SF along with other biological fluids, such as blood, lymph, pancreatic juice, exudates, etc., that comprise protein components. The method is assigned to express analysis since it allows estimation of pathogenesis and severity of different disorders using small quantities of the fluid in question without excessive time, energy and labor consumptions.

4.7.2. Thermostimulated Currents of Synovia

The SF for experimental studies is taken from patients during therapeutic and diagnostic manipulations (joint aspirations or operations). A patient's consent should be received for follow-up experimental study of this biological material.

As first reported elsewhere [81], SF not subjected to any preliminary electric treatment demonstrates TSC spectra within the 20–140 °C range. These findings are of diagnostic value since they were obtained in clinical conditions using pathologically modified joints [6]. The study results are shown in Fig. 4.25. The TSC spectra are taken following the scheme shown in Fig. 4.24. The SF samples (0.2 ml) were heated at a rate of 5 °C/min.

A conventionally healthy SF shows three peaks on TSC spectra, i.e., low-, medium-, and high temperature ones. The low-temperature peak of the negative charge relaxation corresponds to T = 35–50 °C. It is a response to the thermally stimulated destruction of coordination structures that consist of protein formations surrounded by hydrate shells. The hydrate shells result from water molecules linked to polar fragments of macromolecules by hydrogen bonds [75]. The charge relaxation activation energy that corresponds to this peak equals W = 0.25–0.45 eV, which is commensurable with hydrogen bond energy. The charge liberation going hand in hand with thermal structural recombination of SF liquid-crystals [91] based on cholesterol derivatives, occurs at the same temperature range.

The medium-temperature peak (T = 80–100 °C) of the positive peak relaxation presumably corresponds to denaturing of protein-polysaccharide compounds and permolecular formations as well as irreversible changes in tertiary and partially secondary protein structure without breaking polypeptide chains. The activation energy required to charge relaxation to fit the peak falls within W = 0.5–0.7 eV, which conforms to the activation energy of the above-mentioned processes [82].

The high-temperature peak at T = 110–120 °C is the most intensive. It is partially overlapped by the medium-temperature peak so that their set forms a dual peak and corresponds to the phase transition in the SF protein constituent to result in the solid phase. Thermooxidative destruction of protein macromolecules is accompanied by the liberation of charge carriers that are responsible for the high-temperature peak.

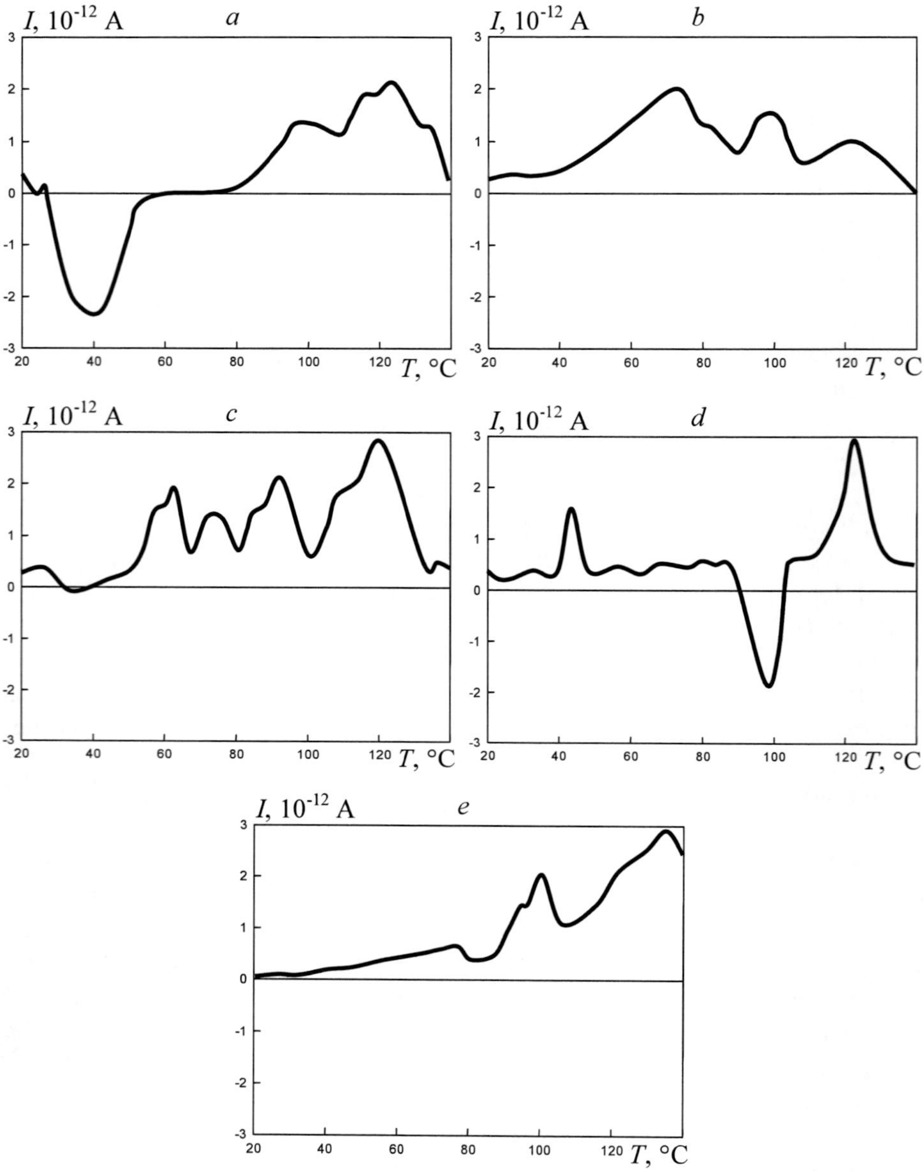

Figure 4.25. TSC spectra of SF samples taken from knee joints: *a* – conventionally healthy; *b* – degenerative-dystrophic lesion; *c* – acute inflammation; *d* – Bekhterev's disease; *e* – rheumatoid arthritis.

Degenerative-dystrophic lesions of joints (*b*) cause SF changes characterized by the disappearance of the low-temperature peak on TSC spectra and appearance of low-intensive medium- and high-temperature peaks at 75, 100, and 120 °C. Chronic joint inflammation is known [83] to be accompanied by a lower molecular weight of SF proteins. Presumably, depending on the molecular-weight distribution of degenerated macromolecules, several types of permolecular structures generate in SF, each of which fits an individual peak on the TSC spectrum. The absence of the low-temperature peak indicates that the degenerative dystrophic process in the joint has caused destruction of hydrate shells and disordering of SF liquid-crystal structures.

Acute joint inflammation gives rise to four positive current peaks on the TSC spectrum (c) within the ranges of medium (60, 70, 90 °C) and high (120 °C) temperatures. Acute synovitis is accompanied by a sharp decrease in the molecular weight of proteins and hyaluronic acid in SF. It is naturally to assume that the peaks on the TSC spectra correspond to the denaturing of four types of protein-polysaccharide compounds consisting of different-length molecules.

Bekhterev's disease is characterized by the TSC spectrum peaks within the same temperature ranges as in SF taken from a conventionally healthy joint; however, low- and medium peaks are of different polarity (*d*). This can be attributed to the fact that Bekhterev's disease initiates pathological forms of protein in SF (C-reactive protein, fibrinogen, seromucoid) with altered macromolecule conformation.

Rheumatoid arthritis can be identified using the ETA technique (*e*) by the degenerated low-temperature peak and displacement of the high-temperature peak to the region of high temperatures (140 °C). The former indicates the destruction of hydrate shells around SF polar structures and recombination of the liquid-crystal phase. An abnormally high intensity of the high-temperature peak can be caused by increased protein amount in SF including its pathological forms (see 3.2). These forms presumably form with hyaluronic acid permolecular structures that are stronger than those in healthy SF. They decay at elevated temperatures with liberation of a great amount of energy.

Thus, SF is a quasi-electret medium that demonstrates TSC spectra. Analysis of the spectra of SF taken from pathologically altered joints give the data on the density of hydrate shells around SF polar components, availability of liquid-crystal phase, relative length of protein macromolecules, and energy saturation of bonds in SF protein-polysaccharide complexes [84]. The TSC spectra can be used to properly assess structural changes in SF that govern the SF performance. The application of this simple and informative technique in clinical practice yields new qualitative data necessary to diagnose joint diseases [85].

4.8. Fluorescence

Luminescence is emission of light by some substances and excited by a source of energy (arises under the action of light, radioactive and X-ray radiations, electric field, during chemical reactions and under mechanical effects). Fluorescence is a short-time luminescence quenching during 10^{-8}–10^{-9} s once excitation has stopped. As for the mechanism of energy transformation, fluorescence is a spontaneous (self-arbitrary) luminescence. Its duration depends on the life span of the excited electron state of sample molecules.

Fluorescent analysis is the set of the quantitative analytical methods based on fluorescence of substances. Qualitative analysis is performed using the color of fluorescent radiation and quantitative analysis measures the intensity of radiation, i.e., takes a fluorescence spectrum. To record the fluorescence spectrum small amounts of a substance are required. This makes fluorescence spectroscopy advantageous over, e.g., absorption spectroscopy. Fluorescence spectra carry information on the structure of luminescence centers, i.e., molecules absorbing the excitation energy. Fluorescent analysis is used to examine the structure of substances and physical processes occurring in them. Fluorescence finds applications in microbiology, medicine, and biophysics to study fluids. By analyzing the fluorescence spectra one can obtain data on macromolecule conformation in solution, binding places, interactions with a solvent, intermolecular distances, and rotational diffusion coefficients of macromolecules.

4.8.1. Theoretical Foundations

The theory of fluorescence does not necessarily allow unambiguous correlation to be set between fluorescent characteristics of an excited molecule and the characteristics of its surrounding. Therefore, the fluorescence capacities are governed by the findings of investigation of model compounds [86].

In line with the zone theory, a molecule of any substance can only have discrete energy values. Transition of a molecule from one level of potential energy to another is a quantum transition. An elementary act of luminescence consists of energy absorption by the molecule and its transition from ground energy state *1* (Fig 4.26) to excitation state *3*, as well as nonradiative *3→2* and radiative *2→1* transitions. A probability of the *3→2* transition is commonly higher than that of the direct *3→1* transition. State *2* lies lower than absorption state *3*. If state *2* belongs to the center of luminescence the luminescence is called spontaneous, or fluorescence. During transition *2→1* part of excitation energy is lost converting to heat and the energy of light emitted is less and wavelength is longer than that of the absorbed light. If the molecule has several radiation sublevels the emitted light has different wavelengths. The fluorescence spectrum carries information on all transitions from the excited state level to each vibration level of the ground state.

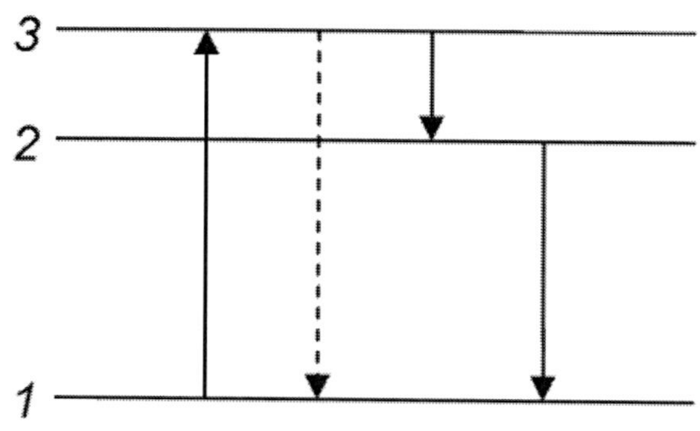

Figure 4.26. Diagram of quantum transitions for an elementary luminescence process: *1* – ground state, *2* – radiation state, *3* – excitation state.

Intensity of fluorescence is evaluated by quantum output *W*, equaling the ratio of photons emitted and those absorbed by the sample. *W* is governed by the factors that are referred to the properties of the molecules in question (internal factors) and their surrounding. Internal factors are responsible for the transformation of the energy of flexible molecules into heat. That is why fluorescent substances (fluorophores) are met rarely and their molecules almost always comprise rigid aromatic rings.

The internal factors are commonly uninteresting for biochemists dealing with the properties of macromolecules in biological fluids. The surrounding factors are of much grater significance. They are responsible for the appearance of nonradiative transitions that compete with fluorescence and decrease *W*. In biological systems, a decrease in *W* commonly results from either the collision of macromolecules accompanied by energy exchange or nonradiative (resonance) energy transfer.

4.8.2. The Measurement Scheme

Figure 4.27 illustrates a standard diagram of a spectrofluorometer – a device used to measure fluorescence.

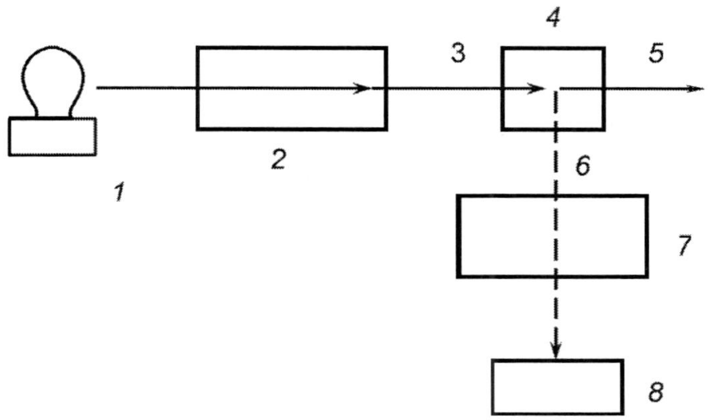

Figure 4.27. Structural diagram of spectrofluorometer: *1* – light source; *2* and *7* – monochromators of excitation and emission; *3* – exciting light; *4* – cell with a sample; *5* – bypassing light; *6* – emitted light; *8* – detector.

A light beam of high intensity moves through monochromator *2* – a device that generates a narrow interval for excitation wavelengths (a fluorescent molecule absorbs efficiently the light of this proper wavelength). After that, exciting light *3* passes through sample-containing cell *4*. Thus fluorescence is emitted by the sample equally in all directions; therefore, in order to exclude the influence of the exciting light on measurement results, fluorescence is commonly observed at a right angle to its beam. Emitted light *6* passes through second monochromator *7* to provide analysis of wavelength and reaches light-sensitive detector *8* (photoelectron multiplier). Modern instruments are equipped with scanning and recording systems to vary wavelengths of the exciting light and build the relationship between intensity of the light emitted and its wavelength.

In fluorescent analysis of macromolecules in solutions two types of fluorophores are used, namely, proper fluorescent macromolecules and those brought in the solution that are bound to the macromolecules under study [87]. They are called fluorescent marks or probes.

Proper fluorescence is demonstrated by the SF proteins that comprise three fluorophores of amino acids class – residuals of tryptophan, tyrosine, and phenylalanine (listed in order of decreasing *W*). Fluorescence of each of them can be identified by the respective excitation wavelength. Commonly, the tryptophan fluorescence is studied since phenylalanine has a low *W* and tyrosine fluorescence is frequently very weak. The main goal of studying SF proper fluorescence is to set the parameters of conformation of protein macromolecules. This is possible because the fluorescence of tryptophan and tyrosine essentially depends on macromolecule surrounding, i.e., on the composition and pH of SF saline solution, concentration of fluorescent molecules in it and their structure.

Nature not always ensures a macromolecule with fluorophores in the convenient for the researcher region. In many cases a fluorophore is introduced in the macromolecule under study by a chemical bond. Usage of such indicator groups in fluorescent analysis is called the "incorporated" fluorescence method or the method of fluorescent probes. Its applicability is limited by several demands to fluorescent molecules: 1) they must be strongly bound to a certain area of the macromolecule; 2) their fluorescence must be susceptible to surrounding conditions; 3) they must have no effect on the properties of the macromolecule in question. The observation of these criteria should be checked. The most widely spread fluorescent probes in proteins are 1-anyline-8-naphthasulfonate-anion (ANS); 1-dimethylamino naphthaline-5-sufonate-anion (DNS) and its acid chloride; dansyl chloride; 2-*n*-toluidyl naphthalene-6-sulfonate-anion (TNS); and rhodamine. Application of probe to detect the SF liquid-crystal phase is exemplified in 2.7.2.

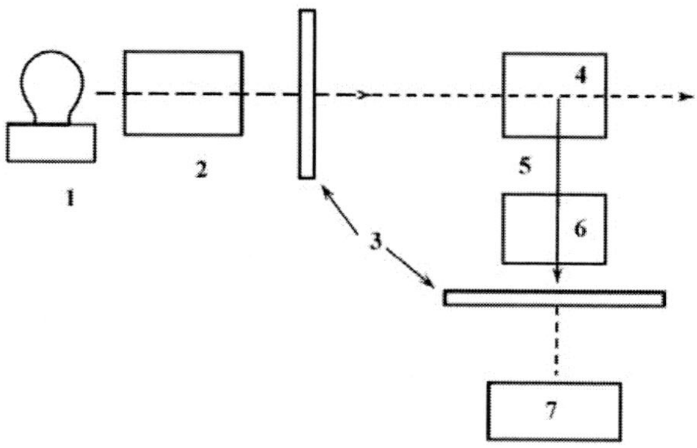

Figure 4.28. Diagram of a device for measurement of fluorescence polarization: *1* – light source, *2* and *b* – monochromators of excitation and emission, *3* – polarizer, *4* – cell with a sample, *5* – light emitted, *7* – detector.

Polarization is one of the variants of fluorescent analysis. Polarization of light is the ordering in the stress vector orientation of electric and magnetic fields in the plane perpendicular to a light beam. A polarizer is a device that produces the polarized light. The intensity of polarized light depends on the polarizer orientation, i.e., passage is maximum and polarization is zero when the plane of light polarization is parallel to the optical axis of the polarizer. In other cases partial polarization is observed. Fluorescence polarization is studied using instruments with a modified scheme of fluorescence measurement (Fig. 4.28): on the path of the exciting light a polarizer is placed to induce the light polarization with polarized light; the second polarizer whose axis is either parallel or perpendicular to the axis of the first polarizer is mounted between the sample and the detector. If the exciting light is polarized then fluorescence is either partially polarized or totally unpolarized. The degree of polarization carries information on the physical state of the emitting group of macromolecules. If the emitting group of SF protein macromolecule rotates rapidly, that is, Brownian motion takes place, and molecule orientation during the life span of its excited state varies significantly the polarization of the SF sample decreases. Depolarization of this type also depends on temperature, SF viscosity, as well as the size and shape of protein macromolecules containing the emitting group.

This makes it possible to obtain the data on SF protein macromolecules that cannot be obtained by other research methods. For instance, by variations in the SF sample polarization one can judge about the movability of not only the molecule as a whole but its parts as well. Commonly, polarization fluorescent analysis studies "incorporated" fluorophores.

ACKNOWLEDGMENTS

Methodology of studying structure and properties of SF includes the multitude of methods to address the complexity of multiphase condensed medium with the hierarchic level of its permolecular arrangement, which synovia presents. Those incorporate both the tests carried out by Hippocrates and Avicenna and novel experimental techniques borrowed from colloid chemistry, electrochemistry, physics of condensed states, and immunology. A special emphasis should be made on the method of thermostimulated current, improved tribological methods that simulate SF friction in the biofield of a natural joint, and immune diagnostics of SF, now under rejuvenation in arthrology. These techniques allow detection of liquid-crystal and quasi-electret states of SF as well as checking of biochemical equilibrium of the synovial medium of joints. Novel knowledge about physicochemical and biochemical nature of SF obtained by means of technologies of the 21st century provides prerequisites for development of up-to-date generation of means for joint treatment.

REFERENCES

[1] Bazarnyi, VV. *Synovial fluid (clinical diagnostic value of laboratory analysis).* Ekaterinburg: UGMA, 1999.

[2] Tepper, EZ; Shilkova, VK; Pereverzeva, GI. *A workshop on microbiology: a handbook for universities.* Moscow: Drofa, 2004.

[3] Kupchinov, BI; Ermakov, EF; Beloenko, ED. *Biotribology of synovial joints.* Minsk: Vedy, 1997.

[4] Muldiyarov, PYa. Scanning electron microscopy of synovial membrane and synovial fluid: a review. *Vopr. Revmat.,* 1981, N 4, 55–59.

[5] RF Patent Application 2173462 G 01N 33/48, 33/68. *Method for Testing Rehumatic Disease.* Sokolova, LA; Malchikova, LP. Publ 2001, http:www.fips.ru.

[6] Cherniakova, YuM. *Optimization of diagnostics and treatment of synovitis by controlling biophysical properties of the synovial fluid.* PhD Med Thesis, Minsk, 2006.

[7] Chernyikova, YuM; Kadolich, ZhV; Pinchuk, LS; Tsvetkova, EA; Nikolaev VI. Effect of electromagnetic field on tribological characteristics of synovial fluid. *J. Friction and Wear,* 2003, Vol 24, N 6, 636-641.

[8] Cherniakova, YuM; Kadolich, ZhV; Pinchuk, LS; Nikolaev, VI; Tsvetkova, EA; Beloenko, ED. Tribological properties of synovial fluid as a criterion of functional deficit of the lubricating medium of joint. *Dokl. NAN Belarus,* 2004, Vol 48, N 4, 75−79.

[9] *Practical scanning electron microscopy.* Ed. Goldstein, J; Yakovits, Kh. Moscow: Mir, 1978.

[10] Remizov, AN. *Medical and biological physics: a handbook for medical universities.* 3rd Ed. Moscow: Vysshaya shkola, 1999.

[11] Chirkin, AA; Okorokov, AN; Goncharik, II. *Diagnostic reference book of a physician.* Minsk: Belarus, 1994.

[12] Dawson, R; Elliot, D; Elliot, W; Jones, K. *Reference book of a biochemist.* Moscow: Mir, 1991.

[13] Klekovkina, EV; Nemtsov, BF. Mediators of immune inflammation in blood and synovial fluid in patients afflicted with osteoarthrosis and rheumatoid arthritis. *Cytokines and inflammation,* 2006, Vol 5, N 3, 55−57.

[14] Beloenko, ED; Slabozhanina, EI; Kozlova, NM; Mamontova, MV; Chernitskii, EA. Spectrophotometric investigation of synovial effucsion in differential diagnostics of pigmented villonodular synovitis. *Orthop. Traumatol. Prosth.* 1990, N 5, 32−34.

[15] Atlas of chemical laboratory procedures. Clinical Chem NJ, 1989, N 5, 235−238.

[16] Gabay, C; Kushner, I. Acute-phase proteins and other systemic responses to inflammation. *N. Engl. J. Med.* 1999, Vol 340, 448–454.

[17] Feldkamp, CS. *Immunological reactions.* In: Clinical Chemistry: Theory, Analysis, Correlation. Ed. Kaplan, L; Pesce, A; Kazmierzak, S. Berlin: Springer, 2003, 216−245.

[18] *Rheumatic diseases.* Ed. Nasonov, VA. Moscow: Medicine, 1997.

[19] Koloskova, SV; Lobachev, AL; Lobacheva, IV. Methods for cholesterol determination (a review). *Clinical laboratory diagnostics,* 2004, N 1, 3−9.

[20] Ronin, VS; Starobinets, GM; Utevskii, NL. *Manual on practical lessons on methods of clinical laboratory investigations.* Moscow: Medicine, 1977.

[21] Kaplan, AV; Makhson, NE; Melnikova, VM. *Purulent traumatology of bones and joints.* Moscow: Medicine, 1985.

[22] *Clinical immunology and allergology.* Ed. Karaulov, AV. MedInform Agency, 2002.

[23] Pavlovich, SA. *Microbiology with virology and immunology.* Misnk: Vysheishaya shkola, 2005.

[24] Ivashkin, VT; Sultanov, VK. *Joint diseases. Propedeutics, differential diagnosis, and treatment.* Moscow: Litterra, 2005.

[25] *Phylogeny of immunological memory.* Ed. Manning, MJ. Amsterdam: Elsevier, 1980.

[26] Mechnikov, I I. *Optimistic essays.* Moscow; Nauka, 1987.

[27] Zamazii, AA; Peredera, RV. Alteration of cellular composition and some enzymes of synovial fluid in aged horses. *Konevodstvo i konnyi sport,* 2002, N 3, 25−26.

[28] Pavlovich, SA; Pyatkim, KD. *Medical microbiology: a practical course. Minsk: Vysheishaya skola,* 1993.

[29] Alekseeva, EI; Zhelobova, ES. Reactive arthritis in children. *Vopr. Sovr. Pediatrii,* 2003, Vol 2, N 1, 51−56.

[30] *Bio-fluid mechanics.* Ed. Power, H. Southampton: Computational Mechanics Publ, 1995.

[31] Pavlova, VN. *Synovial Medium of Joints*. Moscow: Medicine, 1980.

[32] *Biophysics*. Ed. Antonov, VF. 2nd Ed. Moscow: VLADOS, 2003.

[33] Remizov, AN; Maksina, AG; Potapenko, AYa. *Medical and biological physics*. 4th Ed. Moscow: Drofa, 2003.

[34] Vyrva, OE. Artificial synovial fluid in treatment of knee joint pathology. *Orthop. Traumatol. Prosth,* 2000, N 2, 145–150.

[35] Kozhevnikov, EV. Adhesive disease of knee joint. *NN Priorov Vestnik traumatol. and orthop,* 2004, N 3, 62–66.

[36] Bobrysheva, S. Simulation of joint friction mechanism foe creating artificial lubricants. *I Symp IOP'97,* Bialystok, 1997, 235–245.

[37] Nestor, R. *Diagnostics of rheumatic diseases*. Bukharest: Meditsinskoe isdatelstvo, 1975.

[38] Yakovleva, AA. *Infectious nonspecific (rheumatoid) arthritis in children*. Moscow: Medicine, 1971.

[39] Agababova, ER. *Rheumatic Diseases*. Moscow: Medicine, 1997.

[40] RF Patent 2114560 A 61B 6/00. *Method for evaluation of functional hydrodynamics of synovial fluid of joints*. Kozhevnikov, EV; Raspopova, EA; Kolomiets, AA. 1998.

[41] Zimon, AD. Wetting. In: Physical Encyclopedia in 5 Vol. Moscow: Bol'shaya Rossiiskaya Entsiklopedia, 1994, Vol 4, 565.

[42] Pavlova, VN; Kop'eva, TN; Slutskii, LI; Pavlov, GG. *Cartilage*. Moscow: Medicine, 1988.

[43] Ermakov, SF. *Tribophysics of liquid-crystalline materials in metallic and biopolymeric joints. Dr. Sci. Eng. Thesis*. Gomel, 2001.

[44] Summ, BD; Goryunov, YuV. *Physicochemical principles of wetting and spreading*. Moscow: *Khimiya*, 1976.

[45] Pinchuk, LS; Nikolaev, VI; Tsvetkova, EA; Goldade, VA. *Tribology and biophysics of artificial joints*. London: Elsevier, 2006.

[46] Matveeevskii, RM; Lakhshi, VL; Buyanovskii, IA; et al. *Lubricating materials: Antifrictional and antiscoring properties. Test techniques. Reference book*. Moscow: Mashinostroenie, 1989.

[47] USSR Patent 888018 G 01N 19/02. *Setup to study frictional properties of materials*. Baranov, NS; El'kina, TA; Oganesyan, OV; Sosin, SE. 1981.

[48] USSR Patent 347628 G 01N 3/56. *Setup for determining coefficient of sliding friction*. Dvornikov, LT; Velizhanova, NP; Bogomolov, NP. 1972.

[49] USSR Patent 998924 G 01N 19/02. *Setup for determining coefficient of friction at rest*. Avdeev, DT; Chebotarev, PV; Ivanov, AV. 1983.

[50] Oganesyan, OV; Sosin, SE; Maslikova, TA; El'kin, AI. On the method of investigation of friction properties of joints of living organisms. *Orthop. Traumatol. Prosth*. 1985, N 1, 59–63.

[51] Rehbinder, P; Wenström, *E. Sur less effets electrocapillaires de reduction de la rigidite et de la durete des metaux. Acta physicochimica URSS,* 1994, Vol 19, N 1, 36–50.

[52] Clarke, IC; Contini, R; Kenedi, RM. Friction and wear studies of articular cartilage: a scanning electron microscope study. *Trans. ASME,* 1975, Vol F97, N 3, 358 –368.

[53] Rebinder, PA. *Physicochemical mechanics: selective works*. Moscow: Nauka, 1979.

[54] Akhmatova, AS. *Molecular physics of boundary lubrication*. Moscow: Fizmatgiz, 1963.

[55] Unsworth, A; Dowson, D; Wright, V. *The frictional behavior of human synovial joints. Part 1. Natural joints. Trans ASME,* 1975, Vol F97, N 3, 369–376.
[56] Ermakov, SF. Integral calculation method for estimation of small variations of cyclic signal parameters in tribometry. *Mater. Tekhnol. Instr.* 1999, N 2, 92−98.
[57] USSR Patent 1420480 G 01N 19/02. *Electron-counting pendulum tribometer.* Ermakov, SF; Kupchinov, BI. 1988.
[58] USSR Patent 1630033 A 61F 2/76. *Method for investigation of lubricating fluid for joints and device for its implementation.* Ermakov, SF; Kupchinov, BI; Beloenko, ED. 1990.
[59] Ermakov, SF; Parkalov, VP; Shardin, VA. Integral calculation method for evaluation of amplitude oscillation variations and its application in pendulum tribometry. *J. Friction and wear,* 2003, Vol 24, N 2, 166−172.
[60] Patent BY C1 G 01N 11/00. *Method for evaluation of synovia lubricity.* Pinchuk, LS; Cherniakova, YuM; Kadolich, ZhV. 2007.
[61] Pinchuk, LS; Tsvetkova, EA; Kadolich, ZhV Effect of electromagnetic field on friction of joint implants. *J. Friction and Wear,* 2001, Vol 22, N 5, 69−73.
[62] USSR Patent 740242 A 61B 17/18. A device for investigation of surface friction. Maslikova, TA; El'kin, AI; Oganesyan, OV; Sosin, SE; El'kina, TA. 1980.
[63] USSR Patent 1053819A A 61B 17/18. *A device for investigation of surface friction. Maslikova,* TA; El'kin, AI; Oganesyan, OV; Sosin, SE. 1983.
[64] USSR Patent 1205902 A 61B 17/58. *A device for investigation of surface friction. Oganesyan,* OV; Sosin, SE; Maslikova, TA; El'kin, AI. 1986.
[65] Pinchuk, LS; Kadolich, ZV. *On the control of tribological parameters of joint endoprosthesis. Acta of Bioeng and Biomech*, 2002, N 4, 707−710.
[66] Dormidontov, EN; Korshunov, NI; Frizen, BN. *Rheumatoid arthritis.* Moscow: Medicine, 1981.
[67] Peyron, JG. *A new approach to the treatment of osteoarthritis: viscosupplementation. Osteoarthritis Cartilage*, 1993, N 1, 85−87.
[68] Mashkovskii, MD. *Medical Drugs.* In 2 Vol. Moscow: Medicine, 1998.
[69] VIDAL *reference book. Medical preparations in Russia.* Moscow: OVPE – AstraPharmservice.
[70] Lifshits, VM; Sidelnikova, VI. *Medical laboratory analyses. A Manual.* Moscow: Triada-X, 2000.
[71] Cherniakova, YuM; Pinchuk, LS; Kravtsov, AG; Kadolich, ZhV; Nikolaev, VI. *Zh. Tekh. Phys.* 2005, Vol 75, Issue 5, 119−123.
[72] Clinical aspects of Synvisc drug application. *Margo Anterior,* 2002, N 4, 5−8.
[73] Pinchuk, LS; Cherniakova, YuM; Kadolich, ZhV; Nikolaev, VI. Tribological monitoring of preparations used for treatment of joint diseases. *Bull. Exp. Biol. Med.* 2006, Vol 141, N 3, 278−286.
[74] Sharnopol'skii, AI. *Analyzers of fluids.* In: Chemical Encyclopedia in 5 Vol. Moscow: *Sov. Encyclopedia.* 1990, Vol 2, 290−293.
[75] *Electrets.* 2nd Ed. Ed. Sessler, GM. Berlin: Springer-Verlag, 1987.
[76] RF State Standard 25209–82. *Plastics and polymer films. Methods for determining surface charge of electrets.* Moscow: Izdatelstvo standartov, 1982.
[77] Bridelli, R; Capeletti, MG; Mozzarelli, A; Velci, A. Water induced TSCD in hemoglobin and myoglobin. *Proc. 8th Int. Symp. on Electrets.* 1994, 869−874.

[78] Pinchuk, LS; Goldade, VA; Sessler, GM; Kravtsov, AG; Zotov, SV; Tsvetkova, EA. Electret-thermal analysis of blood. *Medical Eng. Phys.* 2002, Vol 24, 361–364.
[79] Kravtsov, AG. *Electric and magnetic fields in polymeric fiber filter elements for fine cleaning of multiphase media.* Dr. Sci. Eng. Thesis. Gomel, 2007.
[80] BY Patent 12206 7 G 01N 33/487. *Method for electret-thermal analysis of biological fluid.* Pinchuk, LS; Cherniakova, YuM; Zotov, SV; Goldade, VA; Kravtsov, AG. 2009.
[81] Kadolich, ZhV. *Physical modification of polymer-metal joints to increase the wear resistance based on simulation of biophysical properties of natural joints*. PhD Eng Thesis, Gomel, 2002.
[82] Hauptman, S; Graefe, J; Remane, H. *Lehrbuch der Organischen Chemie*. Leipzig: VEB Deutscher Verlag für Druntstoffsindustrie, 1979.
[83] Gerasimov, AM; Furtseva, LN. *Biochemical diagnostics in traumatology and orthopedics.* Moscow: Medicine, 1986.
[84] Pinchuk, LS; Cherniakova, YuM; Kadolich, ZhV; Nikolaev, VI; Beloenko, ED. Investigation into structural changes of synovial fluid using electret-thermal analysis. *NN Priorov Vestnik traumatol. and orthop.* 2005, N 3, 57–61.
[85] BY Patent 9451 A 61B 5/05, G 01N 33/487. *Method for diagnostics of rheumatic diseases.* Pinchuk, L S; Cherniakova Yu M; Tsvetkova, EA; et al, 2007.
[86] Lakowich, JR. *Principles of fluorescence spectroscopy*. NY: Plenum Press, 1983.
[87] Freifelder, D. *Physical biochemistry: applications to biochemistry and molecular biology.* NY: WH Freeman, 1976.

Chapter 5

TREATMENT METHODS FOR JOINT DISEASES

Treatment of joints aims to eliminate subjective manifestations and normalize clinical laboratory parameters of damages to synovial medium via complex intervention in the main chains of pathogenesis, such as tissue inflammation and immunopathological disorders in SF. The goal of joint therapy is 1) to relieve or eliminate pain; 2) to reduce or eliminate manifestations of local and general inflammation; 3) to normalize immunity regulation; 4) to prevent from arthritis exacerbations; and 5) to activate the recovery of the damaged synovial medium of joints.

Joint therapy presumes the treatment to start as soon as possible once a disease is diagnosed, along with complex application, stage modality and continuity of medicinal actions. Complex treatment means the usage of pathogenetic and symptomatic pharmacotherapy (anti-inflammatory drugs, basic immunomodulators, and chondroprotectors) in combination with physiotherapy as well as conservative and surgical orthopedics [1]. The rejection of tactics of observation and playing the waiting game after a rheumatic disease has been diagnosed is due to the opportunity of inversing the current of pathology at the initial stage of its manifestation. This is possible if the treatment starts in due time before chondordestruction, joint deformation, osteoporosis, autoimmune pathological mechanisms and other complications occurred [2].

Chapter 5 reviews recent approaches to the treatment of pathology of the synovial medium of joints as well as discusses the concept of chondroprotection and perspectives of this trend intended to correct the composition, structure, and functions of synovia.

5.1. PHARMACOTHERAPY

Pharmacotherapy (disease management with drugs) of joint diseases is based on the data of clinical, laboratory and instrumental examinations of patients. Medication is chosen in each case individually with due regard for previous findings in the therapeutic effects of a drug and patient's individual features (age, body weight, associated diseases, etc.). Optimal joint disease therapy requires an individual choice of single and daily doses, observation of drug administration including its frequency, rhythm, routes, and duration.

5.1.1. Non-Steroidal Anti-Inflammatory Drugs

Historically, this is the oldest group of anti-inflammatory (antiphlogistic) drugs. In 1827, salicine glycoside was obtained from the bark of willow. In 1838, it was used to obtain salicylic acid, and in 1860, full synthesis of this acid and its sodium salt was performed. In 1869, acetylsalicylic acid was synthesized under "Aspirin" trademark.

Over 30 million people throughout the world take non-steroidal anti-inflammatory drugs (NSAIDs) daily to treat joint diseases, 40% of them being over 60 years old [3]. About 30% of patients are treated with NSAIDs in hospitals. The popularity of these drugs is attributed to their anti-inflammatory, analgesic, and antipyretic effects and possibility to relieve such symptoms as inflammation, pain, and fever that can accompany numerous diseases.

Nomenclature and Classification

Medication of joint disorders starts with choosing NSAID. Long-term NSAID therapy is possible thanks to a variety of drug formulations, i.e., tablets, capsules, ampoules, suppositories, and ointments, which permit one to modify drug taking if side effects, for instance, gastropathies occur.

NSAID is chosen in each case based on the list of NSAIDs recommended by rheumatologists for treatment of certain groups of disorders and their nosological forms [2]. The list includes about 30 chemical compounds that are used in practical medicine as constituents of more than 1000 drugs of various brand and trade names. Most NSAIDs refer, according to modern terminology, to "acidous" anti-inflammatory drugs because they are weak acids with pH = 4.0 or derivatives of organic acids. Table 5.1 gives the alphabetical list of most frequently used NSAIDs.

NSAIDs include combined drugs such as acetylsalicylic acid with Vitamin C (Aspirin-C, Aspirin Upsa, etc.), acetylsalicylic acid with paracetamol and coffeine (Tomapyrin), ibuprofen with paracetamol (Ibuclin), phenylbutazone with aminofenazon (Reopyrin, Pyrabutol), etc. Production of combined drugs aims to optimally affect inflammation with minimal drug doses since anti-inflammatory, analgesic, and antipyretic effects of their active substances are different, e.g., one substance can relieve pain without exerting an anti-inflammatory effect while another substance, on the contrary, has an evident anti-inflammatory effect.

NSAIDs are divided into three groups by the duration of their effect on joints:

1) short-term action [the half-period of their elimination (half-life) from blood is 2–9 hours] – Ibuprofen, Ketoprofen, Indometacin, Phenoprofen, Voltaren, Phemates, Tolmetin;
2) medium-term action (the half-life is 10–20 hours) – Naproxen, Sulindac, Diflunizal;
3) long-term action (the half-life is 24 hours and more) – oxicams, phenylbutazone.

Properties

From practical point of view, it is of importance that drugs of the same group and even similar in chemical structure differ in both the power of the effect exerted and the frequency and mechanism of development of adverse reactions. Clinical efficacy of a drug can depend on the kind and pathogenetic features of a disease as well as patient's response. According to [4], all NSAIDs can be ranked according to their positive and negative activity (Fig. 5.1) by comparing it with that of acetylsalicylic acid (ASA), which is taken 1 in all series.

Table 5.1. Non-Steroidal Anti-Inflammatory Drugs

International name of active substance	Some brand names	Drug's chemical group
Acelysin	Lysine acetylsalicylate Aspizol, Laspal	Arylcarbonic acids (salicylic acid)
Acetylsalicylic acid	ASA, Aspirin, Aspro, Colfarit	
Diclofenac	Almiral, Voltaren, Diclac, Diclobene, Dicloberl, Diclomax, Diclonate P, Dicloran, Diclofenac Sodium, Diclofenac-Teva, Voltaren, Difen, Diclonac-Rivopharm, Clofen, Naklofen, Orthofen, Revodina, Sanfinac, Feloran	Arylalkane acids (arylacetic acid)
Ibuprofen	Brufen, Burana, Ibusan, Yprin	Arylpropionic acid
Indometacin	Indovis, Indometacin-Pharmacim, Metindol, L-Metacin, Indocid, Indoretard, Indobene	Indol- and indenacetic acids
Kebuzon	Ketazon	Enolic acids (pyrazolones)
Ketoprofen	Profenid, Knavon, Ketonal,	Arylpropionic acid
Ketorolac	Ketanov, Toradol, Ketrodol	Arylalkane acids (heteroakrylacetic acid)
Lornoxicam	Xefocam	Enolic acids (oxicams)
Meloxicam	Movalis	
Metamizole sodium	Analgin, Baralgin M, Devalgin, Novalgin, Toralgin, Dipyrone	Enolic acids (pyrazolones)
Naproxen	Daprox entero, Naproxen-Teva, Naprosin, Sanaprox	Arylpropopionic acid
Nimesulid	Actasulid, Mesulid, Nise, Nimesil	Sulfonamides
Niflumic acid	Donalgin	Nicotinic acid
Paracetamol	Aldorol, Panadol, Efferalgan, Calpol, Lekadol, Acetominafen, Mexalen	Paraaminophenol derivatives
Pyrprofen	Rengasil	Arylpropionic acid
Piroxicam	Sanicam, Remoxicam, Felden, Pirocam, Erazon	Enolic acids (oxicams)
Sulindac	Clinoril	Indol- and indenacetic acids
Tiaprofenic acid	Surgam	Arylpropionic acid
Phenylbutazone	Butadion	Enolic acids (pyrazolones)
Flufenamic acid	Mobilizin	Arylcarbonic acids (anthranilic acid)
Flurbiprofen	Flugalin, Phtorbiprofen, Anseid, Froben	Arylpropionic acid
Celecoxib	Celebrex	Sulfonamides
Etodolac	Elderin	Indol- and indenacetic acids

A curative effect of NSAIDs depends on the rate of their accumulation and concentration in SF. Kinetic curves of drug concentration in SF lag behind their concentration in blood. However, NSAID concentration in SF is maintained longer than in blood. Different NSAIDs penetrate into SF at different rates and are present in it during different periods.

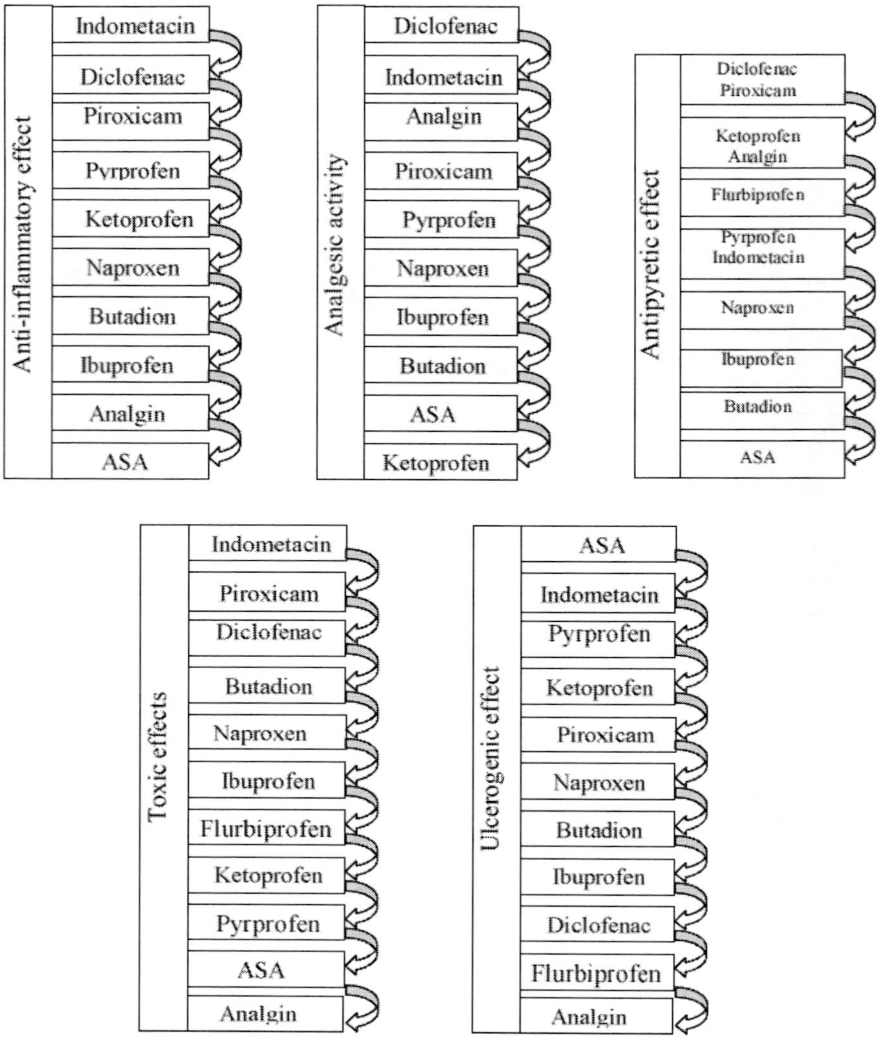

Figure 5.1. NSAID series that exert anti-inflammatory, antipyretic, analgesic, toxic, and ulcerogenic effects.

An anti-inflammatory effect of NSAIDs is due to following biological effects exerted:

- inhibition of synthesis of prostaglandins (hormones) by inhibiting the activity of prostaglandin synthetasis (cyclooxygenase);
- stabilization of lysosome membranes – cytoplasm organoids that disintegrate protein macromolecules;
- inhibition of production of macroergic compounds whose disintegration is accompanied by the liberation of a large amount of energy;
- inactivation of inflammation mediators (histamine, bradykinin, cytokines, components of complement system);

- inhibition of proliferative phase (accompanied by the growth of connective tissue, glands, and lymphatic nodes) of inflammation and retardation of sclerotic changes in synovial medium;
- slowing down of transcription (primary reproduction) of genes resulting in inhibition of the proliferative activity of SM cells;
- stimulation of production of endogenous peptides of endodorfine group having the analgesic effect;
- inhibition of expression (biosynthesis and release) of adhesion molecules (selectins and integrins);
- decreasing permeability of capillaries.

The main and general element of anti-inflammatory mechanism of NSAIDs is inhibition of prostaglandin (PG) synthesis from arachidonic acid via inhibiting the cyclooxygenase enzyme (PG-synthetasis) (Fig. 5.2). PGs can be active in various ways: i.e., they: *a*) mediate inflammatory reaction (cause local vasodilatation, edema, exudation, leukocyte migration, and other effects (PG-E_2 and PG-I_2); *b*) sensibilize receptors to pain mediators (histamine and bradykinin) and mechanical effects lowering a sensibility threshold; and *c*) increase the sensibility of hypothalamic centers to endogenous pyrogens (interleukin-1, etc.) arising in an organism under the effect of microbes, viruses, and toxins (mainly PG-E_2).

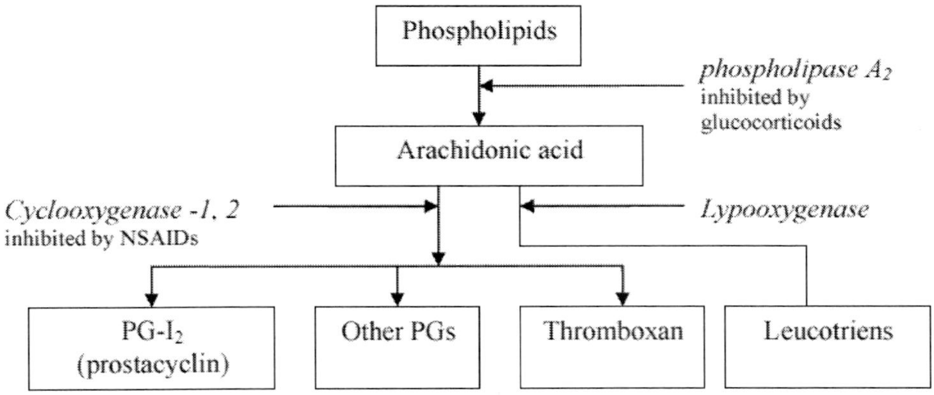

Figure 5.2. Diagram of arachidonic acid metabolism.

At least two isoenzymes of cyclooxygenase exist that are inhibited by NSAIDs. The former – cyclooxygenase-1 (COX-1) – is responsible for the production of prostaglandins, maintains the integrity of the lining of the gastrointestinal tract, and regulates renal blood stream and platelet function. The latter – cyclooxygenase-2 (COX-2) – participates in prostaglandin synthesis in inflammation. Normally, COX-2 is absent in the joint and occurs under the action of some tissue factors initiating an inflammatory reaction (cytokines, etc.). In this connection, it is assumed that the anti-inflammatory effect of NSADs is due to COX-2 inhibition and their adverse reactions are caused by COX-1 inhibition. As reported elsewhere [5], COX-2 is inhibited largely by meloxicam, celecoxib, and nimesulid, and COX-2 – by diclofenac, indometacin, ibuprofen, flurbiprofen, and naproxen. Table 5.2 presents the classification of NSAIDs according to the selectivity of their response to different forms of

COX. As for the COX-1/COX-2 inhibition, the ratio of NSAIDs activity allows assessment of their potential toxicity. The lower the ratio, the more selective the drug is towards COX-2 and thus, less toxic. By way of example, it is 0.33 for meloxicam, 2.2 for diclofenac, 15 for tenoxicam, 33 for piroxicam, and 107 for indometacin.

Table 5.2. NSAID Selectivity Realtive to COX

Degree and kind of selectivity	Drug
Pronounced COX-1 selectivity	Aspirin, indometacin, ketoprofen, piroxicam, sulindac
Moderate COX-1 selectivity	Diclofenac, ibuprofen, naproxen
Approximately equal COX-1 and COX-2 inhibition	Loronoxicam
Moderate COX-2 selectivity	Etodolac, meloxicam, nimesulid, nabumeton
Pronounced COX-2 selectivity	Celeoxicab, rofecoxicab

A potent anti-inflammatory effect of indometacin, diclofenac, and phenylbutazone is complemented with the inhibition of the proliferation phase of inflammation in connective tissues, lower synthesis of collagen, and tissue scleroitization. NSAID does not affect substantially the alteration phase (tissue damages). As for anti-inflammatory activity, all NSAIDs rank below glucocorticoids which while inhibiting phospholipase A_2 inhibit the metabolism of phospholipids and break the formation of both prostaglandins and leucotriens as intrinsic mediators of inflammation (Fig. 5.2).

NSAIDs as analgesics are effective at weak or low-intensive pains localized in muscles, joints, tendons, nerve columns as well as in headache and toothache. At severe pains, e.g., after joint operations, most NSAIDs are low efficient and rank below narcotic analgesics in analgesic effect. A high analgesic activity is typical of ketorolac, ketoprofen, diclofenac, metamisol that are used to relieve after-operation pains. The advantage of NSAIDs over narcotic analgesics is that they do not inhibit the respiratory center, do not cause euphoria and drug dependence and do not exert a spasmogenic effect. The analgesic effect of many drugs is dose-dependent: ketorolac 30 mg > (ketoprofen 25 mg = ibuprofen 400 mg = flubiprofen 50 mg) > AC 650 mg = paracetamol 650 mg = fenoprofen 200 mg = naproxen 250 mg = etodolac 200 mg = declofenac 50 mg = mefenamic acid 500 mg) > nabumeton 1000 mg. In particular, the efficiency of 30 mg of ketorolac injected intramuscularly is equivalent to 12 mg of morphine. Drugs are chosen for analgesic purposes empirically because of the absence of standards, objective and reliable criteria for individual choice of a drug for a patient as well as because most patients are self-treated before visiting a doctor.

An antipyretic effect of NSAIDs manifests only in fever. In arthritis and synovitis, it is related to the inhibition of mediators of inflammation (endogenous pyrogens and proteins with a molecular weight of 10–12 thousands) in phagocytes, monocytes, and reticulocytes of the joint capsule and SM as well as the inhibition of thermoregulation centers and increasing heat emission. The effect of NSAIDs on central thermoregulation is reduced to lower liberation of serotonin, adrenaline, and acetylcholine by hypothalamic cells and inhibition of excitation transmission in hypothalamic nuclei, which was confirmed both electrophysiologically and biochemically. An evident inhibiting effect of salicylates on the post-synaptic signal is revealed (it arises from polarization-depolarization of cell membranes within the synapse region – the contact of nervous cells) in various sections of the brain. These drugs do not exert any effect on the normal temperature of the body, except for amidopyrin and phenacetin, which possess the hyperthermogenous effect.

Toxic effects of NSAIDs may vary. The occurrence and manifestations depends on a system or organ that is most responsive to the effect of toxic products of drug metabolic transformations. If butadion, Indometacin, and aspirin are taken for a long time, a liver disorder may manifest in the form of toxic hepatitis. The markers of toxic hepatitis are high concentrations in blood of alkali phosphatase, aminotransferases, gamma-glutamyltranspeptidase, and other enzymes secreted from the damaged hepatocytes. NSAIDs affect the function of kidneys in patients with accompanying cardio-vascular and chronic renal diseases. The toxicity of drug metabolites leads to uricosuaria (excretion of uric acid with urine), deposition of urates in kidney channels, and acute necrosis of kidney channels. Naproxen and indometacin can reduce the glomerular filtration and slow down the rate of urine formation and excretion of free water and electrolytes. In long-term intake of phenacetin and ACA, toxic nephritis manifests as proteinuria (protein excretion), hematuria (loss of erythrocytes with urine), and polyuria (excessive production of urine during a day) in conjunction with cramps, arterial hypertension, and development of chronic renal insufficiency. Hematological complications such as anemia, leucopenia, agranulocytosis, and thrombocytopenia may also accompany the administration of NSAIDs. A risk of the development of total suppression of haematopoesis – aplastic anemia – during a long-term administration of metamizole sodium (Analgin) has resulted in the prohibition of this preparation in many countries.

The anticoagulation activity of NSAIDs sometimes causes heamarthrosis – periarticular hemorrhage and hemorrhage from the gastrointestinal tract. Neurotoxic disorders occur when taking ACA and indometacin. Patients note headache, noise in ears, sleepiness, depression, nausea, vomiting, etc. Dermatotoxic reactions to mainly pyrasalone preparations are encountered in 20–25% of rheumatoid arthritis patients. A toxic effect of NSAIDs on pregnancy (overcarrying of pregnancy, prolongation of delivery) and fetus in the form of teratogenic factors (congenital heart diseases, diaphragm defects, fetus hypotrophy, and hemorrhagic syndrome) is reported [2].

With duration of NSAIDs therapy, an immunosuppressive effect is revealed. A number of NSAIDs (indometacin, butadion, naproxen, and ibuprofen) inhibit directly the transformation of lymphocytes induced by various antigens, which causes their immunosuppressive effect. Secondary immunosuppression consists in reducing capillary permeability, hindering contacts of immunocompetent cells with antigens and antibodies with the inflammation substrate, and stabilization of lysosome membranes in macrophages. This limitates the breakdown of poorly soluble antigens that is necessary for the development of next stages of immune reaction.

An ulcerogenic effect of NSAIDs is characterized by gastropathies, i.e., erosive-ulcerous lesions of superior sections of the gastrointestinal tract. Such complications as acute gastric bleeding, gastric and duodenal ulceration and perforation are of utmost danger because they can lead to the death of elderly patients afflicted with joint diseases. Below, the toxicity, ulcerogeneity, and some other adverse effects of NSAIDs are discussed in more detail.

Antiaggregatory properties of NSAIDs, i.e., their ability to inhibit the formation of aggregates in the blood, are due to the inhibition of COX-1 in platelets (blood plates, nucleus-free blood cells). As a result, the synthesis of endogenic (arising in the bloodstream) proreagent (precursor of aggregation) thromboxan – factor 2 is inhibited. Different preparations affect in different ways the aggregation of platelets – cells that are initially incapable of protein synthesis, including enzymatic ones because of different mechanisms of COX inhibition. This feature allows us to distinguish three groups of NSAIDs that cause: 1) slow and reversible competitive inhibition (Indometacin, Voltaren), 2) slow and irreversible inhibition (salicylates), and 3) rapid reversible and competitive inhibition of enzyme (brufen, naproxen, butadion). Aspirin exhibits the strongest and longest anti-aggregation activity: it irreversibly inhibits the platelet ability of aggregation during its lifetime (7 days). ACA irreversibly inhibits COX-1 by its acetilzing (reaction of introduction of acetyl group CH_3CO) in platelets. After ACA taken once, a clinically significant reduction of platelet aggregation lasts for 48 hours and more. Synthesis of thromboxan is renewed only due to the appearance of new populations of platelets from marrow. The antiaggregatory effect of other NSAIDs is weaker and reversible. Selective COX-2 inhibitors do not affect the platelet aggregation.

A NSAID dose depends on drug pharmacokinetics, state of organs of biotransformation and secretion (liver, kidneys, lungs, etc.) as well as rate of drug accumulation and its concentration in blood and SF. Drug biotransformation (metabolism) is taken to mean the complex of its physicochemical and biochemical transformations during which water-soluble substances with polar molecules (metabolites) arise. Biologically, they are less active and toxic than the initial preparations and are excreted from the organism more easily than the drugs. However, the biotransformation of some NSAIDs results in more active metabolites than a substance taken. For instance, ACA changes into an active metabolite – salicylic acid, and butadion – into oxyphenbutazone.

The NSAID pharmacokinetics within a body is described by a two-chamber model where one of the chambers is tissues of the synovial medium and the second one is the vascular network of the joint. NSAIDs are well absorbed from the gastrointestinal tract, bound almost totally to plasma albumins squeezing out some other drugs and biliribin in newborns, which can lead to the development of bilirubin encephalopathy (in this relation, salicylates and phenylbutazon are the most dangerous). Protein binding results in a reduced drug concentration in the tissues since only an unbound preparation can pass through biological membranes. A protein-bound substance is deprived of specific acitivity. Free and bound parts of the preparation are in dynamic equilibrium. Sometimes the substances are accumulated in tissues in higher concentrations than it is expected assuming diffusive equilibrium. The accumulation effect depends on pH, binding to intracellular elements, and drug distribution in the adipose tissue. Most NSAIDs penetrate easily into SF. The degree of drug penetration through SM into the joint depends on the route of drug passage (oral, intramuscular, or intravenous) and intensity of degenerative and inflammatory processes in SM. In patients with chronic inflammations of joints, NSAIDs are accumulated in SF more slowly than in healthy people and in lower concentrations than in blood. However, a therapeutic concentration of drugs in SF of affected joints is maintained longer than that in blood [6]. Maximum NSAID concentration in rheumatoid arthritis occurs within 45 min (acetylsalicylic acid), 4 hours (diclofenac), and 6 hours (flugalin).

Adverse Reactions

As has been noted, the gastrointestinal tract lesions are most frequent of other adverse reactions observed in arthritis treatment. In 30–40% of patients dyspeptic (impaired digestion) phenomena, in 10–20% gastric ulcer, and in 2–5% bleeding and perforation of gastric ulcer are observed [7]. Such complications as stomatitis, duodenal or intestinal ulcer, diarrhea, and pancreatitis are also possible. The risk of development of adverse reactions prevails in elderly people, in combination of NSAIDs with glucocorticoids, with duration of therapy are large doses or at a simultaneous use of 2–3 drugs of this group. Smoking, alcohol, and violation of meal regime increase the ulcerogenic effect of NSAIDs.

Today, NSAID-induced gastroduodenopathy is distinguished as a specific syndrome of lesion of stomach and duodenum [8]. It is related to a local damaging effect of NSAID only in part due to inhibition of the isoenzymes COX-1 caused by the systemic effect of the drugs. Therefore, gastrotoxicity can take place at any route of NSAID. A lesion is most often localized in the stomach, mainly in antral or prepyloric parts. Clinical symptoms of NSAID-induced gastroduodenopathy are absent in almost 60% of patients, especially the elderly, therefore, fibrogastroscopy is used in many cases to diagnose the disease. At the same time, the signs of mucous coat damage are absent in many patients having dyspeptic complains. The absence of clinical symptoms in NSAID-induced gastroduodenopathy is related to the analgesic effect of these drugs. Therefore, the patients, especially the elderly, that do not have adverse reactions concerning the gastrointestinal tract under long-term care are considered as a group of higher risk of severe complications of NSAID-induced gastrodudenopathy (bleeding, severe anemia) and need a thorough control including endoscopic examination [3].

To minimize a local irritation of the gastrointestinal tract, NSAIDs should be taken during or immediately after meal. Concurrently, preparations to protect the mucous coat of the gastrointestinal tract are administered, e.g., H_2-receptor antagonists (Famotidine, Ranitidine, etc.). misoprostol, omeprosol, sucralfate, etc. [3, 8] following the algorithm presented in Fig. 5.3.

In order to reduce the ulcerogenic effect of the drugs, the combined drugs containing NSAIDs and gastroprotectors are produced. H_2-blockers are capable of preventing duodenal ulcers, but, as rule, are inefficient in stomach ulcers. However, there are data that high doses of famotidin (40 mg twice a day) reduce the frequency of stomach and duodenal ulcer. Misoprostol, the synthetic analog of PG-E_2 has a high efficiency. Its intake allows one to prevent ulcers in both stomach and duodenum. To minimize the ulcelrogeneity, the NSAIDs referring to selective inhibitors have been developed. They inhibit COX-2 that is responsible for prostaglandin production in inflammation and do not affect COX-1 that controls the production of prostaglandins supporting the integrity of the mucous coat of the gastrointestinal tract, renal blood flow, and platelet function. Rheumatoid arthritis and osteoarthrosis patients are tolerable to them largely compared to diclofenac, ibuprofen, piroxicam, and naproxen while showing a similar efficiency [9].

Nephrotoxicity is the second significant group of adverse reactions of NSAIDs. Two main mechanisms of the negative effect of NSAIDs on kidneys have been revealed.

The first mechanism consists in the inhibition of synthesis of PG-E_2 and prostacycline in kidneys, which causes the vasoconstriction and impaired renal bloodstream. This leads to ischemic disorders in kidneys and the reduction of glomerular filtration and diuresis volume. Disturbances in aqueous-electrolyte exchange are observed such as water retention, hypersodiumaemia, swelling, hyperpotassaemia, growth of creatinine in the serum, and hypertension. Indometacin and phenylabutazone have the most pronounced effect on the renal bloodstream.

The second mechanism consists in a direct effect of NSAIDs on the kidney parenchyma (the tissue incorporating specialized cellular elements and connective tissue composition) leading to interstitial nephritis (so-called analgesic nephropathy). At this point phenacetin is the most dangerous. In addition, a severe renal failure can be potentially developed up to renal insufficiency.

Hemotoxicity characterizes pyrazolidines and pyrazolones. Aplastic anemia and agranulocytosis are the most severe complications.

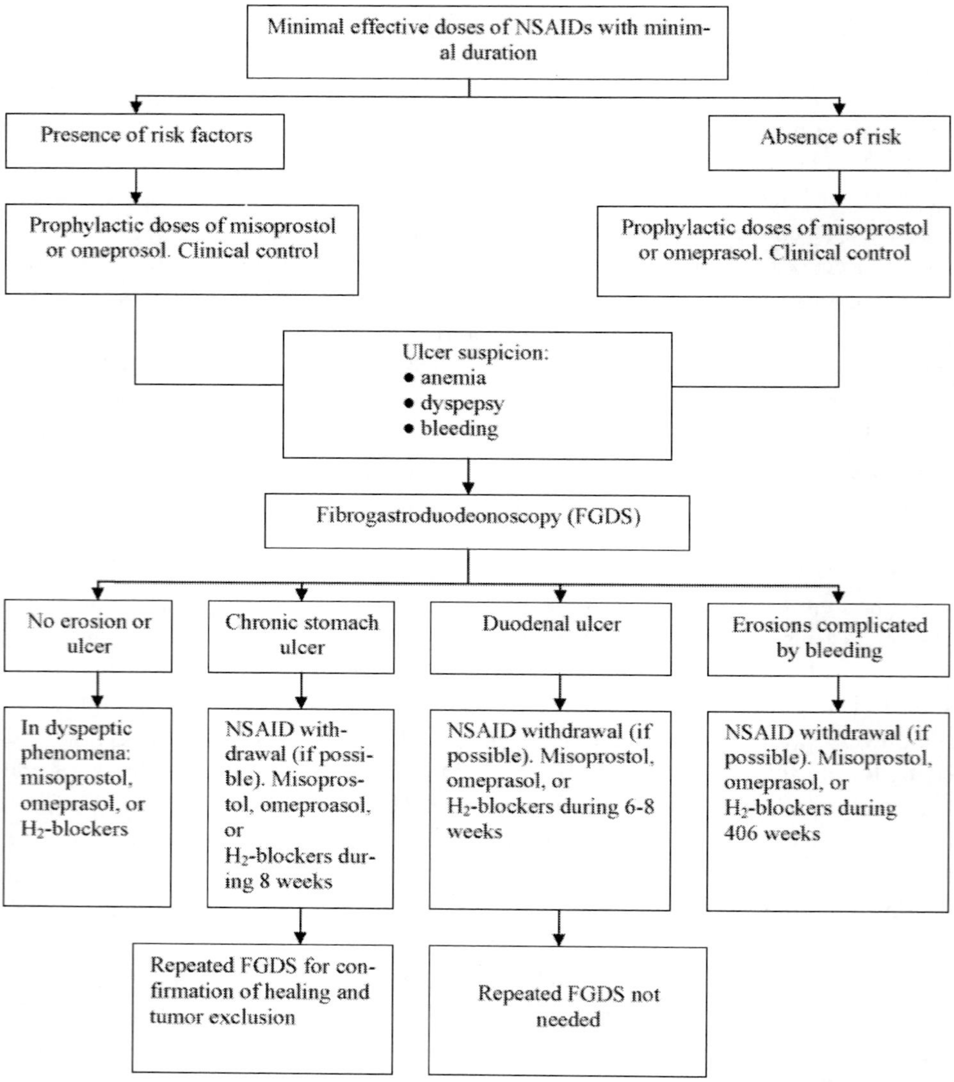

Figure 5.3. Algorithm of prophylaxis and treatement of NSAID-induced gastroduodenopathy [8].

Coagulopathy is the malfunctioning of the coagulating blood system. This NSAID-induced complication is due to the inhibition of platelet aggregation and impairment of prothrombine formation in liver. It results in bleedings, most often from the gastrointestinal tract.

Hepatotoxicity manifests in varying activity of transaminases catalyzing transfer reactions, and some other enzymes. In severe cases jaundice and hepatitis may occur.

Hypersusceptibility (allergy) in the form of rash, Quincke swelling (H.I. Quincke, the German therapeutist), anaphylactic shock, Lyell (A.M. Lyell, the modern Scottish physician) and Stevens-Johnson (A.M. Stevens and F.C. Johnson, the American pediatricians) syndromes, and allergic interstitial nephritis are observed largely when pyrazolones and pyrazolidines are taken. A bronchospasm is commonly developed in bronchial asthma patients and most often with administration of aspirin. This may be due to allergic mechanisms and inhibition of synthesis of PG-E_2 as an endogenic bronchodilator.

Administration and Dosage of NSAIDs

It is recommended to select the most effective well-tolerated drug for each patient individually. The susceptibility of patients to NSAIDs of the same chemical group may vary over a wide range, therefore, inefficiency of one of the drugs does not evidence to the inefficiency of the group as a whole. When replacing one drug with another, it should be taken into account that the anti-inflammatory effect is developed more slowly than the analgesic one. The latter is noted during several hours while the former manifests in 10–14 days of regular intake and in the case of naproxen or oxicams the effect occurs even later, within 2–4 weeks.

Any new drug is first administered to a patient in its minimal dose. Once the drug is well tolerated, later within 2–3 days, the daily dose is increased. Recently, there is a tendency to increase single and daily therapeutic doses of drugs characterized by a sufficient tolerance (naproxen and ibuprofen) along with limitations on maximal doses of aspirin, indometacin, phenylabutazone, and piroxicam. In some patients, the medicinal effect is achieved only at very high NSAID doses.

In rheumatology, in protracted therapeutical course, NSAIDs are taken after meal 2–3 times a day. To achieve rapid analgesic or antipyretic effects it is recommended to take the drugs 30 min before meal or 2 hours after meal. After taking a drug, it is advisable not to go to bed during 15 min to prevent esophagitis. The moment of NSAID intake also depends on the period of maximal manifestation of disease symptoms (pain, joint stiffness). In this case, it is permitted bending the common schemes and indicate NSAIDs at any time of day, which allows achievement of a better curative effect at a lower daily dose. In pronounced morning stiffness, the earliest intake (immediately after awaking) of fast absorbed NSAIDs or indication of preparations of prolonged action for the night are advisable. Naproxen-sodium, Diclofenac-potassium, water-soluble aspirin, and ketaprofen have the highest rate of absorption in the gastrointestinal tract and achievement of the effect.

Simultaneous administration of two or more NSAIDs is not recommended because of the following reasons: there is no evidence of the efficiency of combinations of two or more drugs; in a number of cases a reduced concentration of the drugs in the blood is noted (e.g., aspirin decreases the concentration of indometacin, diclofenac, ibuprofen, naproxen, and piroxicam) and a risk of development of adverse reactions grows. The exception can be made for the administration of paracetamol in combination with another NSAID to maximize the analgesic effect. Sometimes two NSAIDs are taken at a different time of the day, namely, a fast absorbed drug it taken at morning or daytime and that of prolonged action, at night.

NSAIDs interact with drugs of other pharmacological groups. NSAIDs can enhance the action of indirect anticoagulants and peroral hypoglycemic (reducing sugar in blood) preparations, weaken the effect of antihypertensive drugs, and increase the toxicity of antibacterial aminiglycosids, digoxin, and some other drugs. Simultaneous administration of

NSAIDs and diuretics should be avoided because of, on the one hand, weakening of the diuretic effect and, the other, a risk of renal insufficiency. The combination of indometacin with triamteren is the most dangerous.

Many preparations administered together with NSAIDs, can affect the pharmacokinetics of the latter. Thus, aluminum-containing antacids (Almagel, Maalox, etc.) and cholestiramine weaken the absorption of NSAIDs in the gastrointestinal tract. In this case, NSAIDs are administered at increased doses, and at least 4-hour intervals are required between the intakes of cholestiramine and NSAIDs. Sodium bicarbonate enhances the absorption of NSAIDs in the gastrointestinal tract. The anti-inflammatory effect of NSAIDs is enhanced by glucocorticoids and anti-inflammatory drugs of slow action (basic) such as gold preparations and aminocholines). Narcotic analgesic and sedative drugs enhance the analgesic effect of NSAIDs.

Nsaids with Evident Anti-Inflammatory Activity

Acetylsalicylic acid (ASA) is the oldest NSAID. In clinical trials, it serves a reference for other NSAIDs in efficiency and tolerance. Aspirin as a trade name proposed by the Bayer Company (Germany) has become identical to the name of its active substance in efficiency all over the world. Aspirin is manufactured in tablets 100, 250, 300, and 500 mg and in the form of combined preparations Aspirin C, Aspro-C forte, Citramon P, alka-zeltzer, etc.

The effect of ASA is due to lower energy supply of inflammation because of inhibition of oxidative phosphorylation and ATF synthesis, suppression of glycolysis enzymes, tricarbonic acid cycle, and proteolysis. The drug reduces the permeability of capillaries. Salicylate suppresses immunity by binding SH-groups of the proteins of immunocompetent organs.

Aspirin is one of the preparations to treat rheumatoid arthritis including juvenile arthritis. According to recommendations of most manuals on rheumatology, anti-inflammatory therapy should start with Aspirin. It should be noted that its anti-inflammatory effect manifests at high doses that are poorly tolerated by many patients. Aspirin is used as an analgesic and antipyretic. Systematic small doses (up to 325 mg per day) of Aspirin often reduce the frequency of development of colorectal cancer [10].

Pharmacodynamics of Aspirin depends on a daily dose: low doses (30–325 mg) induce the inhibition of platelet aggregation, moderate doses (1.5–2 g) have the analgesic and antipyretic effects, and high ones (4–6 g) have the anti-inflammatory effect. An Aspirin dose higher than 4 g enhances the excretion of uric acid (uricosuric action) while in lower doses its excretion is retarded.

The preparation is absorbed well from the gastrointestinal tract. Its absorption is improved if the tablets are refined and taken with warm water as well as if water-soluble tablets are used. Coffein and metoclopromide stimulate the absorption of Aspirin from the gastrointestinal tract. The half-life of Aspirin is 15 minutes. Under the action of esterases of the mucous membrane of the stomach, liver, and blood, salicylate having the main pharmacological activity segregates from aspirin. Maximal concentration of aspirin and period of its half-excretion is 4–6 hours. Salicylate is metabolized in the liver and excreted with urine. When pH of urine increases (e.g., when taking antacids), the excretion of the drug enhances. At very large Aspirin doses, the saturation of metabolizing enzymes and increase of the period of salicylate half-excretion within 15–30 hours is possible. Glucocorticoids accelerate the metabolism and excretion of aspirin. Aspirin inhibits the gastric alcogoldehydrodenase, which leads to increasing level of ethanol in the organism even at its moderate doses (0.15 g/kg) [11].

An adverse gastrotoxic effect is possible even when using aspirin as an antireagent at low doses, 75–300 mg per day. The risk of bleedings is dose-dependent: in administering 75 mg per day, it is by 40% lower than at 300 mg, and by 30% lower than at 150 mg [12]. Even insignificant bleeding from an erosion or an ulcer can lead to systematic blood loss with feces (2–5 ml per day) and development of iron-deficient anemia. Officinal formulations with a coating soluble in the gastrointestinal tract have lower gastrotoxicity. Some patients who take Aspirin adapt themselves to its gastrotoxic effect. The co-administration of Aspirin doses of more than 5 g per day and anticoagulants is dangerous because of broken platelet coagulation, inhibition of prothrombine synthesis in the liver, and increased bleeding.

Hypersensitivity reactions manifest as skin rash or bronchospams. Specific nosological forms are distinguished called a Fernan Widal's syndrome (Fernan Widal, the French therapeutist and infectionist) or "aspirin triad", i.e., combination of polyposis of nose and (or) paranasal sinus, bronchial asthma, and full intolerance to aspirin. Therefore, Aspirin and other NSAIDs are recommended very carefully to the bronchial asthma patients.

In mild cases, overdosing or intoxication manifest as "salicylism" symptoms, that is, noise in ears (points to the saturation with salicylate), obnubilation, reduced hearing, headache, sometimes nausea and vomiting. In severe intoxication, abnormalities of the central nervous system and water-electrolyte metabolism are developed. Dyspnea (as the result of the respiratory center stimulation), abnormalities of acid-base state (first respiratory alkalosis due to carbonic acid losses and afterwards metabolic acidosis due to inhibition of tissue metabolism), polyria, hyperthermia, and fluid loss are observed. Myocardial oxygen consumption rises, and cardiac insufficiency or pulmonary edema can arise. Children before 5 years old are the most responsive to the toxic effect, which, the same as in adults manifest as abnormalities of acid-base state and neurological symptoms. The degree of intoxication depends on Asprin dose. At 150–300 mg/kg the intoxication is mild or moderate, a 300–500 mg/kg dose leads to severe intoxications, and a dose of more than 500 mg/kg is potentially lethal.

In aspirin intoxication, the assistance is in washing the stomach, taking activated carbon within 15 g, plenty fluid (milk or juice) within 50–100 ml/kg per day, and intravenous injection of polyion hypotonic solutions (1 part of 0.9% sodium chloride and 2 parts of 10% glucose). In collapse, an intravenous infusion of colloidal solutions is administered while in acidosis (after determining pH of blood) sodium bicarbonate is prescribed. Hemosorption and hemodialysis (in renal insufficiency) are also used.

The Aspirin dosage for adults in non-rheumatic diseases is 0.5 g 3–4 times a day, in rheumatic diseases the initial dose is 0.5 g 4 times a day, then the does increases by 0.25–0.5 g every day each week. Aspirin is administered as an antireagent at doses 100–325 mg per day taken once.

Children within 1-year-old take 10 mg/kg 4 times a day, after 1 year old – 10–15 mg/kg 4 times a day in non-rheumatic diseases. In rheumatic diseases, with a body weight within 10–15 kg they take 80–100 mg/kg per day and at a body weight above 25 kg – 60–80 mg/kg per day.

Lysine acetylsalicylate is an Aspirin derivative for pareneteral injection (omitting the gastrointestinal tract). The drug surpasses Asprin in rapidity and power of the analgesic effect. Adverse reactions are similar to those of aspirin. It is administered to discontinue acute pain syndrome (rheumatic pains, radicultitis, postoperative and posttraumatic pains, colics) as well as in hyperthermia and trombophlebitis.

Doses for adults are as follows: a single dose is 2 g, maximal dose is within 10 g per day. Children take 20–50 mg/kg per day in 2–3 injections.

Diflunisal (Dolobid) refers to the nonacetylized salicylates. It is prescribed in rheumatoid arthritis, osteoarthrosis, and pain syndrome. Diflunisal does not cause salicylism, since it is not metabolized to salicylate. It has potent anti-inflammatory and analgesic effects and exhibits the uricosuric action. Dislike aspirin, Diflunisal is not an antipyretic since it does not penetrate into the central nervous system. It reversibly inhibits the aggregation of platelets only when maximal doses (2 g per day) are prescribed.

The drug is readily absorbed from the gastrointestinal tract. Its maximum concentration in blood develops in 2–3 hours, and the analgesic effect is exerted within 1 hour, especially at the maximal dose (1000 mg). It has a longer than Aspirin half-life period of 8–12 hours.

In rheumatoid arthritis and osteoarthrosis, adults take 0.5–1 g every 12 hours. To stop the pain, the first dose is 1 g, then 05 g every 8–12 hours. The drug is not prescribed to children.

Phenylbutazone surpasses aspirin in the power of the ant-inflammatory effect. It enhances the excretion of uric acid from an organism. Its maximum concentration in blood develops within 2 hours of oral administration and within 6–8 hours after intramuscular injection (phenylbutazone is bound by tissues at the place of injection). The half-life is about 70 hours. One of metabolites of phenylabutazone – oxyphenbutazone – is manufactured in the form of an independent preparation that is equal to phenylbutazone in all parameters (including toxicity).

Phenylbutazone is one of the most potent "displacement agents" of other drugs from the blood albumin bonding, which results in increased concentration of active free fractions of this drug in blood. In addition, it can inhibit the metabolism of some preparation in the liver. Therefore, the effect of indirect anticoagulants, tableted anti-diabetic drugs, sulfanilamides, etc. is enhanced with co-administered phenylbutazone. By impairing the renal bloodstream, phenylbutazone weakens the action of diuretic and antihypertensive drugs.

About 45% of patients treated by phenylabutazone report the adverse reactions. The depressive effect of the drug on the marrow is the most dangerous since it leads to the hematotoxic reactions such as leucopenia, thromobocytopenia, pancytemaia, hemolytic anemia, aplastic anemia, and agranulocytosis. The risk of aplastic anemia is high in women, people after 40 years old, and in protracted drug administration. However, even during short-term administration aplastic anemia can develop in young people. Adverse reactions of the gastrointestinal tract (erosions, ulcer, bleeding, and diarrhea), fluid retention in organism followed by edema, disoroders of the central nervous system (slow response, excitation, and tremor), hematuria, proteinuria, and liver abnormalities are observed. Phenylbutazone possesses the cardiotoxicity (cardiac insufficiency might exacerbate) and can cause an acute lung syndrome manifesting in short breath and fever. In a number of patients, the hypersusceptibility in form of bronchospasm, generalized lymphadenopathy, and skin rash is revealed. Phezone and especially its metabolite oxyphenbutazone can lead to exacerbated porphyria. Regarding the risk of development of these hematological complications, it is necessary to tell the patient about their early manifestations and observe the rules of indication of pyrazolones and pyrazolidones.

Phenylbutazone is used as a reserve NSAID in short-term courses if other preparations turn to be inefficient. The drug is the most efficient in the Bekhterev's disease and gout. The drug and phenylbutazone-containing preparations (Reopyrin and Pyrabutol) are not recommended for wide usage in clinical practice as analgesic and antipyretic drugs. Phenylbutazine is contradicted to the patients with disorders in blood formation, erosions and ulcers in the gastrointestinal tract (including their presence in the history), cardiovascular diseases, thyroid gland pathology, abnormalities of the liver and kidneys, and allergy to aspirin and other NSAIDs. It can impair the condition of patients with systemic lupus erythematosus.

The initial dose is 450–600 mg 3–4 times per day in adults. Upon achieving the therapeutic effect, maintaining doses of 150–300 mg 1-2 times a day are prescribed. The drug is not administered to children below 14 years old.

Clofezone (Perclusone) is an equimolar composition of phenylbutazone and clofexamide. Clofexamide possesses the analgesic and anti-inflammatory (to a lesser degree) effects thus supplementing the effect of phenylbutazone. The Clofezone tolerance is somewhat better than that of phenylbutazone. Adverse reactions develop more rarely if the precautions are followed. Indications are the same as for phenylbutazone.

Adults are given 200–400 mg 2–3 times a day perorally or rectally. Children of body weight of no more than 20 kg are given 10–15 mg per day.

Indometacin is one of the most potent NSAIDs. Its maximum concentration in blood develops within 1–2 hours after taking ordinary forms and within 2–4 hours after taking prolonged (retarded) forms. Meal impedes its absorption. When taken rectally, it is absorbed worse and its maximum concentration in blood comes later. Its half-life is 4–5 hours.

Pharmacological effects of Indometacin are due to blocking prostaglandin synthesis and inhibition of leucocyte migration into nidus of inflammation. Indometacin impairs the renal bloodstream to a grater extent than other NSAIDs; therefore, it can weaken the action of diuretic and antihypertensive drugs. The combination of indometacin and potassium-saving diuretic triamterene is very dangerous since this combination provokes the development of acute renal insufficiency.

The main shortcoming of indometacin is frequent adverse reactions (in 35–50% of patients) depending on daily dose. Neurotoxic reactions including headache (due to brain edema), dizzying, obnubitation, impaired reflector activity; nephrotoxic (recommended to avoid in renal and cardiac insufficiency), and hypersensitivity (crossed allergy with Aspirin) are the most frequent.

Indometacin is the most efficient in ankylosing spondylarthritis and acute gout; also, it is used in the treatment of rheumatoid arthritis and active rheumatism. In juvenile rheumatoid arthritis, it is a reserve drug. Due to its potent anti-inflammatory effect, indometacin can maximize clinical symptoms of infections; therefore, it is not advisable for infectious patients. There is a long-standing experience in using indometacin in osteoarthrosis of hip and knee joints. However, as has been shown recently, the drug accelerates the destruction of articular cartilage in osteoarthrosis patients. Having a potent anti-inflammatory effect indometacin can varnish clinical symptoms of infections; therefore, it is not recommended to infectious patients.

The initial dose for adults is 25 mg 3 times a day, maximum doze is 150 mg a day. The dose is increased gradually. Retarded tablets and rectal suppositories are administered 1–2 times a day. Sometimes they are taken at bedtime with another NSAID during daytime. The ointment is used topically. Children are administered 2–3 mg per day in divided doses.

Sulindac is converted to an active metabolite in the liver. Maximum concentration of the metabolite in blood occurs within 3–4 hours after its administration. The half-life of sulindac is 7–8 hours and that of its active metabolite is 16–18 hours, which provides a prolonged effect and can be taken 1–2 times daily. It is used in rheumatic and nonrheumatic diseases.

Dislike indometacin, sulindac is less gastro- and nephrotoxic, has a significantly weaker effect on the renal bloodstream and glomerular filtration (since the active metabolite of sulindac does not inhibit PG synthesis in the kidneys), scarcely interacts with diuretic and antihypertensive drugs. It causes crystaluria and is not recommended to urolithiasis patients. Its hepatotoxicity is higher than that of indometacin.

Adults are administered 400 mg per day orally in divided doses and children – 4.5–6 mg/kg per day in divided doses.

Etodolac is rapidly absorbed from the gastrointestinal tract. The half-life is 7 hours. The drug is tolerated better than indometacin and its gastrotoxicity is weaker.

The indications are rheumatoid arthritis, Bekhterev's disease, osteoarthrosis, pain syndrome of different localizations. A single dose of 200 to 400 mg provides postoperative analgesia for 6 to 8 hours [13].

In internal use, the dose for adults is 200 to 400 mg every 6–8 hours. The maximal daily dose is 1200 mg. The drug is not administered to children.

Diclofenac-sodium is the most widely used NSAID. Diclofenac combines high anti-inflammatory activity and good tolerance in prolonged administration, has a potent and rapid analgesic effect, and is widely used in rheumatology. In severe pain syndrome (renal or hepatic colic, post-operative pains, traumatic pains) it is injected intramuscularly.

Diclofenac is well absorbed from the gastrointestinal tract. Bioavailability (the fraction of the medication that reaches the systemic circulation) is 50–60%. Its maximum concentration in blood occurs in 0.5–2 hours after internal intake and in 10–30 minutes after intramuscular injection. Te half-life is 1.5–2 hours. In SF, maximal concentration occurs in 4–6 hours. The half-life in the joint is 8 hours, i.e., diclofenac stays in SF longer than in blood and its concentration exceeds the therapeutic one in blood 4–5 times.

Diclofenac is tolerated well. Adverse reactions develop more rarely than when using major other NSAIDs. In protracted therapy, the drug can have negative effect on the gastrointestinal tract and especially on the liver; therefore, the clinical and laboratory control is required.

Adults take diclofenac-sodium 25–50 mg 2–3 times a day orally or rectally. Retard tablets 100 mg are administered 1-2 times a day. The intramuscular injectable dose is 75 mg 1–2 times a day; if the first dose is inefficient, the second one can be injected within 30 minutes. Children over 1.5 years old take 2–4 mg/kg in 2 intakes orally or rectally.

D*iclofenac-potassium* (Voltaren rapid) compared to diclofenac-sodium is absorbed more rapidly, mainly from the stomach and has a faster analgesic effect – within 20–30 minutes after oral taking. It is used to rapidly stop the pain.

Doses for oral administration are 100–150 mg per day in 2–3 intakes. For children the doses are not set.

Piroxicam has strong anti-inflammatory effect, which develops slowly within 1–2 weeks of continuous administration. The maximal effect is observed within 2–4 weeks. It exerts a rapid and pronounced analgesic effect, especially when injected intramuscularly.

Piroxicam is well absorbed from the gastrointestinal tract. Food inhibits the absorption. Maximal concentration in blood develops in 3–5 hours. The half-life is 45–60 hours. The equilibrium concentration in blood occurs within 7–12 days. It can develop faster if the saturation dose is taken.

As for adverse reactions, the gastrotoxicity (higher than that of Indometacin, especially in prolonged treatment with doses 30 mg and higher), hematotoxicity (thrombocytopenia, aplastic anemia, reduced hemoglobin and hematocrit level, bleedings not associated with gastrointestinal location), nephrotoxicity, and skin reactions (rash, photodermatitis) are reported.

Piroxicam is used as an anti-inflammatory drug including juvenile rheumatoid arthritis and gout. It can be used as an analgesic in postoperative and posttraumatic pains.

The drug is administered to adults 20 mg per day orally or rectally. For a rapid effect the saturation dose can be administered – 40 mg per day in one or several doses. In acute gout attack, 40 mg is taken once per day and during next 4–6 days 40 mg per day once or in divided doses. Children of a body weight within 15 kg should take 5 mg per day, 16–25 kg – 10 mg per day, 26–45 kg – 15 mg per day, and above 45 kg 20 mg per day.

Tenoxicam (Tilcotil) is similar to piroxicam in activity and pharmacokinetic parameters. Its maximal concentration in blood occurs within 1 to 2.5 hours if taken on an empty stomach and within 4-6 hours if taken after meal. The half-life is 60–75 hours. A full clinical effect develops in 2 weeks. The drug penetrates in SF well and exhibits lower gastrotoxicity than piroxicam.

For adults the recommended doses are 20 mg per day in a single dose rectally or intramuscularly. For children the doses are not set.

Lornoxicam is a NSAID belonging to the oxicam group (chlortenoxicam) and used in rheumatology to treat rheumatoid arthritis, psoriatic arthritis, and osteoarthrosis. As for the COX inhibition, it surpasses other oxicams and almost equally inhibits COX-1 and COX-2 taking the intermediate position in the NSAID classification based on the selectivity principle. It has the pronounced analgesic and anti-inflammatory effects. Its analgesic effect consists in inhibiting pain impulses and increasing the threshold of pain sensitivity if the receptors (especially in chronic diseases). In intravenous injections, the drug increases the level of endogene opioids (chemical compounds synthesized in the organism and having the opium properties) activating physiological antinociceptive system of organism (reduced sensitivity to pain). Indications for lornoxicam are acute and chronic pains including oncological. In intravenous injection of 8 mg it is not inferior to narcotic analgesics (promedol). When taken perorally, 8 mg of Lornoxicam is equivalent to 10 mg of ketorolac, 400 mg of ibuprofen, and 650 mg of aspirin in the patients with post-operative pains. In severe pain syndrome, lornoxicam is co-administered with opioid analgesics to reduce the dose of these latter.

Lornoxicam is well absorbed from the gastrointestinal tract. Food reduces to some extent the bioavailability of the drug. Maximum concentrations in blood plasma occur within 1–2 hours. In intramuscular injections, its maximum content in plasma is reached in 15 minutes. It penetrates easily in SF where its concentration is 50% of the concentration in blood plasma and is maintained in it for 10–12 hours. It is metabolized in the liver and excreted mainly through the bowels and kidneys. Its half-life is 3–5 hours.

Lornoxicam has a lower gastrotoxicity than first-generation oxicams (piroxicam, tenoxicam). This is due to a short half-life period which makes it possible to recover the protective level of PG in the mucous coat of the gastrointestinal tract. As for tolerance, lornoxicam surpasses indometacin and is not inferior to diclofenac.

For adults, the doses in pain syndrome are 8 mg twice a day orally, also the single impact dose 16 mg can be taken orally, and 8–16 mg intramuscularly or intravenously (1–2 doses with an interval of 8–12 hours); in rheumatology, it is taken orally 4–8 mg twice a day. Doses for children are not set.

Meloxicam, a selective inhibitor of COX-2, belongs to new-generation NSAIDs used to treat rheumatoid arthritis and osteoarthrosis. It selectively inhibits PG formation involved in inflammation. At the same time, meloxicam inhibits much weaker COX-1; therefore, it affects less the synthesis of PG regulating the renal bloodstream, production of protective mucus in the stomach and aggregation of tromobocytes. Meloxicam is not inferior to piroxicam, naproxen, and diclofenac in anti-inflammatory activity and causes less adverse reactions in the gastrointestinal tract and kidneys [14].

The bioavailability of meloxicam taken orally is 89% irrespective of meal. Maximum concentration in blood occurs within 5-6 hours and equilibrium concentration is achieved in 3–5 days. The half-life is 20 hours, which makes it possible to administer the drug once a day. Meloxicam passes well through histogematogeneous barriers, penetrates into SF where its concentration is 50% of that in blood plasma.

For adults, the dose is 7.5–15 mg once a day orally or intramuscularly. The efficacy and safety of the drug for children has not been studied.

Nabumeton (Relafen) selectively inhibits COX-2 in rheumatoid arthritis and osteoarthrosis similarly to meloxicam. It is well absorbed and food accelerates absorption. Active metabolite arises in the liver with the half-life about 24 hours. Adverse reactions in the gastrointestinal tract are encountered more rarely compared to other NSAIDs.

Adults are administered 1000 mg once a day and in individual cases 1500–2000 mg a day taken twice irrespective of meal. For children the doses are not set.

Ibuprofen is inferior to many other drugs of the group in question in anti-inflammatory activity. When taken 1200 mg and more, it yields satisfactory anti-inflammatory effect. Analgesic and antipyretic activity prevails over anti-inflammatory activity.

Maximum concentration of the drug in blood develops within 1-2 hours after oral administration. Ibuprofen is rapidly metabolized and excreted from the organism. Its half-life is 1.8–2.5 hours due to which the analgesic and antipyretic effects are maintained within 8 hours. Its advantage is good tolerance and rare adverse reactions. Ibuprofen is one of the least gastrotoxic NSAIDs.

It is largely used as an analgesic and in mild rheumatoid arthritis and osteoarthrosis. For adults the dose is 400–600 mg 3–4 times a day, retarded formulations – 600–1200 mg twice a day. Children are prescribed 20–40 mg per day. In the USA ibuprofen has been available over-the-counter since 1995 to children above 2 years old in fever and pains 7.5 mg/kg up to 4 times a day, maximum 30 mg/kg per day.

Naproxen is one of NSAIDs most often used in rheumatism, ankylosing arthritis, and rheumatoid arthritis in adults and children. The drug inhibits the activity of proteoglykanase enzyme thus preventing degenerative changes in the articular cartilage in osteoarthrosis.

Naproxen surpasses ibuprofen in anti-inflammatory activity. The anti-inflammatory effect develops slowly and reaches maximum within 2 to 4 weeks. It has potent analgesic and antipyretic effects. The antiaggregatory effect manifests only when high doses are administered. The drug is well absorbed when taken orally or rectally. Maximum concentration occurs in 2–3 hours after oral administration. The half-life is 12–15 hours, which allows its administration 1–2 times a day.

Its gastrotoxicity is lower than that of indometacin, Aspirin, and piroxicam. Nephrotoxicity is observed, as a rule, in patients with renal pathologies and in cardiac insufficiency. Allergic reactions and cross allergy with aspirin are possible.

For adults, it is recommended to take 500–1000 mg per day orally or rectally. The daily dose can be increased up to 1500 mg for a limited period (within 2 weeks). In acute pain syndrome (bursitis or tendovaginitis), the first dose is 500 mg, then 250 mg each 6–8 hours. For children the doses are 10–20 mg/kg in divided doses; as antipyretic a single dose is 15 mg/kg.

Naproxen-sodium (Aliv, Apranax) differs from naproxen in more rapid absorption from the gastrointestinal tract and higher bioavailability. The analgesic effect develops within 15 minutes and maximum concentration in blood occurs within 1 hour. The half-life is 13 hours, which allow it to be taken once or twice a day.

Naproxen-sodium is taken as a fast-acting analgesic and anti-inflammatory drug in rheumatology, in postoperative pains and traumas. It is similar to naproxen in anti-inflammatory activity.

The dose for adults is 220–550 mg 1–2 times a day, for children – 10–20 mg/kg per day in divided doses.

Flubiprofen is close to naproxen in pharmacodynamics. Adverse reactions are possible in the gastrointestinal tract, in the form of skin rash, and bronchospasms. Maximum concentration in blood develops 1.5 hours after oral administration. The half-life is within 3–9 hours. In adults, the dose is 50–100 mg 3–4 times daily, and in children 4 mg/kg in 2–4 intakes.

Ketoprofen has evident anti-inflammatory and analgesic effects being not inferior to indometacin, diclofenac, and better than ibuprofen and piroxicam. The doses 50–100 mg have a stronger analgesic effect than combined drugs such as Paracetamol/Codeine and Aspirin/Codeine.

Its indications are rheumatoid and gouty arthritis, osteoarthrosis, pain syndrome (postoperative and posttraumatic pains, pains in oncological diseases). In acute closed traumas of soft tissues, ketoprofen can be used topically in gel form. It is better than similar formulations of diclofenac and piroxicam in efficacy. In severe pains, ketoprofen is often co-administered with narcotic analgesics.

It is well absorbed at different routes of administration. It is capable of crossing rapidly the hemato-encephalic barrier owing to its absolute fat solubility. The drug has a central analgesic affect at the level of posterior columns of the spinal cord via inhibition of depolarization of their neurons. Maximum concentration in blood develops 1–2 hours after oral administration, 2.4–4 hours after rectal administration, and 15-20 minutes after intravenous injection. The half-life is 1.6–1.9 hours.

Gastrointestinal side effects are possible. In rare cases the renal and kidney impairment, headache, ringing in the ears, and visual disorders are noticed. Also, allergic reactions may occur.

Adults are prescribed 100–300 mg daily in 2–3 doses orally or rectally (one can combine tablets and capsules with suppositories, e.g., 1 capsule (50 mg) in the morning and at daytime and 1 suppository (100 mg) at bedtime) and intramuscularly 100 mg 1–2 times a day. Short-term infusions (100–200 mg of ketaprofen in 100 ml of physiological sodium chloride solution every 8 hours) are executed intravenously and take from 0.5 to 1 hour: Infusions are executed during 8 hours (100–200 mg in 500 ml of physiological sodium chloride solution (or glucose solution)) every 8 hours. In prolonged infusion, ketoprofen can be mixed with 10–20 mg of morphine but not with tramadol because of sediment. The doses for children are not set.

Tiaprofenic acid is similar to naproxen in anti-inflammatory activity and has an evident analgesic effect. It is well absorbed from the gastrointestinal tract when taken orally. Maximum concentration in blood develops in an hour. The half-life is 3 hours. The data are available on the positive effects of this drug on the metabolism of articular cartilage.

It can irritate the bladder lining and lead to cystitis, which manifests in hematuria and dysuria. Therefore, it should not be used in patients with the diseases of the urinary tract and prostate especially if they are indicated in the history.

The recommended doses for adults are 300 mg twice a day. In patients with renal, kidney, and cardiac impairment the dose is 200 mg twice a day. For children the doses are not set.

Fenoprofen (Nalfon) is identical to naproxen in anti-inflammatory activity and to Aspirin in analgesic activity. Maximum concentration in blood occurs in 2 hours after oral administration. The half-life is about 3 hours.

For adults the doses are 200–300 mg 3 to 4 times daily. For children the doses are not set.

Celecoxib is a new-generation NSAID, a selective COX-2 inhibitor, referring to a group of nonacid derivatives (is a derivative of sulfonamide). It selectively breaks the formation of PG involved in inflammation reaction and does not affect the production of PG regulating the renal bloodstream and integrity of the mucous coat of gastrointestinal tract. It does not inhibit the synthesis of thromboxane and aggregation of platelets. It is recommended in rheumatoid arthritis and osteoarthrosis.

The drug is well absorbed from the gastrointestinal tract and its peak concentration in blood develops within 3 hours. Food, especially fatty, retards absorption but increases the dose by 10–20%. It is metabolized in the liver and excreted with feces and urine. The half-life is 11 hours and can be longer in impairment of hepatic function.

As a selective COX-2 inhibitor, celecoxib leads more rarely to side effects in the gastrointestinal tract than other NSAIDs. Headache, dizzying, rashes, rhinitis, and dyssomnia) can occur. No data on nephrotoxic reactions are available.

Celecoxib interacts with fluconasol with the concentration of the former in blood plasma increasing twice due to its metabolism in the liver. Celecoxib increases the lithium concentration in plasma. There are no data on Celecoxib interaction with diuretics, antihypertensive drugs, indirect anticoagulants, and methotrexate.

For adults the dosage is 100–200 mg daily in divided doses. The doses for children below 18 years old are not set.

NSAIDs with mild anti-inflammatory activity are used mainly as analgesics and antipyretics.

Mefenamic acid (Ponstel) is inferior to the drugs of the previous group in anti-inflammatory effect. The treatment course should not last more than a week.

It is slowly absorbed from the gastrointestinal tract and metabolized in part in the liver; its half-life is 4 hours. It is known to cause side effects (in 25% of patients), especially upset stomach. Other side effects include diarrhea associated with colitis, hepatotoxicity, hemolytic anemia, and allergic reactions. In elder patients, nonoliguric renal insufficiency can develop, especially in dehydration.

For adults the first dose is 500 mg, then 250 mg 4 times a day. For children above 14 years old the single dose 6.5 mg/kg is used. The drug is not administered to children below 14 years old.

Etofenamate (Reumon gel, Etogel) is a topical drug. It has local anti-inflammatory and analgesic properties. The indications are bursitis, tendovaginitis, articular syndrome, myositis, lumbago, sprains, displacements, and bruises.

A column of 5–10 cm of 5% gel is applied directly to an inflamed tissue and slowly rubbed into it 2–3 times a day. It is not recommended to apply the gel to the damaged skin.

Metamizole is used as an analgesic and antipyretic. Despite its structural affinity to phenylbutazone, its anti-inflammatory effect is much lower. This is due to a weak effect of metamizole on PG synthesis in inflammations. It has an evident analgesic effect due to mainly blocking the passage of pain impulses in the spinal cord. Dislike other NSAIDs it possesses antispasmodic activity. The drug is well and almost fully absorbed. Maximum concentration develops within 1–2 hours. The half-life is 2.5 hours. The pareneteral route is used to provide a quick effect. There is a risk of hematological complications characteristic of all pyrazolones and pyrazolidines.

The metamizole dose administered to adults is 0.5–1 g 3 to 4 times daily intramuscularly and 2–5 ml of 50% solution intravenously 2 to 4 times daily. For children the recommended dose is 5–10 mg/kg 3 to 4 times a day. In hyperthermia 0.01 ml/kg of 50% solution is injected intravenously or intramuscularly to infants below 1 year old and 01. ml/kg per injection to infants above 1 year old.

Aminofenazone (Amidopyrin) has been used for many years as an analgesic and antipyretic. It is more toxic than metamizole and cause severe skin allergic reactions, especially in combination with sulfanilamide. Presently, aminofenazone is prohibited to use and its manufacture is declined since its interaction with food nitrites can give rise to cancerogenic compounds. Nevertheless, aminofenazone-containing preparations are still sold in drugstores (Omazol, Anapyrin, Pentalgin, Pyrabutol, Pyranal, Pyrcophenum, Rheopyrin, Theophedrin H).

Propiphenazone displays powerful analgesic and antipyretic properties. It is well absorbed from the gastrointestinal tract and its maximum concentration develops 30 minutes after oral administration.

It is the safest drug compared to other pyrazolone derivatives. Agranulocytosis is not reported in its administration. In rare cases the platelet and leucocyte reduction is reported.

It is not used as a mono-drug but is a constituent of combined drugs such as Saridon and Plivalgin.

Phenacetin is well absorbed from the gastrointestinal tract, metabolized in the liver with its part transforming into active metabolite paracetamol. Its other metabolites are toxic. The half-life is 2 to 3 hours.

Phenacetin has high nephrotoxicity. It can cause tubulointerstitial nephritis due to ischemic lesions in the kidneys that manifest in lumbar pains, dysuria, hematuria, proteinuria, cylindruria (analgesic nephropathy, phenacetinic kidney), and severe renal damage. Nephotoxic effects are evident in protracted treatment when co-administered with other analgesics and are encountered most often in women. Phenacetin metabolites can cause formation of methemoglobin and hemolysis. The preparation exhibits cancerogenous properties, i.e., a risk of bladder cancer. In many countries is it prohibited for usage.

It is administered to adults 250−500 mg 2 daily in divided doses. It is not used in children.

The drug enters the combined preparations such as Pyrcofen, Sedalgin, Theophedrin H tablets, and “Cefecon” suppositories.

Paracetamol is an active metabolite of phenacetin. It is less toxic compared to phenacetin. It inhibits the PG synthesis in the central nervous system and to a lesser degree in peripheral tissues and exhibits mainly “central” analgesic and antipyretic effects with a very low peripheral anti-inflammatory activity. The anti-inflammatory effect can be seen only at a low peroxide compound content of tissues, e.g., in osteoarthrosis, acute trauma of soft tissues, but not in rheumatic diseases.

Presently, paracetamol is classified as an efficient analgesic and antipyretic for wide applications. It can be used in the absence of contradictions to aspirin and other NSAIDs by patients with bronchial asthma, ulcerous history as well as by children with viral infections. Paracetamol is close to aspirin in analgesic and antipyretic activity.

Paracetamol is well absorbed in oral and rectal administration. Paracetamol absorption from the gastrointestinal tract is enhanced by metoclopramide and coffeine. Its maximal concentration in blood develops within 0.5 to 2 hours. The drug is metabolized in the liver in two stages, i.e., first under the action of enzymatic systems of cytochrome P-450 intermediate hepatotoxic metabolites arise which afterwards are splitted with glutathione involved. An amount of less than 5% of paracetamol is excreted in invariable form by the kidneys. The half-life is 2 to 2.5 hours. The effect lasts 3 to 4 hours.

Paracetamol is one of the safest NSAIDs. It does not display gastrotoxicity, does not affect platelet aggregation and does not induce agranulocytosis and aplastic anemia. However, it poorly inhibits intensive pain syndrome in joints. According to the data of work [15], in long-term administration of paracetamol more than 1 tablet daily (1000 and more tablet during a lifetime) a risk of severe analgesic nephropathy increases twice, which leads to terminal renal insufficiency. It is due to nephrotoxic effect of paracetamol metabolites, especially paraaminophenol that is accumulated in renal papillae inducing severe cell dysfunction and structure damages that make them die. At the same time, systematic administration of aspirin is not associated with the similar risk. Hepatoxicity of paracetamol becomes evident in very high doses. A single administration of a dose more than 10 g in adults and more than 140 mg/kg in children results in intoxication followed by severe hepatic abnormalities. This is due to exhausted glutathione and accumulation of paracetamol metabolites having hepatotoxic effect.

Inducers (activators) of hepatic enzymes (barbiturates, rifampicin, difenin, etc.) accelerate the splitting of paracetamol into hepatotoxic metabolites and increase a risk of hepatic lesions.

The intoxication with paracetamol can be observed in individuals taking paracetamol systematically. Even therapeutic doses of the drug can cause hepatotoxicity, especially if the drug is taken in shortly after taking alcohol [16].

In intoxication with paracetamol, the stomach washing, vomiting, activated carbon, 20% solution of Acetylcysteine, intravenous glucose, and intramuscular vitamin K_1 1−10 mg are recommended.

For adults the doses of paracetamol are 500−1000 mg 4 times per day. For children 10−15 mg/kg 4 to 6 times a day are administered.

Ketorolac has a potent analgesic effect exceeding many NSAIDs. A dose of 30 mg injected intramuscularly is identical to 12 mg of morphine with the side effects characteristic of morphine and other narcotic analgesics (nausea, vomiting, aspiration inhibition, stool and urinary retention) being observed more rarely. Taking of ketorolac does not lead to drug dependence. In combination with opioid analgesics the analgesic effect is enhanced which leads to lower dosage. Intravenous or intraarticular injections of ketorolac co-administered with local anesthetics (Lidocaine, Bupivacaine) enhance the analgesic effect after traumas, operations on extremities, and in oncological patients (in metastases in bones). Ketorolac has antipyretic and antiaggregation effects.

The drug is well and almost fully absorbed from the gastrointestinal tract, and its bioavailability is 80–100%. Maximum concentration in blood develops within 35 minutes after oral administration and 50 minutes after intramuscular injection. It is excreted by the kidneys. The half-life is 5 to 6 hours.

Benefits of ketorolac administration prior to operations in combination with morphine or fentanyl are reported. This allows reduction of opioid analgesic doses by 25–50% during first 1–2 days after operation, facilitates the recovery of gastrointestinal tract functioning, leads to lower vomiting and nausea, and reduces the terms of in-patient period [17].

Ketorolac is not advisable in operations with a high risk of bleeding, in labor pain relief, and reduction of pain syndrome in myocardial infarction.

For adults, the dose is 10 mg every 4 to 6 hours orally, the highest dose is 40 mg, the duration of therapy is within 7 days. The intramuscular and intravenous dose is 10–30 mg, the highest dose is 90 mg, the duration of therapy is within 2 days. For children the first dose is 0.5–1 mg/kg, then 0.25–0.5 mg/kg every 6 hours.

Combined products contain in addition to NSAIDs other drugs, which enhance the analgesic effect of NSAIDs, increase their bioavailability, and reduce the risk of adverse reactions.

Saridon consists of paracetamol, propiphenazone, and coffeine. It is administered to relieve pain syndrome of different localization (rheumatic diseases, headache, toothache, fever, etc.).

The analgesics act as synergists in the drug, i.e., they enhance the effect of each other and, in addition, paracetamol increases the bioavailability of propiphenazone. Coffeine in the recommended dose normalizes brain vascular tonus and accelerates the bloodstream without stimulating the central nervous system; therefore, it enhances the analgesic effect in headache. Moreover, it improves the absorption of paracetamol. Saridon is characterized by high bioavailability and rapid development of analgesic effect.

Plivalgin is produced in the form of tablets each of which contains paracetamol and propinfenazone 210 mg, coffeine 50 mg, phenobarbital 25 mg, and codeine phosphate 10 mg. Its analgesic effect is enhanced by analgesic codeine and sedative phenobarbital. The indications are articular and muscular pains, head- and toothaches, neuralgia, and fever.

Plivalgin is administered orally 1 to 2 tablets 3 to 4 times daily. In frequent use, especially in elevated doses, fatigue and sleepiness can occur. Drug dependence can develop as well.

Reopyrin (Pyrabutol) contains aminofenazone (amidopyrin) and phenylbutazone (butadion). During many years, the drug was widely used as analgesic. However, it does not have any benefits over modern NSAIDs but surpasses them considerably in the severity of side effects. Hematological complications are especially high probable, therefore, precautions should be observed in reopyrin administration and other analgesics are preferable. In intramuscular injections phenylbutazone is bound by tissues in the place of injection and is poorly absorbed, which retards the analgesic effect and leads to infiltrates, abscesses, and damages of sciatic nerve. The doses for adults are 1 to 2 tablets 3 to 4 times daily or 2–3 mg intramuscularly 1 to 2 times daily. The drug is not administered to children.

Presently, combined products consisting of phenylbutazone and aminophenazone are forbidden in most countries.

Baralgin is a combination of metamizole (Analgin) and two antispasmodics one of which – pitofenone has a myotropic effect and another – fenpiverinium – has an atropine-like effect. It is indicated in pains due to spasms in smooth muscles (renal colic, hepatic colic, etc). Like other drugs with atropine-like activity, it is not used in glaucoma and prostate adenoma.

Therapeutic doses are 1 to 2 tablets 3 to 4 times a day, or 3–5 ml intramuscularly or intravenously 2 to 3 times a day. The rate of intravenous injection is 1.1.5 ml per minute.

Artropotec consists of diclofenac and mizoprostol (synthetic analog of PG-E_1), which allows reduction of frequency and power of gastrotoxic reactions characteristic of diclofenac. Artrotec is equal to diclofenac in efficiency, while erosions and ulcers are reported much more rarely.

Adults take 1–2 tablets daily in divided doses. One tablet of artrotec contains 50 mg of diclofenac and 200 mg of mizoprostol.

In conclusion, we should note that these drugs are contradicted to individuals with intolerance to drug components and allergic reactions. Relative contradictions are ulcerous disease of stomach and duodenum, acute stages of chronic gastritis, bronchial asthma, asthmatic bronchitis, pollinosis, and other conditions associated with damaged reactivity of immunity system. When choosing a drug to treat joints, activity and pharmacological effects of NSAIDs are taken into account. At the initial stage of therapy, less toxic drugs are preferred in minimal doses, afterwards the dose increases up to efficient or maximal. The monotherapy principle should be followed since co-administration of several drugs increases the risk of adverse reactions and competition for protein binding.

5.1.2. Glucocorticoid Anti-Inflammatory Drugs

The adrenal cortex of mammals and man produce steroidal hormones called corticosteroids. They are derivatives of pregnan (following IUPAC nomenclature the corticosteroid name includes a root "pregn" with different endings, e.g. with "-an" for saturated steroids) and are divided in three groups in chemical c composition: 11-desoxysteroids, 11-oxysteroids, and 11-, 17-oxysteroids. In their effect on the metabolism, corticosteroids are divided into mineral corticosteroids and glucocorticosteroids (GC) [18].

GCs are believed to be biological hormones of the second-stress phase produced by the organism to mobilize all forces after the first-phase stress hormone – adrenalin – has been exhausted. Adrenalin stops its activity since it decays very rapidly. The first GC hormone – cortisone was extracted in 1948 from bile acids. Afterwards, it was found that cortisone was biologically inert and hydrocortisone (cortisol) was an active natural hormone of adrenal cortex. Cortisone is converted into biologically active cortisol in the hepatic cells. In addition to cortisol, the adrenal cortex also produces corticosteron, mineral corticoids, androgens, estrogens, and progesterone. As for chemical composition, they are related to 11, 17-oxysteroids.

Cortisol is secreted rhythmically corresponding to the influence of stress mechanisms and negative feedback in hypothalamic-pituitary-adrenoctortical axis. In the absence of additional stimulation (stress, hormones, etc.) impulse secretion of cortisol occurs 8–12 times a day with maximum early in the morning (cortisol concentration in blood is 140–500 nmol/l) and minimum at midnight (15–20% of maximum). Normally, 10–30 mg of cortisol and 1–4 mg of corticosterone are secreted daily. Within a body, GCs are found in free (5–7%) and protein-bound forms. The main binding protein – transcortin – is α-globulin. Biological activity of bound hormones decreases, however, they break and are excreted more slowly. Enzymatic decomposition of GCs occurs in hepatic cells with formation of cortol, cortolone, and 17-ketosteroids that are excreted by the kidneys and intestines in the form of glucuronic and sulfuric acids.

The adrenal gland work is regulated with corticotropin (adrenocorticotropic hormone – ACTH), i.e., a peptide neurohormone produced by the anterior pituitary. ACTH is a polypeptide in chemical structure consisting of 39 amino acids, 15 of which have immunological activity inducing allergic reactions. Adrenal cortex reacts to ACTH production for 2 minutes, its half-life in blood plasma is within 10 minutes. ACTH accelerates cholesterol synthesis and its transportation from blood plasma to tissues, stimulates synthesis of progesterone and pregenolone, which are constituents of sex hormones, gluco- and mineralocorticoids. In the absence of ACTH, the adrenal cortex is atrophied.

Synthesis of corticotropin is controlled, in turn, by hypothalamus through corticoliberine polyopeptide. Its production depends on the level of circulating glucocorticoids and external factors. A high concentration of GCs in blood plasma inhibits the liberation of corticoliberine and further ACTH and gydrocortisone, which leads to hypofunctioning and atrophy of adrenal cortex.

Pharmacological Properties of GCs

In joint therapy anti-inflammatory, immunosuppressive, anti-allergic, antitoxic, and antimitotic biological properties of GCs performed at the molecular and cellular levels are of importance. GCs cross the cellular membranes and form complexes with specific cytoplasmic receptors. These complexes, in turn, penetrate into cell nuclei and depress genes regulators of protein synthesis. As the results of this suppression, the regulation of carbohydrate, lipid, protein and water-saline metabolism is impaired. Clinically, metabolism impairment is shown in increasing glucose level in blood (stimulation of glucogenesis, reduced transportation of glucose to cells) and atrophy of protein-rich tissues, namely, muscular and bone. Reduced activity of vitamin D results in reducing absorption of calcium ions and their enhanced excretion (negative balance of calcium within a body), which leads to retardation of growth in children, and osteoporosis in adults. In this case bloating around the hips, stomach, back and face, the so-called Itsenko-Cushing's syndrome, occurs (N.M. Itsenko, the Soviet neuropathologist and H.W. Cushing, the American neurosurgeon).

Cortisol and corticosteron have a mineralocorticoid activity. Similarly, to mineralocorticoids, they increase the resorption of sodium, chloride, bicarbonates and water ions in distant channels of the kidneys. Uric excretion of potassium and hydrogen vice versa increases. This explains the occurrence of electrolyte imbalance within the body in treatment with GC.

The nonspecific anti-inflammatory effect of GC is associated with induction of lipocortin synthesis, which results in inhibited activity of phospholipase A_2 and inhibition of anti-inflammatory PG and leucotriene synthesis that favors dilatation and increasing exudation, i.e., escape of the protein-rich fluid from capillaries to surrounding tissues. Stabilization of the membranes of cells and lysosomes, reduction of permeability of capillary endothelium, improvement of microcirculation, reduced bloating of leucocytes and fatty cells, and reduced amount of serum proteins and hydropic fluid in inflamed tissues favor the inhibition of inflammation.

The immunosuppressive action of GC is due to the inhibition of immunogenesis stages, i.e., migration of stem cells (cells of bone marrow), movability of leucocytes and functional activity of macrophages. The number of B- and T-lymphocytes (mainly T-helpers) decreases in the blood, their interaction and antibody formation is broken. GCs reduce the adhesion of leucocyte to vessel endothelium, synthesis of cyclic endoperoxides, and formation of free radicals. The compelement system, formation of immune complexes, and their fixation to cell membranes are inhibited. At the same time, synthesis of anti-inflammatory cytokines (interleukins-1, -2, and -8) and tumor necrosis are inhibited.

The antimitotic effect of GC is due to the inhibition of fibroblast division and decreasing effect of histamine, serotonin, and kinins whose formation is also inhibited by GC. In high doses, GCs inhibit the development of lymphoid and connective tissues including macrophage-containing reticuloendothelium. However, a period of therapeutic remission in joints does not exceed 4 weeks and within 6–8 weeks the therapeutic effect disappears [19].

GCs under usage in modern medicine are synthetic analogs of natural human and animal hormones produced by the adrenal cortex.

Systemic local (see 5.3.1) therapy of joint inflammation with GCs is performed following strict indications. Their administration is recommended in active arthritis with effusion into the joint cavity (in rheumatoid arthritis, seronegative spondylarthritis, systemic diseases of connective tissue, etc.), reactive synovitis of different genesis (in osteoarthrosis, gouty arthritis, traumas, etc.), inflammations of periarticular connective and synovial tissues (periarthritis, tendinits, tendovaginitis, bursitis, enthesitis) of non-infectious genesis. These drugs are administered in the case of NSAID inefficiency as well as in rapid progress and development of systemic manifestations of a disease.

Prior to GC administration, it is recommended to determine the ACTH and cortisol level to detect a glucocorticoid hypofunction and once is diagnosed to test ACTH to determine functional reserves of the adrenal gland. [2]. After long-term GC treatment, the functions of the pituitary and adrenal cortex as producers of ACTH and natural GC recover during 6 to 9 months. During this period, the risk of acute adrenal insufficiency is very high in patients. Therefore, GC doses should be tapered. During first 3 to 4 days after GC withdrawal, small doses of corticotrophin are administered (10–20 units of activity) to stimulate the function of the adrenal cortex [18]. In order to reduce side effects, a sufficient amount of protein, reduced amount of chlorides, and increased amount of potassium are required. Also, arterial pressure, blood glucose, blood coagulability, diuresis, and body weight should be controlled.

GC Nomenclature

Presently about 70 trade names of GC hormones are available. Depending on the duration of biological activity (duration of ACTH inhibition) of the active substances of GC, the drugs are divided into three groups: short-term action – 24 to 36 hours (hydrocortisone, prednisone, methylprednisolone), medium-term action – within 48 hours (triamcinolone), and long-term action – more than 48 hours (dexamethasone, bethamethazone).

Hydrocortisone (hydrocortisone acetate, Cortisol, sodium hydrocortisone succinate, Solu-cortef, etc.) is used to treat non-infectious arthritis of different etiologies, synovitis in osteoarthrosis, humeroscapular periarthritis, bursitis, epicondylitis, and tendovaginitis.

Hydrocortisone in tablets is well absorbed. Its maximum concentration in blood occurs within an hour. After intramuscular injection, the absorption occurs slowly (24 to 28 hours). Up to 40–60% of the injected drug is bound to blood plasma proteins, and readily cross the mucous membranes and SM. The medicinal effect in intra-articular injection occurs within 6 to 24 hours and lasts within several weeks. It is metabolized in the liver and excreted with urine and bile. In local administration in form of applications, it is accumulated mostly in the grainy layer of epidermis.

The initial dose of hydrocortisone is 20 to 240 mg in tablets daily. The maintaining dose is found by gradually decreasing the initial dose to a minimum to achieve the desirable effect. 125–250 mg of the drug is injected intramuscularly deep into the buttock. Depot-forms of GCs in form of suspensions are injected intra- and peri-articulalry 25–50 mg in major joints (shoulder, hip, or knee) (in acute conditions up to 100 mg) and 5–20 mg once in small joints (elbow, middle carpeal, and interphalangeal joints). Injections are repeated within 7–10 days. In children within 3 months to a year old hydrocortisone is injected intra- or peri-articulalry 25 mg, within 1 to 6 year old 25–50 mg, and from 6 to 14 years old – 50–75 mg. The effect occurs within 6–25 hours and lasts several days or weeks. In combination with NSAID, a GC dose can be reduced because of the cumulative therapeutic effect.

The interaction of hydrocortisone with other drugs can lead to adverse reactions. Hydrocortisone increases a risk of hepatotoxic action of paracetamol (induction of hepatic enzymes and formation of a toxic metabolite of paracetamol). Indometacin increases a risk of adverse effects because of displacing GC from the bond with albumins. Hydrocortisone weakens the influence of vitamin D on the absorption of Ca^{2+} in the bowels. In combination with amphotericin B and carbonic anhydrase inhibitors, a risk of osteoporosis increases. Estrogen-containing drugs prolongate the half-life of GCs and their therapeutic and toxic effects. Co-administration of GCs with m-cholinoblockers (including antihistamine drugs and tricyclic antisuppresssants) or with nitrates increases intraocular pressure. Hydrocortisone increases the toxicity of cardiac glycosides (a risk of arrhythmia is due to hypokaliemia). The co-administration of hydrocortisone and living viral vaccines as well as against the background of other immune events increases a risk of microorganism activation and development of infections. Antacids that neutralize hydrochlocric acid of the gastric juice reduce the absorption of GC from the gastrointestinal tract. The curative effect of GCs decreases under the effect of barbiturates, ephedrine, theophylline, rifampicin, and other inducers of hepatic microsomal enzymes.

Prednisolone (Medopred, Prednisolone Hafslund Nycomed, Prednisolone-Rivopharm, etc.) has a potent anti-inflammatroy effect. The anti-inflammatroy action of 5 mg of prednisolone is equivalent to 4 mg of methylprednisolone or triacinolone, 0.75 mg of dexamethazone, 0.6 mg of betamethazone, and 20 mg of hydrocortisone. The mineralocorticoidal cativity of prednisolone is about 60% of that of hydrocortisone.

Prednisolone is well absorbed from the gastrointestinal tract. Maximum concentration in blood plasma occurs within 90 minutes. Its major part is bound to transcortin (cortisol-binding globulin). The drug is mainly metabolized in the liver, 20% of prednisolone being excreted with the kidneys. The half-life is about 200 minutes.

The dosage is set individually according to indications, therapy efficacy, and patient's condition. According to the daily rhythm of endogenous GC secretion, the drug is recommended to take once in the morning. In some cases, the drug is administered more than once a day. In acute conditions and as a suppressing dose 20–30 mg per day (4 to 6 tablets) cane be taken with maximum daily dose 200 mg. irrespective of its unique structure, properties, and functions. The maintaining dose is 5–10 mg daily (1–2 tablets). In children, prednisolone is administered based on 1–2 mg/kg of body weight in 3–4 intakes (in acute cases it may be 1–2 mg/kg per day). After achieving a desirable medicinal effect, the dose is reduced down to minimally efficient.

Methylprednisolone (Depo-Medrol, methylprednisolone acetate, Metipred, Solumedrol, Urbazon, etc.) is a synthetic analog of prednisolone and has more evident and faster anti-inflammatory and anti-allergic effects, delayed immunosuppressive action, and low mineralocorticoid activity.

The anti-inflammatory activity of methyprednisolone is 5 times higher than that of hydrocortisone. 8 mg of methylprednisolone is identical to 40 mg of cortisol. Since the mineral corticoid activity of methylprednisolon is not so much evident, the electrolyte concentrations in blood serum remain unvaried and maintained within the normal values even when high doses of the drug are used. In protracted treatment with methylprednosolone, the same as other GCs a sufficient potassium and lower sodium amounts should be provided.

In oral administration, more than 70% of the drug is absorbed. In deep intramuscular injections the absorption is full and rapid (from hip muscles more rapidly than from buttocks). The bioavailability in intramuscular injection is 89%. The binding with proteins (only with albumin) is 62% irrespective of the dose injected. Maximum concentration in blood serum occurs within 1.5 hours in oral administration, within 0.5–1 hour in intramuscular, and within 15 minutes in intravenous injections. The half-life is 3 to 4 hours. Methylprednisolone is metabolized mainly in the liver; metabolites (11-keto- and 20-oxyconjugates) do not have hormone activity and are excreted mainly with urine and feces. The duration of action exceeds the duration of the drug life (12 to 36 hours) in blood. Methylprednisolone readily crosses vascular and tissue barriers. Methyprednisolone acetate (Depo-Medrol) intended for intramuscular injections is absorbed more slowly and has longer action. In particular, the effect of an injection of 80 mg lasts for 12 hours and the suppressive action of the systemic reaction to the cortisone level in blood is observed during 17 days.

A methylprednisolone dose depends on the kind and severity of a disease as well as individual patient's reaction. A daily oral dose can be 4 to 96 mg. In the beginning of treatment, high doses are used, afterwards reduced to a maintaining one (4 to 6 mg). After protracted administration, the drug is tapered. If a high dose is used for several days, an instantaneous withdrawal is permitted. If the treatment lasts for 3 to 4 weeks 12 mg daily, the dose is reduced by 4 mg daily, with a daily dose of above 12 mg – by 2 mg every 2–3 days or by 4 mg every 4–6 days. In longer treatment with a maintaining dose, it should be tapered by

2 mg each 2–3 days and 2 mg should be taken every other day during the last week of administration.

Depo-forms of methylprednisolone of prorogated action are prescribed intramuscularly. The week dose 40 to 120 mg equivalent to sevenfold daily dose is injected once intramuscularly in rheumatoid arthritis. The effect occurs within 6–48 hours and lasts within 14 days. The depot-forms are prescribed for intra-articular, peri-articular, and intrabursal in injections doses are 20 to 40 mg for major joints, 20 mg for medium, and 10 mg for small joints. Peri-articular injection of 20–100 mg of the drug should have an interval of 4 to 6 days.

Triamcinocolone (Aristocort, Kenalog, Kenacort, Polcortolon, Triamcinolone acetonide, Flogicort, etc.) produces an anti-inflammatory effect by inhibiting T-lymphocytes and acidophilic granulocytes in the connective tissue. The mechanisms of immune therapy are as follows: reduced binding of immunoglobulins to the cell receptors; inhibited synthesis and liberation of anti-inflammatory cytokines; less pronounced immune response; reduced concentration of the complement system and immunoglobulins at the site of inflammation. In therapeutic doses, the drug does not lead to retention of sodium ions and swellings, increasing potassium ion liberation, and elevated arterial pressure.

After oral administration, the bioavailability of triamcinocolone is 20–30%. It is metabolized in the liver, is excreted by the kidneys in the form if inactive metabolites. In adults, the oral dose is 4 to 40 mg per day once or in divided doses. In the case of single administration, the daily dose should be taken in the morning after meal according to the daily rhythm of endogenous GC secretion. After improvement, the daily dose should be tapered gradually by 1-2 mg every 2–3 days to achieve minimum maintaining dose or withdraw the drug. An ointment or cream is applied as a thin layer to the damaged skin sites 1 to 3 times a day.

Dexamethasone (Dexasone, Dexamethasone phosphate, Dexaven, etc.) is superior to hydrocortisone in anti-inflammatory activity 30 times and does not demonstrate mineralcorticoid activity. It is metabolized in the liver and is excreted by the kidneys. The half-life is 2 to 3 hours.

In acute cases, the initial oral dose is within 10–15 mg per day and the maintaining dose is 2 to 4.5 mg and more per day. The amount it taken in divided doses. In low doses, dexamethasone is taken once in the morning.

In pareneteral administration dexamethasone is slowly stream- or drop-injected intravenously (in acute and emergency conditions) or intramuscularly 4 to 20 mg (not more than 80 mg) per day as well as within 4 mg peri-articularly and intra-articularly. During a day, 4 to 20 mg of dexamethasone can be injected 3 to 4 times. The duration of parenetral administration is commonly 3 to 4 days and then the tablet formulations are used as maintaining therapy.

Betamethasone (Diprospan, Celeston, Betamethasone dipropionate, Diprolen, Floreston, etc.) has a greater vasoconstricting effect and lower mineralocorticoid activity in comparison to other GCs.

Binding to plasma proteins achieves 64%. Bethametasone is metabolized in the liver and metabolites are excreted mainly by the kidneys and in part with the bile.

In adults, the daily dose is 0.25–8 mg in tablet form in the morning taken once or in divided doses, in children the dose is 17 to 250 mg/kg. After protracted therapy, betamethasone is withdrawn gradually by tapering the dose by 250 μg every 2–3 days. A single dose of slow stream or drop introduction is 4 to 8 mg (if necessary, the dose is increased up to 20 mg). The maintaining dose in intravenous therapy is 2 to 4 mg. The dose 1–2 ml is injected intramuscularly deep in the buttocks every 2–4 weeks. A single dose for intramuscular injection is 4 to 6 mg. For intra- and para-articular injection, a single dose is 0.4 to 6 mg depending on the size of the joint and damaged region. If necessary, betamethasone can be mixed in a syringe with a local anesthetic (novocaine or lidocaine solutions).

Duodenal and gastric ulcer, severe forms of arterial hypertension, Itsenko-Cushing's disease, psychoses, nephritis, evident systemic oseoporosis, severe forms of diabetes mielitus, acute infectious diseases, pregnancy, tuberculosis, and syphilis are general contradictions for GC therapy. If "absolutely necessary", the only contradiction for short-term GC administration is hypersensitivity. Contradictions for intra-articular injections are precursor arthroplasty, pathological bleeding (including anticoagulant-induced), intra-articular bone fracture, infection in the joint and peri-articular infections (including those in the history), as well as general infectious disease, marked peri-articular osteoporosis, absence of inflammation signs in the joint ("dry" joint, e.g., in synovitis-free osteoarthrosis) evident bone destruction as the result of arthritis, epyphisial aseptic necrosis. In local administration, the contradictions are hypersensitivity, postvaccinal period, bacterial (including tuberculosis) viral and fungal skin disorders, disintegration of skin, syphilitic damages of skin, skin swelling, and age below 2 years old.

5.1.3. Slow Acting Drugs

Slow acting (or basic) drugs are used in serious immune disorders of joints and connective tissues irresponsive to standard treatment. Presently, it is advisable, once an immune disease is diagnosed, to avoid expectant management using NSAIDs, GCs, and physiotherapy. In these cases basis treatment starts with gold, immunosuppressors, sulfalazine, D-penicillamine, aminocholines or their combinations with each other, with NSAIDs, and GCs [2]. Imunomodulation methods with cyclosporine (in combination with methotrexate or chlorbutin), human placental immunoglobulin as well as selective immunotherapy with monolocal antibodies to cytokines and lymphocyte antigens are under development.

A French physician, J. Forestier first used **gold medication** in rheumatoid arthritis in 1929. Active rheumatoid arthritis was the first object of gold medication. Aurotherapy is used to treat young and middle-aged patients, active seropositive juvenile rheumatoid arthritis, and pronounced synovitis. Aurotherapy is efficient in psoriatic arthropathy and Reiter' chronic syndrome (see 3.2.1).

The therapeutic properties of aurotherapy have not been established definitely. It is believed that gold complexes are capable of inhibiting macrophages interacting with antigens of class II histocompatibility (HLA-DR) on the cell surface. As gold drugs and DR molecules interact, the spatial configuration of the latter varies in such a way that they are unable of binding to antigen peptides and T-lymphocyte receptors. Thus, the development of autoimmune reaction is inhibited. Allergic reactions in aurotherapy are because DR present gold comps as antigens to T-lymphocytes which can cause allergy.

Tauredon inhibits antigen-induced stimulation of lymphocytes, monocytic and granulocytic phagocytosis, stabilizes lysosome membranes, strengthens collagen fibers, and occupies immunologically active areas capable of provoking the autoimmune process.

Its maximum concentration in blood occurs within 3 to 6 hours after deep intramuscular injection. The active agent (sodium aurothiomalate) is almost totally bound with plasma albumins. The drug is accumulated in the tissues of the reticulo-endothelial system. Relatively high concentrations occur in adrenal glands and renal cortical layer while low concentrations occur in muscles and bones. The half-life of the drug is about 27 days. It is excreted by the kidneys and from 10 to 17% is excreted through bowels. The clinical effect occurs between 9th and 17th weeks after injection when the total dose of aurum accumulated in the body is within 300 to 800 mg.

At the initial stage, adults take 10 mg of the drug. A week later, the dose is 20 mg. The third and subsequent doses of 50 mg are injected with a week interval. Afterwards, depending on the effect achieved, the dose and injection regime are corrected. The doses for children depend on body weight.

Treatment with *crysanol* (oil suspension of calcium-aurothiopanol-sulfonate) and *myocrisin* (sodium salt of thiomalic acid) does not differ from tauredon medication. The drugs are introduced intramuscularly once a week each time increasing the dose by 10–15 mg up to reaching 50 mg. Once a patient's state has improved, the intervals between the injections are extended up to 2 and then 3 weeks. Before each injection, urine and blood are tested. Accurate dosing is based on checking of the gold concentration in blood serum bearing in mind that optimal concentration is 250–300 μg in 100 ml of serum [20]. A crisotherapeutic effect commonly occurs at 200–400 mg of gold injected and rises gradually. Per treatment course a patient should get at least 1 g of gold. The gold accumulated in the body is excreted by the kidneys during a year. In the absence of the marked improvement, another basic therapy is advised after 4 months.

Auranofin (Auropan, Riadura, Actyl) is a gold drug for parenteral use. It has anti-inflammatory, desensibilizing (preventing or inhibiting the development of ellergic reactions), and immunosuppressive properties. It blocks the output of lysosome enzymes in tissues. It decelerates the occurrence of rheumatoid arthritis.

Auranofin is administered to adults 6 mg per day in a single dose or twice a day during a meal. If the effect is not marked enough within 4 to 6 months of treatment the daily dose is increased up to 9 mg. Auranofin can be taken in combination with NSAIDs.

The advantages of gold preparations is that they can be administered (in contrast to immunosuppressant) to patients with accompanying chronic infections including those in the history.

The side effects of the gold preparations manifest in the form of "golden" dermatitis, i.e., pink spotty popular rashes accompanied by itching, eosinophilia (increasing number of acidophilic granulocytes in the peripheral blood) and increasing amount of immunoglobulin E in the blood. This can result in stomatitis, cytopenia, and kidney damage caused by the deposition of immune complexes in the glomerules whose antigen is gold complex with autologic protein. Gold medicines are discontinued at the more than 0.2 g/l of protein in urine and microhematuria of more than 10 erythrocytes on the field of vision.

Cytostatic immunosuppressants that inhibit immune reactions in rheumatic diseases have been used since the 1950s. The ability of cytostatic drugs of inhibiting the synthesis of nucleic acids and proteins has initiated their application in oncology. However, with accumulation of clinical experience it was found out that they also suppressed the activity of the immune system. This oncologically undesirable effect was afterwards investigated in detail and used successfully in treating diseases wherein the autoimmune mechanisms were of major importance [21].

There are several classes of cytostatic substances, namely, antimetabolites, alkaloids, antibiotics, enzymes, and radioactive drugs. Cytostatics exert an immunosuppressive action on the cells of the lymphoid tissue characterized by increased proliferative activity that causes the growth of connective and glandular tissues.

Alkylating agents (myelosan, chlorbutin, cyclophosphan, cyclophosphamide, thiophosphamide, etc.) break the synthesis of nucleic acids (DNA and RNA) and inactivate (make inert) a number of enzymes.

Antimetabolites are chemicals similar to natural products of metabolism (metabolites) in structure, which inhibit transformations and physiological activity of these endogenous compounds. An antagonist of folic acid, methotrexate, which inhibits the activity of folatreductase enzyme, is an antimetabolite. This enzyme favors the transformation of folic acid in its active form – tetrahydrofolic acid that is involved in biosynthesis of nucleic acids. Azathioprine and 6-mercaptopurine are antagonists of purine bases and 5-ftoruracyl and cytarabin are antagonists of pyrimidine bases.

Alkaloids – vincristin, vinblastin, vindesin – affect the cells in mytosis (division phase).

Antibiotics with cytostatic effect are actinomycin D, bleomycin, adriamycin, rubidomycin, cyclosporine, sandimmune, etc.

Cytostatic enzymes are presented by asparginase and kolspase, radioactive agents include radioactive phosphor (^{32}P), radioisotopic gold (^{198}Au) and yttrium that are used as an alternative to synoviectomy, i.e., excision of joint SM.

Indications to cytostatics are progressive diseases, intolerance or inefficacy of NSAID and GC treatment, development of steroid dependence with daily maintaining doses of prednisolone more than 20 mg.

Methotrexate does not have side effects and is tolerated better in protracted therapy compared to gold preparations.

Cyclophosphane as an immunosuppressive drug is taken 1.0–1.5 mg/kg (50–100 mg per day) and with good tolerance, the dose can be 3 to 4 mg/kg. Its side effects are depression of leucopoiesis, i.e, leucocyte formation. It is contradicted to start treatment at less than 3.5×10^9/l of leucocytes and 120×10^9/l of platelets. During treatment, it is necessary to control blood count at least twice a week. With leucocytes reduced down to 2.5×10^9/l and platelets down to 100×10^9/l the treatment is discontinued. The drug is most often excreted by the kidneys. To prevent from hemorrhagic cystitis, reduction of concentration of cyclophosphane in urine, and contact with the epithelium of the urinary tracts, plenty drinking and frequent urination are recommended.

In intra-articular therapy of major joints 2 to 3 injections of 100–200 mg of cyclophosphane with a week interval are administered.

Azathioprine (Imuran, Immunal, etc.) was used the most often as the drug of choice in rheumatoid arthritis before methotrexate was approved. The drug is administered either independently or in combination with prednisolone.

The influence of cytostatics on immunity is not reduced to their influence to pathogenetic mechanisms of a main disease. Depression of cellular and humoral immunity deteriorates responses to infections and immune reactions as a whole. Recently there is a trend to direct the action of medicines to the factors responsible for the development of a main disease without involving the mechanisms of immune protection. One of such drugs is cyclosporine.

Cyclosporine (Cyclosporine A, Sandimmune, Sandimmune Neoral, Cyclorine) is a cyclic polypeptide consisting of 11 amino acids. It was first obtained from fungus *Tolypocladium intlatum*. The drug acts as immunosuppressant selectively at the lymphocyte genome level through depression of interleukyne-2 synthesis (T-lymphocyte growth factor), damages the interaction of T-helpers and T-killers which results in the production of anti-inflammatory cytokines and enzymes. Dislike other cytostatics, it does not suppress hemopoiesis and phagocytosis.

The pharmacological effect of Sandimmune also aims to depress the cellular type reactions including immunity towards allograft; "graft against host" disease, arthritis due to Freund's adjuvant (adjuvant is an agent that increases antibody immunogenicity, J.Th. Freund, the American pathologist); skin hypersensitivity of delayed type, etc.

A cytostatic immunodepressant, its doses, and management scheme are selected in rheumatologic in-patients' clinics. Further prolonged treatment is performed under rheumatologist's control in outpatients' clinics or diagnostic centers.

The drugs of several pharmacological groups outlined below in general use as basic differ from each other by mechanism of their impact on immune inflammation.

Sulfasalazine (Salas Sulfapyridine, Azopyrine, Salazopyridine, etc.) is an antimicrobe and antiparasitic sulfanilamide agent. Its anti-inflammatory effect is due to depression of cyclooxygenase and inhibition of prostaglandin synthesis. Suppression of humoral and cellular immunity manifests in inhibition of monocytes and blocking of lymphocyte transformation. The drug is accumulated in the connective tissue as well as in synovial, peritoneal and pleural fluids.

Sulfasalazine is a delayed-action drug of reserve and administered in adult rheumatoid arthritis if gold preparations and methotrexate are inefficient or intolerable. The clinical effect occurs within 6-10 weeks. Treatment is efficient during 6 months and longer.

Penicillamine (D-Penicillamine, Cuprenyl, Metalcaptase, Distamine, etc.) is the product of penicilline hydrolysis. The drug has high complex-forming activity relative to metal ions binding largely ions of copper, mercury, iron, lead, gold, arsenic, and calcium. Chelate complexes arising are excreted by the kidneys. In rheumatology, penicillamine is used in immunopathological processes. Under its effect, the level of pathological macroglobulins including rheumatoid factor is reduced. Penicillamine depresses T-helpers, inhibits chemotaxis of neutrophils from lysosomes and stimulates macrophages. It breaks the synthesis of collagen separating crossed links between tropocollagen molecules to be synthesized and normalizes the relation between soluble and insoluble fractions, which favors inhibition of tissue sclerotization. When taken orally, penicillamine is readily absorbed and present in blood plasma for a long time. In adults, penicillamine is administered in various kinds of rheumatoid arthritis and in the absence of response to conventional anti-inflammatory remedies. It is taken orally within 2–2.5 hours after meal. The treatment starts from 150–300 mg per day, each 2–4 weeks the dose increases by 150 mg up to a total daily dose of 500 mg. First signs of clinical benefits (reduced arthralgia, morning stiffness, excudative phenomena in joint, etc.) commonly appear within 2–3 months. Once the therapeutical effect is achieved, the maintaining daily dose of the drug 140–300 mg is taken. The treatment lasts one year and longer.

In treatment with penicillamine, adverse reactions are possible, such as allergy, dyspepsia, leucopenia, thrombocytopenia, agranulocutosis, myalgia, arthalgia, myasthenia, nephrotoxicity (proteinuria and hematuria). Complete blood cell count, urine test, and liver function should be performed periodically to monitor the progress or check for side effect.

Aminocholine preparations traditionally treating malaria have been used in rheumatology since 1951. Active agents are chloroquine and hydroxychloroquine.

Chloroquine (Delagil, Quingamine, Resoquine) is derivative of 4-aminoquinoline. The immunosuppressive effect manifests in inhibition of metabolism of immune-competent cells and connective tissue in rheumatoid arthritis and Bekhterev's disease.

Adults are given 250 mg per day. Therapeutic effect occurs as a rule within 4-week treatment. Once maximum effect is achieved, the dose is tapered.

Hydroxychlorquine (Plaquenil, Oxychlorquine) is indicated in rheumatoid arthritis, juvenile arthritis, systemic and discoid lupus erythematosus.

The drug stabilizes lysosome membranes and prevents enzyme output from them, breaks doubling of DNA and synthesis of RNA. It has moderate immunosuppressive and nonspecific anti-inflammatory properties, inhibits the formation of prostaglandins, weakens activity of proteases and collagenases available in the rheumatoid nodes, and inhibits the cellular proliferative phase of immune inflammation.

In rheumatoid arthritis, the initial dose for adults is 400–600 mg a day and the maintaining dose is 200–400 mg a day. In juvenile arthritis, the dose should not exceed 6.5 mg/kg or 400 mg daily. In discoid and systemic lupus erythematosus, the initial dose for adults is 400–800 mg daily and the maintaining dose is 200–400 mg daily.

5.1.4. Some Other Medicinal Preparations

In complex treatment of the synovial medium of joint metabolic, microcirculatory, antioxidant, derivant, nonspecific medicinal therapy aimed at inhibiting symptoms of main disease and favoring the general patient's condition [18] is of great significance.

Metabolic therapy aims to improve metabolism in articular cartilage. As monotherapy it does not have a great effect on osteoarthrosis but if co-administered, is efficient. The following drugs can be mentioned as the most popular metabolic preparations:

Riboxin (Inosine) stimulates synthesis of protein, increases the activity of several enzymes of Krebs cycle The Kerbs cycle (H.A. Krebs, the German biochemist, awarded Nobel prize in 1953) also known as tricarboxylic acid cycle refers to a series of enzymatic reactions resulting in carbohydrate, protein, and fat oxidation with liberation of energy in the organism. Riboxin is a purine derivative, precursor of ATP. The drug is taken orally by 400 mg 3 times daily during a month. Riboxin can be also introduced intravenously 10 ml of 2% solution in 10 ml of isotonic solution of sodium chloride or 10 ml of riboxin in 200–250 ml 5% of glucose solution or isotonic sodium chloride solution drop-by-drop intravenously. With satisfactory tolerance, the dose can be increased up to 20 ml per infusion. The treatment course is 10 to 15 days.

Sodium adenosine triphosphate (ATP) (Sodium ATP, Atriphos, Phosphobion) improves the function of transversal striated muscles and activates the metabolism in tissues. Sodium ATP is introduced intramuscularly 1 ml of 1% solution daily for 20–25 days. Also intra-articular injections are possible.

Phosphaden (Adenosin-5'-monophosphoric acid) is an ATP fragment and constituent of a number of co-enzymes regulating redox processes and possessing antiaggregant properties. The drug essentially improvers metabolic processes in tissues and microcirculation and therefore, can be recommended in complex therapy of osteoarthrosis. Phosphaden is taken orally 50 mg 3 times a day for 3–4 weeks or intramuscularly 2–4 ml of 2% solution 2–3 times a day for 2–4 weeks. It is well-tolerated though sometimes nausea, dizziness, tachycardia, and allergic reactions are reported. Adenyl is its analog.

Pyridoxalphosphate is a co-enzyme (a supplementary factor of enzyme activity being part of it) of vitamin B_6. It is involved in decarboxilation and over-amination of amino acids having a positive effect on the metabolism in tissues including articular cartilage. The drug is taken orally 20–40 mg 3 times daily during 3–4 weeks. It also can be taken intramuscularly 10 mg 3 times a day (the ampule content is diluted in 1–2 ml of water for injections). Usually the drug is well-tolerated although allergic reactions are possible.

Potassium orotate is a potassium salt of orotic acid. Orotic acid is one of the precursors of pyrimidine nucleotides being a constituent of nucleic acids involved in the synthesis of protein molecules. Thanks to this, orotic acid and its salt are anabolics. Tablets are taken orally 500 mg 3 times daily for 3–4 weeks before meal. It is well-tolerated although sometimes allergic and dyspeptic reactions are observed.

Anabolic steroids improve the synthesis of proteins in tissues including articular cartilage and provide reparative processes in it. They are indicated in osteoarthrosis to individuals of normal body weight. *Retabolil* is taken intramuscularly once every 2 weeks 2 or 3 injections total, or *methandrostenolone* (Nerobol) is taken by 5 mg 2-3 times a day for a month.

Wobenzym comprises a combination of herbal or animal high-active enzymes with rutin. The drug is used in treatment of joint inflammations, injuries of joints and tissues, irrespective of its unique structure, properties, and functions and during postoperative period since it stops inflammation and swelling of soft tissues, reduces stiffness and improves joint mobility [22]. It is recommended to take 3 tablets 3 times a day for 5 weeks.

To improve the microcirculation in subchondral parts of bones and in joint capsule, the drugs called “antiaggregants” are administered. They are inhibitors of particle aggregation in the biological fluids of organism.

Curantil (Dipyridamol) is produced in tablets 25 mg and 3 tablets 3 times a day for 1–2 months are recommended.

Trental (Agapurin) is administered at a dose of 100 mg 3 times a day for 1 month.

Teonicol (Xantinol Nicotinate) combines the properties of theophylline and nicotinic acid, has spasmolitic and antiaggregant properties, and improves microcirculation. Its dosage is 1–2 tablets (150–300 mg) 2–3 times a day for 2 months after meal.

Antioxidant drugs inhibit peroxide oxidation of lipids and reduce formation of free radicals in tissues thus slowing down cartilage destruction. In complex treatment of joints, the following antioxidant agents are used.

Vitamin E (Tocoferol acetate) is produced in capsules containing 0.2 ml of 50% solution. Patients are administered 1-2 capsules a day for a month or intramuscularly 1–2 ml of 10% solution once a day for 20 days.

Orgotein (Superoxid dismutase) is a drug of the main enzyme of antioxidative protective system and actively blocks peroxide oxidation of lipids. The drug is indicated in reactive synovitis due to its marked anti-inflammatory effect. Orgotein is introduced intra-articularly 4 mg once a week for 6 weeks. The effect is maintained for 3 months.

Drugs containing honeybee and snake venom relieve pain in polyarthritis, myositis, and radiculitis. Sometimes they are administered as desensibilizers in allergic conditions. Their action refers to irritation of receptors and stimulation of reflector reactions. Specifically, this is due to high-active substances (histamine, enzymes, microelements, and organic acids) available in venom that affect the regulatory processes including immune reactions, microcirculation, and blood coagulation. A local effect is due to hyaluronidases and phospholipase A found in venom that penetrate deep in the skin when applied topically.

Apifor tablets comprise 1 mg of lyophilized honeybee venom. It is used in electrophoresis after dissolving one tablet in 20 ml of water. The number of procedures is 15 to 20.

Apisatron is an ointment in tubes by 20 and 100 g to be applied to painful areas. In 100 g 200 units of activity of honeybee venom (1 unit of activity equals 10 μg of honeybee venom) are found.

Vipraxin, an aqueous solution of adder venom in 1 ml ampules is introduced subcutaneously in most painful places.

Viprosal is an ointment based on blunt-nosed viper venom (16 units of activity in 100 g of the ointment) is used for local applications in tubes.

Diverse abnormalities of the synovial medium of the joint assume a wide set of pharmacological means available to treat a specific nosological kind of a disease with account for its symptoms and etiopathogenetic mechanisms of progress. More detailed data on the management of joint diseases using these medicinal preparations can be found in handbooks on rheumatology and pharmacology [23, 24, 25, 26].

5.2. NON-DRUG THERAPY

5.2.1. Physiotherapy

Physiotherapy (Greek *physis* – nature and *therapeia* – treatment; synonyms: physical therapy, physiatria) is a medical science dealing with physiological and medicinal action of natural and artificially produced physical factors and developing methods for their application for prophylactic and curative goals.

Main kinds of physiotherapy are electric therapy, heat therapy, water therapy, and treatment with mechanical effects. SPA therapy is an independent division in physiotherapy. Electric therapy unites the largest diversity of medicinal methods with utilizing electric field, direct, alternating, continuous and discontinuous electric currents, and electromagnetic fields. Light therapy includes methods based on the utilization of the energy of light (including ultra-violet and infrared) radiation. The methods for hydrotherapy assume utilization of sweet water (shower, baths, and other water procedures) as well as natural and artificially prepared mineral water. Heat therapy uses hot paraffin, mineral wax, therapeutic mud, sand, vapor, dry air, etc. Treament using mechanical effects includes ultrasound, vibrotherapy, and massage.

Physical therapy procedures improve peripheral, regional, and central blood circulation, relieve pain, improve cellular nourishment, and normalize neurohumoral regulation and immune processes.

Physical therapy of joints commonly supplements medicinal and orthopedic therapy, but in a number of cases, it might become a major method and alternative to medication. A course of physiotherapy stimulates responsive mechanisms of reaction to external irritators. According to the theory of the Russian physiologist, Nobel Prize winner (1904) I.P. Pavlov, receptors (sensitive nervous endings of skin and viscera) are specific transformers that transform an irritator energy into a specific form of nervous activity, i.e., excitation.

Receptors are related anatomically and physiologically to vegetative formations of the medulla oblongata and spinal cord. These vegetative formations innervate (link to the central nervous system by means of nerves) viscera, endocrine system, muscles and skin. This interaction gives rise to skin-visceral and visceral-visceral reflexes. In addition, subcortical vegetative formations and cerebral cortex are involved in reflex interactions. Irritation of the cerebral cortex enhances excitation and inhibition. Therefore, the effect of physical factors on skin and hypodermic tissues modifies the trophism and blood supply not only within the region of exposure but in viscera as well. Each of physical factors has a characteristic specific effect [27].

The following physiotherapeutic methods are the most popular in treating pathologies of synovial medium of joints.

*Inductothermy (*Lat. *inductio* – introduction and Greek *therme* – heat) or short-wave diathermia is a method in electric therapy when definite parts of a human body are heated when exposed to alternating current, largely, high-frequency and ultra-high-frequency electromagnetic field. It induces vorticity currents in the tissues with a power proportional to electroconductivity of the tissues. Currents are the most intensive in biological fluids having a considerable electroconductivity (blood, lymph, SF, etc.). The regions exposed to vorticity currents demonstrate temperature elevation of the tissue, better blood circulation due to arteriole dilatation, improved metabolism and tissue trophism, and lower tension of muscle fibers. Under the effect of inductothermy, the excretion of corticosteroids and a catecholamine (adrenaline) and neuromediator content of blood and urine increase. At the same time, intensity of phagocytosis rises, redox processes are stimulated, and inflammatory lesions even deep located are absorbed better.

In inductothermy generators of high-frequency electric oscillations are used. The energy is supplied through a flexible cable (cable electrode) or a flexible applicator to the patient. The cable is shaped as a cylindrical or flat spiral, and the applicator is a flat spiral of copper tube. A person has a feeling of a pleasant heat during the procedure.

Indications for inductothermy in orthopedics and traumatology are subacute and chronic inflammatory and metabolic-dystrophic diseases, bone fractures, joint traumas, and commissures.

Inductothermy is contradicted to patients with skin defects as well as those having dry plaster and hygiene bandages. Cloth (free of metallic parts) and hair do not prevent inductothermy. Metallic, especially, ringlike things, which are found within the inductor projection field and at a distance of 8–12 cm from it cause skin burning. During one procedure, only 2–3 patient's joints can be subjected to inductothermy. The total duration of the procedures is 10–30 min and the treatment course consists of 10–15 procedures.

A simultaneous usage of inductothermy and galvanization is called galvanoinductothermy, co-treatment with inductothermy and drug electrophoresis is called inductothermic electrophoresis. Combination of inductothermy and mud therapy is called mud inductothermy. Inductothermy can be immediately followed by galvanization, drug electrophoresis, medium-frequency magnetotherapy, impulse current, and ultrasound therapy.

Ultrasound therapy is based on the biophysical interaction of ultrasound with biological tissues. In physiotherapeutic practice, ultrasound vibrations from 800 to 300 kHz are used. Doses depend on ultrasound intensity, duration of action, and ultrasound generation regime (continuous or impulse). As a rule, for medicinal effects, ultrasound intensity should not exceed 1 Vt/cm^2 (intensity below 0.4 Vt/cm^2 is considered low, 0.5–0.8 Vt/cm^2 – medium, and 0.9 Vt/cm^2 and higher - high). Under continuous condition the flow of ultrasonic waves is generated during the entire period of action. The impulse regime assumes the release of impulses at a frequency of 50 Hz and lasting 2, 4, and 10 ms.

The absorption of ultrasound with pathologically modified tissues depends on their acoustic characteristics and frequency of ultrasonic oscillations. Ultrasound intensity of 800–900 kHz frequency reduces in soft tissues twice at a depth of 4–5 cm and at a frequency of about 3000 kHz at a depth of 1.5–2 cm. Adipose tissue absorbs ultrasound ~ 4 times more effectively than blood, 10 times than muscular tissue, and 75 times than osseous tissue. Ultrasound is absorbed best of all at the interface of the tissues with different acoustic parameters (skin-subcutaneous fat, fascia-muscle, periosteum-bone). Ultrasound absorption varies markedly with varying state of the tissue due to pathological processes (swelling, infiltrate, i.e., local sclerosis of tissue with augmented volume, fibrosis, etc.).

Ultrasound primarily exhibits its influence on the tissue and intracellular processes via varying the kinetics of diffusion and osmosis, permeability of cellular membranes, intensity of enzymatic processes, oxidation, acid-base balance, and electrical activity of cells. Under the effect of ultrasound, the metabolism is activated, the amount of nucleic acids rises, and tissue respiration is stimulated [28].

Since the permeability of vessel walls increases under the effect of ultrasound, therefore, ultrasound may accelerate pathological process in inflamed tissues with evident exudative events. A resorption effect of ultrasound on inflammation allows it to be used in subacute and chronic inflammations.

One of specific properties of ultrasound is its "disfibering" effect on tissues that promotes softer scarring and results in resorption (softening) of already formed scar tissue because of the splitting of the collagen fiber bundle into fibrils and their detachment from the amorphous intercellular substance of connective tissue. This is the basis of ultrasound therapy of locomotor system, nerves, as well as scarring after surgical interventions and inflammations.

Low doses of ultrasound stimulate the regeneration of tissues and large doses inhibit these processes. The ultrasound effect on the human organism is referred to the blocking of pain impulse in ganglion nerve cells (nerve nodes) and dissipation of the impulse in nerve fibers. This effect is effective in treating diseases accompanied by marked pain syndrome (neuralgia, osteochondrosis, myositis, etc.).

In physiotherapy, drug phonoresis (ultraphonoresis, sonophonoresis) that combines the action of two agents, namely, ultrasound and drug introduced. Under the action of ultrasound, a drug invades in epidermis and afterwards diffuses in blood and lymph. Procedures of 12–15 min duration are performed daily or every other day, the course consists of 6 to 12 procedures.

Diadynamotherapy (Bernard's diadynamic currents, sinusoidal modulated currents) consists in the effect of direct pulsed electric current. It was proposed by a French physician R. Bernard. Diadynamic currents are pulsations of medium-frequency alternating current (2–5 kHz) modulated with respect to amplitude. The modulation frequency range lies within 10–150 Hz. The effect on tissues depends on current frequency and power as well as modulation amplitude.

Diadynamic currents activate the blood circulation and metabolic processes in tissues, including deep located, and relieve pain. With increasing intensity, they cause local titanic (prolonged tonic) reduction of muscles that is not accompanied by irritation or unpleasant sensations.

In the regime of rectified current, the sinusoidal modulated currents are used in medicinal electrophoresis to affect the deep located tissues and skin receptors. The treatment course is 8 to 12 procedures.

Laser therapy is treatment using low-energy laser light in red spectrum. Helium-neon lasers with a radiation power of 10–25 mVt are used as sources of light energy.

The mechanism of laser biological effect consists in, primarily, enzymatic decomposition of ATA nucleotide, which increases its concentration and secondly, in decreasing intensity of peroxide oxidation of lipids thanks to activation of antiperoxide protective enzymes, which prevents the damage of the barrier function of membranes, This, in turn, enhances antioxidant properties of blood and improves the organisms's resistance [29]. Laser therapy normalizes the sympatic and parasympatic innervation and tissue and capillary circulation; the number of unaltered capillaries increases and aggregation of erythrocytes and permeability of capillaries decrease.

A method has been developed of combined laser therapy of severe lesions of extremities' major joints in adults and the elderly that can be used in concurrent cardiovascular and endocrine diseases [29]. The laser effect in combination with corticosteroids and drug blocking essentially reduces adverse effects and extend opportunities for assistance to such patients. Invasive (intra-articular and intraosseal metaepiphyseal) laser therapy is used in severe pain syndrome and lesions of osteochondral and ligamentous systems of the knee and hip.

Laser therapy is effective at the initial stages of osteoarthrosis, osteochodrosis, periarthritis (including cases complicated by calculous bursitis), trophic changes in extremities as well as pathological processes due to disturbances in neuro-trophic tissue regulation.

Magnetotherapy is a physical therapy method based on the interaction of variable magnetic field on the whole organism or its part. Biological tissues exposed to the magnetic fields are not magnetized but experience a structural reconstruction. A medicinal effect of magnetotherapy manifests at the molecular, submolecular, and subcellular levels. Magnetic fields cause concentration changes in biologically active matters, namely, enzymes, proteins, and nucleic acids. Liquid crystals (cholesterol, lipoproteides, etc.), free radicals of proteins and metalloproteides such as hemoglobin, catalase, vitamins are subjected to the effect of magnetic fields [30].

Magnetic fields improve microcirculation and intensify regenerative and reparative processes in tissues. Magnetotherapy is effective in the treatment of hematoms, inflammations, and pain syndrome in traumas and arthritis. A good tolerance of magnetotherapy by the elderly is reported.

Ultra-high frequency therapy (uhf-therapy) is a method of electric therapy via exposing the organism to mainly high-frequency electromagnetic field. It is employed in the continuous or pulsed regime. During the procedure, a part of the body or a joint is disposed between two capacitor electrodes so that an air gap is formed between the electrodes whose size should not change in the course of the procedure. The physical action of the electromagnetic uhf-field is in active absorption of its energy by the tissues and transformation into heat energy to produce an oscillatory effect characteristic of hf electromagnetic exposures. Heat effect of uhf-therapy is not essentially pronounced since the main heat is formed in the tissues that conduct the current poorly (nervous, bone, etc.). The heat effect depends on the power and degree of energy absorption by tissues [27].

The uhf electromagnetic field has an anti-inflammatory effect owing to improvement of blood and lymph circulation and tissue dehydration and intensifies the metabolism of connective tissue, which allows localization of inflammatory focus. At the same time, the sensitivity of nervous receptors deteriorates, the tonus of capillaries and areterioles decrease, and blood circulation in tissues improves.

Drug electrophoresis (ionophoresis) is a method in physical therapy consisting in simultaneous effect of direct current and medicine ions introduced with its help (through skin or mucous membranes). Electrophoresis (Greek *phoresis* – application, transfer) is a directed motion of colloid particles or macroions under the influence of an external electric filed. It was discovered by professor F.F. Reuss (Moscow State University) in 1807 and is referred to electrokinetic phenomena.

In electrophoresis, nervous fibers and specialized cells become more susceptible to a drug with its pharmacological properties maintained. Low-dosed drug electrophoresis displays a pronounced prolonged therapeutic effect due to "intracutaneus depots" saving drugs during 1–3 days. This provides a local effect in pathological cases (e.g., in local vascular disorders) when there is a difficulty to deliver a drug to the lesion from blood. In electrophoresis about 90% of drug is introduced in tissues owing to electrogenic motion, 1–3% owing to electric osmosis, and 5–8% via diffusion. Most often electrolytic drugs dissociating to form ions in solutions are introduced by this method. It is possible to simultaneously use several drugs. In a number of cases, direct pulsed current is used to augment the therapeutic effect of the method.

Application of heat-carriers (heat treatment, thermal therapy) is the influence of heat on the organism to provide a therapeutic effect. Heat therapy includes medicinal procedures with involvement of heat as the main or governing factor. This can be provided by using heated peloid-like substances such as naphthalane, ozokerite, and paraffin [31].

For naphthalane therapy petroleum mined in Naphthalan health resort, Azerbaijan and petroleum-based preparations are used at 37–38 °C. Medicinal properties of naphthalene oil are due to naphthens predominating over other hydrocarbons. A small amount of benzene and kerosene fraction in oil allows its application in bathing. Outside health resorts, naphthalane therapy in the form of application is combined with other physiotherapeutic methods.

Ozokerite is a mineral from the group of oil bitums. Its high heat capacity, minimal conductivity, and slow heat release make it high efficient as a heat carrier to be used at 40–50 °C (first layer) and 60–70 °C (second layer) without any risks of burns. Along with thermal factor, also mechanical and bioxhemical factors are involved. Mechanically, ozokerite has a compression effect onto underlying tissues due to a significant decrease in its volume in solidification. A biochemical effect is due to biologically active substances found in ozokerite that penetrate through skin and exert a parasympaticotonic effect. Parasympaticotonia or vagotonia is predomination of the tonus of parasympatic nervous system and the vagus nerve over the tonus of its sympathetic part. It manifests in reduced muscle and vessel tonus, increasing threshold of excitation of nervous endings, etc. Ozokerite treatment in used as applications, baths in combination with other physiotherapeutic methods (galvanizing, electrophoresis, ultrasound therapy, massages, etc.).

A medicinal effect of paraffin (wax substance, mixture of saturated hydrocarbons obtained from oil) is based on heat and mechanical effects onto tissues. Like with ozokerite, paraffin is melt on water bath at 65–100 °C when used in form of baths and applications.

The mechanism of action of thermotherapy is due to changes in local and general blood circulation (skin hyperaemia, enhanced blood flow, increasing number of functioning capillaries). A local enhancement of the blood flow is accompanied by improved metabolism, formation of biologically active substances, and intensified regeneration. Heat relieves pain and weakens spasms. Response of tissues to heat irritation is due to intensification of neurohumoral mechanisms governing the functional state of organs and systems. Therefore, heat therapy is implemented with account for general capabilities of the organism.

Applications of heat carriers are indicated in stage I and II osteoarthritis without synovitis or with its slight signs, pain syndrome, proliferative phenomena, and reflector muscular disorders.

Mud therapy (peloid therapy) is a method of heat therapy with the use of therapeutic muds (peloids). They are natural products (sediments of water reservoirs, peat sediments of bogs, eruptions of mud volcanoes, etc.). Peloids are formed under the influence of microorganisms, as a result, they are saturated with biogenic components (compounds of nitrogen, serum, carbon, etc.). According to organic elements content the medicinal mud are separated to organic (peat and sapropels) and non-organic ones (sulphide slit and hill mud).

A healing effect of mud is the combination of heat, mechanical, and chemical factors and depends on the physicochemical properties [32]. Mud therapy is efficient in chronic arthritis such as traumatic, infectious, and dystrophic without exacerbations, rheumatoid arthritis, articular form of rheumatisms in inactive stage (in 8–9 months after exacerbation), osteochondrosis, spondylarthritis without exacerbation, and other diseases and traumas of the locomotor system.

Balneotherapy uses natural or artificially prepared mineral water. It has a positive effect on metabolism as a whole and cartilage metabolism in particular, peripheral haemodynamics and microcirculation on joints. Baleneotherapeutic procedures include radon, hydrogen sulfide, chlor-sodium, iodine-brome, and turpentine baths.

Bischofite therapy, when used in joint diseases, has anti-inflammatory, pain-relieving, and resorption effects. Bischofite is a natural bromine-chloride-magnesium brine with increased amount of potassium, sodium, bromine, iron, and some other elements. The product is obtained in drilling. Once it has been found out that the workers of drills (Nizhne-Kamsk petroleum mine, RF) reported pain relief in joints after washing hands with this brine.

Bischofite is used in form of compresses to joint, baths for hands and legs, general baths at any osteoarthrosis stage without synovitis. The duration of a procedure is 15–30 min. Medicinal baths can be used every day; the course is 15–20 baths. After 2-3 weeks the course is repeated and then the therapy is discontinued for 2–3 months. Baths for hands and legs can be combined with bischofite compresses.

The physiotherapeutic methods of the locomotor system are diverse and described in more detail in special manuals. Physiotherapy supplements other kinds of treatment, but in a number of cases, it may become the leading method and alternative to medication. In joint disease, both monotherapy and combination of two or more procedures can be applied.

Physiotherapy is forbidden in fever, exacerbations of inflammations, cachexia, infectious diseases at acute stage, active tuberculosis, malignant tumors or when they are suspected, systemic blood diseases, bleeding sickness, cardio-vascular diseases with insufficient blood circulation, aneurism of aorta and large vessels, and central nervous system disorders at acute excitation. Physiotherapy is not administered at elevated body temperature, unfixed fractures, and "fresh" haemarthrosis.

5.2.2. Orthopedic Therapy

Orthopedic therapy methods are divided into conservative and surgical ones.

Conservative methods provide immovable fixation of joints and facilitate the recovery of joint functions after traumas and operations.

Provision of sparing orthopedic regimen is an important condition in joint therapy. Mechanical unloading of joints is of particular significance in cases of lower limb pathologies. For this purpose, orthopedic means such as soft and rigid dressings, tutors, ortheses, sticks, crutches, etc. are used.

For soft dressings, one can use a kerchief, elastic and gauze bandage, self-adhesive bandage, pipe elastic bandage, gauze, cotton wool, etc.

Taping, namely, strengthening of joints by means of adhesive plaster is a kind of "soft" immobilization of joints. This preventive measure traditionally used in sports traumatology aims to strengthen and secure the injured locomotorium. Taping is able to compensate the defect of ligamentous system in traumas and insufficient (or ineffective) treatment of joint ligaments. The disadvantage of taping is the necessity to use special plasters and prepare skin in advance [33].

Rigid immobilizing facilities aim to secure body parts in a certain immovable position and provide favorable conditions for healing injuries. The limbs are secured in the most advantageous (physiological) position. Such position for the hip joint is 8-10° abduction and 20° flexion, for the knee joint it is a slight flexion of joint (8−15°), for the ankle joint it is plantar 5° flexion. In the region of bony prominences, the cotton wool pads should be provided to avoid pressure ulcers. Optimal immobilization of the limb is achieved when two or more nearby joints are secured.

Rigid bandages are divided into splint and hardening ones. *A splint* is a lining of a hard material to reinforce the bandage. Splint bandages are divided into securing (to secure the limb in a certain position) and extending (combining the securing and extension of the limb). Irrespective of its unique structure, properties, and functions. The former splint can be exemplified by Cramer's stair splint (F. Cramer, the German surgeon) made of soft wire. In treatment and rehabilitation of orthopedic patients (after arthroplasty, arthrolysis, etc.), extending splint devices are used to simultaneously unload major joints and start their early mobilization. The limb motion in this device is provided by muscular movement of system members or with help of installed electromotor. The devices allow regulation of movement volume and duration.

Hardening bandages include a substance that sets rapidly and takes the shape of the surface to be applied to. For this goal, plaster is common-wide. It is an absorbent substance kept in sealed reservoirs and its condition is checked periodically. Plaster casts include circular, removable, fenestrated ones, bridges, splints, slab bars, body casts, and plaster beds. The founder of plaster casting is A. Mathysen, Netherlands, who published his works on the techniques of plaster casting in the 1850s.

A slab bar consists of 6−8 layers of plaster bandage placed on the table. The roller bandage is impregnated with water, excess water is removed, the bandage is applied to the joint and smoothened thoroughly. The plaster bandage sets within 10−12 min and is secured to the joint with soft or plaster bandage. The immobilization of joint depends on the number of layers and technique for slab application.

If some part of the body is required to keep open then a "window" is cut with a special knife or scissors designed to work with plaster. Through this window, it is possible to observe the pathological focus and treat it. A bridge bandage is used to make some part of the joint open. It consists of two plaster sleeves located above and below the joint and connected with plaster or metallic arcs. Sometimes a common plaster cast is transformed into a bridge one. For this, a window is cut from both sides before the plaster sets.

Plaster casts can have cotton-gauze pads. A properly put bandage reduces pain in the joint. During first days after putting bandage it is necessary to examine open parts of the limb and determine skin sensitivity. In case of pains, limb numbness, cyanosis, and edema of distal parts the bandage should be immediately removed.

Splints made of rigid polymeric material Scotchcast™ and polymer modeling bandages Primacast™ do not have these shortcomings. They get solidified rapidly after wetting or exposed to air, have high strength and low radiodensity.

A tutor is an alternative to plaster cast. It is a fixing orthopedic device to provide joint immobilization (Fig. 5.4). It consists of a rigid sleeve and soft clamps. It is indicated in such joint disorders as spastic and flaccid paralysis of lower limbs, pareses (reduced power or amplitude of motion amplitude in the joint as the result of disorders in muscle innervation), looseness and dislocation of joints, false joints, knee recurvation (overextension), joint arthrosis, clubfoot, and shortening of limb.

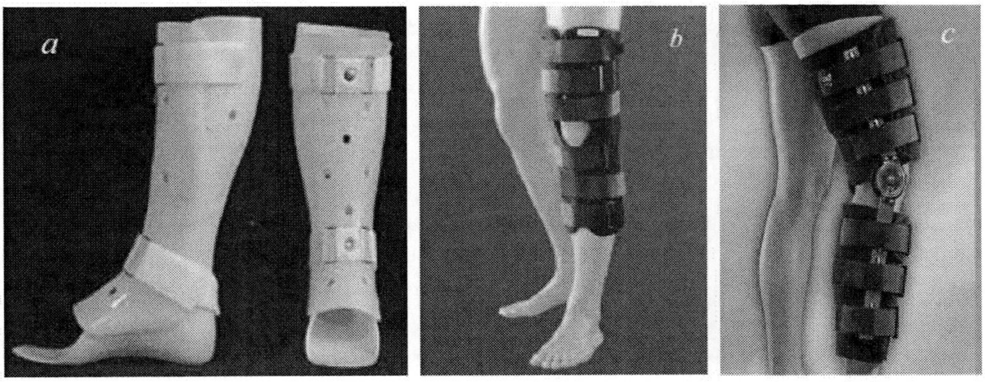

Figure 5.4. Tutors: *a* – for the ankle joint; *b* – for the knee joint; *c* – orthesis for the knee joint.

To restore normal motions after joint traumas and operations, ortheses are used whose main objective is to compensate the broken functions. Most often, the ortheses consist of two sleeves secured on the hip and ankle and connected to each other with a hinge at the level and in the plane of joint motion. As compared to plaster casts this method demonstrates a number of advantages including early mobilization, protection of injured ligaments, prophylaxis of muscle atrophy, reduction of treatment and rehabilitation periods (the restoration period of muscle power is 7–10 times longer than that of joint immobilization).

In order to decrease the load to the damaged joint, sticks or crutches are used in walking. Their length is chosen and regulated individually depending on the patient's height. The stick is taken by a healthy hand with its handle at the level of greater trochanter of the hip, the arm flexion angle at elbow being about 45°. If the stick is chosen incorrectly, functional overloading of the upper limb muscles can occur. In case of incorrectly chosen crutches, the shoulder tissues can be compressed and crutch plexitis (lesion of shoulder nervous plexus) can develop.

Orthopedic surgical treatment aims to restore disease-induced changes in the anatomy and functions of joints. Various variants of arthroplasty, i.e. operation to restore or correct joint functions at evident degenerative-dystrophic or traumatic changes of bones and cartilages [34] are known.

Endoprosthetics or replacement of the synovial joint or its parts with a hinge member or its parts made of engineering materials is the most serious and traumatic intervention in the structure of a damaged joint. This operation is optional. If endoprosthetics is advisable the patient should give a voluntary informed consent. Below, methods for surgical joint treatment not associated with endoprosthetics are considered.

Arthroscopy (low-invasive penetration into joint cavity with optical and surgical tools with displaying the image) makes it possible to diagnose intra-articular changes and treat them surgically accurately and as untraumatically as possible. The up-to-date level of arthroscopic surgery of larger joints allows trimming of defective edges and excrescence of cartilage with oscillating cutter, joint cavity lavage, syndesmoplasty, resection and suture fixation of menisci, chondroplasty, etc.

Arthroplasty including tunneling of subchondral (located beneath the cartilage) bone layer, transplantation of periosteal and perichondral elements result in a defect-structured cartilage. Biomechanical properties of a new cartilage are insufficient to resist loads to the joint under natural conditions. This has provided the basis for development of new approaches to treatment of cartilage defects based on chondrocyte culturing [35].

The procedures consist in the following actions. During arthroscopy of the damaged joint, a cartilage sample 300–500 mg in weight is taken from the unloadable region of medial condyle of femur. The cartilage is kept in a special reservoir with sodium chloride. Within 2–5 hours the cells are isolated, i.e., the cartilage is refined and undergoes threefold washing with HEPAS with gentamicin, amphotericin, and ascorbinic acid. The refined cartilage is placed into a flask with collagenase (an enzyme belonging to hydrolases catalyzes hydrolytic peptidolysis) and desoxycarbonuclease. The cells are filtered with a filter with 25 μm pores, mixed with patient's blood serum, and grown on the medium. The medium is replaced twice a week with obligatory bacteriological control. The suspension of chondrocytes is treated with tripsin (digestive enzyme) and then washed threefold in the patient's blood serum. On the last centrifugation, a suspension is formed from 50 to 100 μl in volume containing from 2 to 5 mln cells. The chondrocyte suspension is ready to repair a cartilage defect within 2–3 weeks after taking the cartilage sample. In culturing, the amount of chondrocytes rises 10–20 times. Under histologic control of implantation results, it was found that a new cartilage is placed near the underlying bone and differs somewhat from the autologous cartilage in collagen stricture, which, nevertheless, allows functional recovery of the joint.

In cartilage transplantation we should pay attention to the following [36]:

1) in joint trauma cytokines and stromelizin enzyme appear in SF that largely cause cartilage regeneration rather than its recovery;

2) local cartilage lesions might not necessarily be cured by regeneration and can stay unchanged for a long time;

3) a full-thickness chondral defect is repaired with fibrous cartilage whose mechanical properties are insufficient to hold normal loads to cartilage;

4) a chondral defect less than 2 cm^2 in area can exist asymptotically without any progress (its treatment has a more favorable prognosis);

5) a chondral defect more than 2 cm^2 in area can progress and cause synovitis, pain, and functional disorders;

6) deformation or instability of joint should be corrected simultaneously with cartilage defect repair;

7) articular cartilage replacement is an efficient and safe procedure.

International Cartilage Repair Society, ICRS has developed a program and proposed a document called "International Cartilage Repair Society Documentation and Classification System" [37]. The document includes 12 main points. Each of them consists of the explanation and several below-listed questions a physician should answer before chondrocytes transplantation.

1. Etiology of the process. Is the chondral defect acute or chronic? Is the chondral defect the result of acute trauma or chronic overloading? As a rule, chondral defects result from combination of unfavorable factors.

2. Defect depth. What is a defect depth of the chondral cover? The Outerbridge (R.E. Outerbridge, the English arthrologist, 1961) classification is the most validated technique for determining chondral defect depth. According to it, there are four grades of cartilage degeneration: 0 – normal cartilage; 1 – cartilage with softening and swelling, 2 – a partial-thickness defect with fissures on the surface; 3 – incomplete cartilage fissuring to the level of the bone; and 4 – full breakdown of chondral cover and exposed subchondral bone. Grades 1 and 2 are considered as partial degrading lesions and grades 3 and 4 as complete degradation. In order to evaluate the lesion grade one should take into consideration the availability of aseptic necrosis of subchondral bone or infarction of bone tissue.

3. Defect size in square centimeters, commonly measured with use of an arthroscopic probe. A defect sized below 2 cm^2 is considered small, from 2 to 10 cm^2 – mean, and larger than 10 cm^2 – large.

4. A degree of stability of defect edges. Are they stable? A regular defect with dense edges is capable of holding a significant load. If the cartilage edges are disfibered or thinned the defect tends to spread and develop. In this case, the narrowing of the articular fissure is seen on the X-ray picture.

5. Defect localization. Where is the chondral defect located? Is it a single defect or several defects? The \data influences the disease prognosis.

6. The state of joint ligaments. Is their integrity retained? Or are they partially or entirely broken down? Is the joint stable? Was the joint stabilized surgically before?

7. Menisci state. Is their integrity maintained? Did they undergo partial or subtotal resection or were they sewed?

8. Position of femur and crus. Are they disposed at the same axis? Is there an angle between them? If yes, is this varus or valgus deformation? How large is the angle? Is there a corrigent osteotomy in the history? If yes, specify. One should pay attention to the state of patella-femoral joint. Is there a need to correct the position of patella?

9. Previous treatment. Is any in the history? If yes, specify. Was it trimming of chondral defects, tunneling, transplantation, etc.?

10. Data of X-ray examination in the anteroposterior projection under load. Main features are the degree of articular fissure narrowing and presence of osteophytes and bone cysts.

11. Magnet-resonance imaging (MRI) data. Determination of the state of chondral cover and subchondral bone. Evaluation of defect depth, bone exposure, availability of osteochondrosis dissecans (flaking of osteochondral area of articular surface in inflammation) or aseptic bone necrosis.

12. Life and family history. One should exclude a specific rheumatoid process, systemic lupus erythematosus, and positive reaction to HLA B-27 antigen. The state of endocrine system (endrocrine gland pathology, diabetes, obesity, etc.) is assessed. Availability of family forms of osteoarthrosis, inherited collagen pathology of Ehlers-Danlos syndrome (hyperextensibility of skin, revealed by dermatologists E. Ehlers and H.A. Danlos) or Marfan syndrome (systemic lesion of connective tissue revealed by a French pediatrician, B.J.A. Marfan) types is taken into account. Chondrocyte grafting is the most effective procedure in the case of cartilage defect of femoral condyle, less efficient in patella, and almost inefficient on the tibial plateau. The efficiency of the procedure is evaluated by the following changes observed: a) the defect is substituted with hyaline rather than fibrous cartilage; b) pains, synovitis, and dyskinesia are discontinued; c) patient's physical activity is recovered. The procedure gives less exacerbations due to this surgical intervention (cartilage damage, inflammation, thrombosis, etc.) and general effects (allergic reactions). As concluded in [38], autologous chondrocyte grafting is a safe procedure although its higher efficacy compared to other treatment methods is not proved.

5.3. Local Therapy

Local (peri- and intra-articular) therapy is an essential part of complex treatment of inflammatory and degenerative joint diseases. Medicinal and diagnostic punctures are indicated when a great amount of blood or inflamed fluid is accumulated in the joint cavity. Exudate removal results in significant weakening of pain. The procedure is combined with injection of drugs in the joint cavity or peri-articular tissues.

5.3.1. Injection of Drugs

Up-to-date injection therapy of joints pursues the following goals: reduction or removal of total and local inflammatory activity, prevention from disease exacerbations, and functional recovery of affected joints [1].

Conditions and requirements to intra-articular and peri-articular drug injection are strictly regulated [39]. According to these standards, the procedure is performed by a physician skillful in intra-articular and peri-articular injections. A drug kind and dose and a room are planned in advance. The room should meet sterility requirements. The procedure is performed with patient's consent.

The hip joint is aspirated from the anterior or lateral surface of the joint. The following procedure is used to find a point of needle introduction: a straight line is marked from the top of greater trochanter to the midpoint of inguinal ligament and in the middle of this line a needle is introduced. The needle is first introduced normally to skin surface up to femoral neck (about 4 to 5 cm) and then directed inside the joint cavity [34]. The hip joint is aspirated by introducing the needle above the greater trochanter top and advancing it normally to the long axis of hip in the frontal plane. Reaching the neck the needle goes upward and enters the joint cavity. With effusion available, the manipulation is easier to implement and effusion indicates that the needle has reached the joint.

The knee joint can be aspirated from four points at the bottom or top of patella. With much effusion, the upper torsion is aspirated without injuring the cartilage. If at the same time the joint cavity should be washed with antiseptic solution, the aspiration is performed with two needles from the outside of and inside the patella. Upon evacuation of the cavity content through the second needle the solution is introduced with a clean syringe that upon effusion removal leaks through the first needle. The same principle is used to wash the knee joint cavity by connecting the hemotransfusion system with an antiseptic solution to one of the needles [40].

The ankle joint is aspirated from the point located 2 cm above and inwards from the lateral malleoulus top or from the point placed 1.5 cm above and outwards from the medial malleoulus top. At these points, retraction of soft tissues is palpated. The needle is advanced from front position backwards passing between ankle and talus [34].

The shoulder joint is aspirated from the anterior, posterior or outward surface. In outward aspiration, one should orient at the coracoid process of scapula. Immediately under it, the needle is inserted and advanced between the process and shoulder head. At posterior aspiration, the needle is inserted backwards from the top of acromion process in the fossa formed by the contours of the rear edge of deltoid muscle and inferior edge of supraspinous muscle and then the needle goes to the coracoid process.

The elbow joint is aspirated from behind or on the outside. The aspiration is perfomed with the joint bent at straight or obtuse angle. The needle is inserted at the top of the elbow process and advanced downward and forward. In correct position, the needle overcomes the elastic obstacle (joint capsule) and penetrates the joint cavity. The outside aspiration point is positioned between the head of radius and articular surface of shoulder.

Aspirations of minor joints are easier to perform since the anatomy and small volume of surrounding soft tissues allow palpation of the joint fissure or its localization in motions.

Methods for intra-articular therapy presume the usage of most of the drugs considered in 5.1.

Standard indications for intra-articular corticotherapy are as follows [41]: 1) infectious non-specific polyarthritis with evident exudative phenomena in one or several joints and with stable remission on most joints; 2) generalized infectious non-specific arthritis and Bekhterev' disease with evident arthritis and predominant exudative process in several major joints where despite complex therapy exudative phenomena persist; 3) contradictions to hormonotherapy in patients with inflammations in functionally important joints; 4) joint flexion deformities persisting for up to 10–12 months; 5) arthritis exacerbation in orthopedic surgical treatment of joint deformities; 6) exacerbation of chronic synovitis in deforming osteoarthrosis; 7) other arthritis forms under exacerbation (psoriatic arthritis, Reuter syndrome) as well as tendovaginitis with evident pain syndrome.

About 1/2 of pharmaceutical drug dose is injected in medium-size joints (e.g., elbow, ankle, or wrist) and 1/4–1/5 of the dose in small joints (interphalangeal, metatrasophalangeal, etc.). The dose can be repeated upon evaluating the result of the previous procedure in each individual case. Intra- or peri-articular injections of GC drugs in the course dosage is contradicted. If the first injection displays a short-time effect, it can be repeated within 4–5 days. If the repeated injection turns out to be inefficient, further GC therapy should be refused. A period between injections of long-term action drugs should be at least 1–2 months, medium-action – 2–3 weeks, and short-term action – 5–7 days. Once this rule is violated, there is a danger of manifestation of undesirable systemic effects of GC and development of dystrophic processes in the articular cartilage and underlying bone including aseptic necrosis. At evident exacerbations of polyarthritis, it is possible to perform a series of 2–3 intra-articular injections during 2–3 weeks (one procedure per week) in different inflamed joints. Local introduction of GC drugs as a supplementary method for treatment of rheumatic diseases allows reduction of in-patient period down to 5–10 days. Up to 50–70% of patients with inflammations localized in 1–2 joints recover after 1–2 procedures.

Injections of *solutions* of Novocain, Lidocaine, and Procain in the joint cavity or infiltrations with anesthetics of peri-articular tissues cause a satisfactory analgesic effect, especially in chronic posttraumatic arthritis. Degenerative joint diseases accompanied with synovitis exacerbations show an essential increase in SF volume and proteolytic enzyme content, as well as nonspecific inflammatory SM changes. In the absence of the effect of general NSAID treatment, local therapy with *anti-inflammatory drugs* is used (orgoteinm dimexide, peroxinorm) as well as inhibitors of proteolytic enzymes (Contrical, Trasylol) [42]. In order to inhibit SM proliferation and chronic inflammation chemical synoviectomy or intra-articular introduction of drugs breaking down the synovial layer and having an antipmytotic effect on plasmatic (immunocompetent) cells is used. The introduction of colloids of gold, yttrium or osmium tetroxide results in prolonged remission of local inflammation. The combination of general antibioticotherapy and introduction of antibacterial drugs of wide or directed spectrum in joints in bacterial arthritis allows effective inhibition of the development of cells of a disease causative agent directly in the site of infection.

Efficacy of local therapy depends on not only drug but also the place of its introduction, i.e., joint cavity, edge zone of painful meniscus, painful zone of epycondyle projection, etc. The injections in the most painful zones show the hihhest efficacy (especially with GC) [43].

After this procedure, especially if it is performed on a support joint, a rest for 3–4 hours should be provided for the limb.

Complications after intra-articular injections of drugs are largely due to violation of rules and technique of drug introduction. Local joint therapy can be followed by purulent inflammations, aseptic necrosis of bones [44], and development of local and systemic (in long-term therapy) osteoporosis that increases the risk of fractures of hip neck and vertebrae [45].

Local therapy can be improved by creating drugs and their combinations that prevent side effects and degradation of joint lubrication in medication. To solve the problem, tribological monitoring of drugs intended for intra-articular therapy (see 4.6.4) and evaluation of drug susceptibility to the biophysical field using the technique outlined in 4.7.1 can be helpful. The findings of work [46] confirm the assumption on the correlation between drug lubricity and coordinating nature of the relation between its components that provide its quazi-electret properties. The drugs comprising structures susceptible to electromagnetic field, in spite of different pharmacological groups, show the best lubricity.

Chondroprotectors are specific drugs intended for decelerating the degeneration of articular cartilage and improving its nutrition and antifriction characteristics.

A concept of disease-modifying therapy of joints has recently shaped. It consists in application of drugs that make it possible not only to monitor osteoarthritis symptoms (pain, joint dysfunction, etc.) but also stop its development and, in an ideal case, gain cartilage recovery (structural modification) [47]. To substantiate the structure-modifying drug effect it is required to quantitavely estimate structural changes in the joint including joint fissure stenosis and changes in cartilage volume and thickness.

Rentgenography (X-ray examination), ultrasound examination, magnet-resonance imaging (MRI), computer tomography (CT), and densitometry of subchondral areas of bone are main radiographic methods for joint examination making it possible to estimate these parameters.

MRI, one of the "youngest" diagnostic methods, has been used in clinical practice since 1981 [48] although the first experience of magnetic resonance application for examining human organism refers to 1967 [49] and the first two-dimension magnet-resonance imaging appeared in 1972 [50]. A necessity to diagnose joints with use of MRI is due to shortcomings of traditional examination techniques. Standard X-ray examination is insensitive to revealing early signs and short-term progress of osteoarthrosis. Ultrasound examination allows assessment of defects in peri-articular tissues and detection of fluid in the joint cavity, but it does not provide data on cartilage thickness and its intial damages. MRI is more sensitive than CT to the assessment of joint cartilage loss and pathologies of menisci and crusicate ligaments. Densitometry of local areas of the bone tissue gives information about the causes of osteoarthritis progress only in combination with other examination techniques.

Arthroscopy serves a criterion of validity of MRI data concerning cartilage defects. The classification of the defects based on comparison of MRI and arthroscopy findings is given in Table 5.3. It corresponds to the classification of histopathological cartilage changes proposed by Osteoarthritis Research Society International [51]. Most orthopedists agree that MRI is inferior to arthroscopy in detecting initial cartilage damages, however, with disease progress MRI sensitivity increases [52, 53]. Presently, MRI is believed to be a valid noninvasive method for measurement of cartilage thickness and volume capable of recording changes in these parameters during a short period. High measurement accuracy and availability of automated techniques for data processing [48] makes it possible to use MRI to prove the structure-modifying drug effect.

Table 5.3. Chodropathy Gradation by MRI and Arthroscopy Data [48]

MRI Stages	Arthroscopy Stages
1 – increased cartilage hydration (increasing signal intensity)	1 – cartilage swelling
2 – cartilage fibrillation or focal loss of < 50% of cartilage thickness	2 – superficial flaking and cracks
3 – erosions with focal loss of 50%< cartilage thickness<100%	3 – deep flaking and cracks
4 – deep erosions with exposure of subchondral bone	4 – deep erosions reaching subchondral bone

Chondroprotective drugs are biological or synthetic analogs to natural components of cartilage (hyaluronic acid, glucosamine, chondroitin).

Hyaluronic acid (glucosamine glucuronoglycan, hyaluronate) is part of SF substitutes considered in 5.3.2. and referring to structure-modifying drugs. Hyaluronic acid (HA) is a polysaccharide or a polymer whose monomer is a disaccharide consisting of N-acetylglucosamine and D-glucuronic acid (see 2.1). A HA macromolecule binds many water molecules owing to a large number of hydroxyl groups. In a synovial joint HA is synthesized by synoviocytes, fibroblasts, and chondrocytes. The molecular weight of natural HA reaches $(6-7)\times10^6$. Together with proteins, it forms large complexes with the molecular weight up to 3×10^8. As part of proteoglycans, HA is found in vitreous body, SF, cartilage tissue, and skin. Owing to its large molecular weight, the HA solution has an increased viscosity.

An exogenous HA recovers the SF viscosity and lubricity, normalizes the synthesis of endogenous proteoglycan with chondrocytes, and has an anti-inflammatory effect. The anti-inflammatory effect of HA preparations is due to inhibition of inflammation mediators (cytokines and PG), stimulation of anabolic (intended for formation and renewal of cells and tissues), and inhibition of catabolic (enzymatic splitting reactions) processes in cartilage matrix [54, 55]. The preparation is synthesized from chicken comb or via bacterial fermentation. It has a molecular weight from 0.7 to 7×10^6 (high- and low-molecular HA). Despite a significant difference in mass and half-life (within 28 days), therapeutic properties of its trade names do not differ essentially.

Presently, HA serves a means to modify disease symptoms and is recommended to patients who do not response to other kinds of therapy or are intolerable to NSAIDs. Therapeutic effects in arthrosis of major joints include pain relief or pain discontinuity, recovery of SF properties, augmenting functional capacities of the joint, decrease or disappearance of objective signs of synovitis, lowering dose or withdrawal of NSAIDs. The pain-relieving effect occurs after several days then the state is stabilized for several weeks and often maintained for several months. The findings of clinical trials performed in different countries substantiate the efficacy of HA drugs in osteoarthritis [56].

The treatment course includes from 3 to 5 intra-articular injections with a one-week interval. HA is introduced into a "dry" joint (with minimum effusion or without it). If the effusion is present it should be removed before injection.

Side effects include local pains in the place of injection and rarely enhancement of synovitis after injection.

Glucosamine is a monosaccharide $C_6H_{13}NO_5$. It is synthesized from glucose and has a molecular weight 179. The medicinal preparation is obtained from crustacean chitin wherein 83% of pure glucosamine is found [57]. Its second kind is crystalline glucosamine sulfate $C_6H_{13}NO_5{\cdot}H_2SO_4$ with the molecular weight 277 which is obtained synthetically. The glucosamine content is 79% [58]. Taken perorally, they both are well absorbed and found in SF in high concentrations. The mechanism of their structure-modifying action is similar to that of HA. The data are available on their capability of inhibiting the formation of superoxide radicals and synthesis of nitrogen oxide, which explains their analgesic effect.

Glucosamine is spread in many tissues and organs including the cartilage. It is not bound with blood proteins and, consequently, does not squeeze the drug out of this bond. Its high doses are safe. Glucosamine has been used in Europe since the 1960s. This drug is believed to be the only preparation in osteoarthritis management at whose long-term administration the risk of arthroplasty of legs is reduced [59].

In work [60], the opinion is suggested that the clinical efficacy of original glucosamine sulfate produced by the Rottapharm Co. cannot be extended to other glucosamine preparations, such as glucosamine hydrochloride, glucosamine-containing over-the-counter medicines and biologically active supplements.

Chondroitin sodium sulphate (ChS) is a group of polysaccharides consisting of sulfated and nonsulfated residues of glucuronic acid and N-acetylglucosamine. The preparation consists of eight components in different proportions. The mechanism of action of ChS is probably due to its physicochemical rather than biological activity [61]. Its use in treatment results in a significant pain relief, improved joint functions, and reduced NSAID dosage. In *in vivo* experiments it has been found that in rabbits oral or intramuscular chondroitin sulphate (with cartilage degeneration caused by chimiopain) essentially increased the amount of cartilage proteoglycans when compared to the control group of animals, which is an evidence of drug's protective ability in damages and ability of maintaining synthesis of proteoglycans [62].

The drug is well tolerated and does not have side effects [63]. At the European Congress of Rheumatologists held in Stockholm in 2002 the results were reported of long-term (2-year) administration of CS in 800 mg dose by 300 gonarthrosis patients that proved the drug ability to slow down the progression of osteoarthritis [64].

In Russia, a combined therapy with glucosamine and chondroitin uses "Artra" preparation comprising these active substances in equal amounts. It stimulates the regeneration of the cartilage tissue. Glucosamine enhances the production of cartilage matrix and ensures the protection of the affected cartilage from metabolic destruction caused by NSAID and GC. Chondroitin sulphate serves a supplementary substrate for formation of cartilage matrix, stimulates the formation of HA and protects it from enzymatic splitting by inhibiting hyaluronidases activity and damaging action of free radicals of SF. In osteoarthritis treatment the drug relieves disease symptoms and reduces the needs in NSAIDs. In 2005, in order to assess the structure-modifying effect of the combined glucosamine and chondroitin preparations the National Institute of Health, USA conducted an independent study called Glucosamine / Chondroitin Arthritis Intervention Trial (GAIT).

Up to recent time, orthopedists have used a group of drugs including Rumalon, Artheparon, Arthron, and Mucarthrin to provide chondroprotection. They were introduced intramuscularly after preliminary evaluation of local and general reactions to the injection of 0.3 mg of the drug.

Rumalon (International name is glucosaminoglycans-peptide complex) is the extract of cartilage and bone marrow of young animals. It comprises biologically active ingredients of cartilage matrix, i.e., peptides, proteoglycans, amino acids, chondrocytes, and cells of bone marrow. The drug stimulates the synthesis of glucosamines with chondrocytes in the affected cartilage, increases HA production, inhibits the destruction of glycoasamines and chondrocytes, and normalizes the SF composition. Indications are degenerative changes in synovial joints stages I and II, spondylosis, spondylarthrosis, meniscopathy, and patella chondromalacia.

The treatment includes a 0.3 ml intramuscular injection of Rumalon on the first day, 0.5 ml on the second day, and afterwards, 1 ml every other day. The course of treatment is 25 injections. The course can be repeated in 6 months following the same scheme.

Arthron (chondroitin sulphate) is similar to Rumalon in action mechanism. It is administered intramuscularly 1 ml every other day, the treatment course is 25 injections. In all, 2 treatment courses are administered during a year. It is superior to Rumalon in efficacy.

Artheparon (mucopolysachcaride polyester of sulfuric acid) is similar in structure to cartilage mucopolysaccharides, is distributed in the affected cartilage tissue, breaks the degradation of the base substance as the result of competitive inhibition of the enzymatic system that decomposes proteoglycan, and stimulates the SF formation.

The indications are similar to Rumalon. It is injected deeply in the gluteus muscle 1 ml 5% solution twice a week during 7–8 weeks (in all 15 injections). The course is repeated if necessary 3 months later. In maintaining therapy, several injections with a 1-week interval are made. In local therapy 0.5–1 ml of Artheparon is introduced into the joint cavity The injections are repeated twice a week (with 3–4 day intervals) during 3 to 5 weeks.

Mucartrine (mucopolysaccharide ether sulphate) is similar to Artheparon in mechanism of action. The treatment includes intramuscular injections 2 ml every other day, in all 10 injections, then twice a week during 4 weeks, and once a week during 4 weeks. The total course consists of 25 injections. During a year, two courses are administered with a 6-month interval.

In Russia, registration of some of these drugs pretending to have structure-modifying effects is canceled. Since 1997, Artheparon has not been used, in 2000 Rumalon prescription was discontinued. This was due to the side effects such as immune and allergic reactions, hemorrhagic complications because of their heparin-like structure, the risk of prionic disease transmission (since the drug is made of animal tissues) as well as the absence of serious evidences of structure-modifying action in clinical trials [65].

In addition, the drugs for external application described in 5.1.4 and 5.2.1 potentially affecting the cartilage do not refer to structure-modifying ones because a degree of their penetration into joints through skin is unknown.

A number of drugs also refer to structure-modifying ones, although the authors of work [66] believe that their medicinal effect is not proved with validity. Nevertheless, they are registered and used in orthopedics. Some of them are listed below.

Alflutop, a sterile extract of sea organisms (4 kinds of small sea-fish) consisting of glycosaminoglycans, polypeptides, amino acids, and microelements was proposed in the mid-1990s. It is assumed that it regulates the permeability of capillaries, inhibits the activity of hyaluronidases, prevents the destruction of the base substance of connective tissue, and stimulates the cartilage recovery. However, the serous evidences of the efficacy and safety of Alflutop are absent.

Piascledine 300 is a compound drug comprising avocado oil (1/3) and soya oil (2/3) fractions. Its application leads to decreasing NSAID doses and improves joint functions. Its role in osteoarthritis therapy is not still understood.

Repisan is a drug of plant origin for osteoarthrosis treatment. It relieves pain, retains and improves joint functions, leads to reduced NSAID doses, is characterized by the absence of side effects, and is combined with the drugs of other pharmacological groups [67].

The nomenclature of the above-listed drugs registered in Russia as structure-modifying is given in Table 5.4.

Recently, Osteoarthritis Research Society International (OARSI) has developed recommendations for management of this disease based on evidence-based analysis of efficacy of structure-modifying drugs (Table 5.5). Only three preparations among them are considered as structure-modifying, namely, glucosamine sulphate, chondroitin sulphate (in osteoarthritis of knee joints), and diacerin (in OA of hip joints). Administration of other drugs the experts believe to be unadvisable.

Table 5.4. Structure-Modifying Drugs in the Treatment of Osteoarthritis [66]

Drug	Active agent	Producer	Registration No.	Registration date	Formulation
Dona	Glucosamine sulfate	Rottarpharm S.r.l., Italy	П No.13737/01-2002	14.02.2002	Solution for intramuscular injections, amp. 2 ml
		Rottapharm Ltd., Ireland	П No.013659/01-2002	25.01.2002	Powder for oral solution, packs 1.5 g
Aminoarthrin	Glucosamine	Moscow Pharmaceutic Plant, Russia	P No.003621/01	08.07.2004	Tablets 300 mg
Structum	Chondroitin sulphate	Pierre Fabre Medicament Production	П No.13685/01-2002	05.02.2002	Capsules 0.5 g and 250 mg
Chondroitin-ACOS		OAO Syntez, Russia	P No.000545/02-2002	18.10.2002	Capsules 250 mg
Arthra Chondroitin 750		Unipharm Inc., USA	П No.015517/01	12.04.2004	Tablets obductae 0.75 g
Arthra	Chondroitin sulphate + glucosamine		П No.014829/01-2003	12.03.2003	Tablets obductae 1 g
Teraflex		Segmel Inc., USA	П No.015287/01	09.10.2003	Capsules
CHONDRO-nova		Panacea Biotec, India	П No.013982/01	27.11.2003	
Alflutop	Extract of sea-fish	BIOTEHNOSS.A., Romania	П No.012210/01-2001	14.12.2001	Solution for injections ampoules 1 ml
Piascledin 300	Oils of avocado and soya	Laboratoires Pharm., France	П No.015127/01-2003	30.06.2003	Capsules 300 mg
Repisan	Plant extract	Bittner Richard AG, Germany	П No.014182/01-2002	28.06.2002	Oral drops 20, 50, or 100 ml

Table 5.5. OARSI Recommendations on Osteoarthritis Treatment [68]

Proposition	Level of evidence (LoE)	ES for pain	Frequency recommended in existing guidelines	Level of consensus, %	Strength of Recommendation SOR, %
Paracetamol up 4 g per day can be an effective initial analgesic for mild to moderate pain syndrome in HJ and KJ OA. In the absence of an adequate response or in the presence of severe pain and/or inflammation, alternative pharmacological therapy should be considered based on relative efficacy and safety as well as comcommitant medications and diseases.	Ia (KJ) IV (HJ)	0.21 (0.02 to 0.41)	16/16	77	92 (88-89)
In patients with symptomatic KJ or HJ OA NSAIDs should be used in the lowest effective doses and their long-term use should be avoided if possible. In patients with high GI risk either a COX-2 selective agent or nonselective NSAID with co-prescription of protone pomp inhibitor PPI or misoprostol may be considered but NSAIDs including both COX-2 selective and non-selective should be used with caution in patients with increased cardiovascular (CV) risk factors.	Ia (KJ) Ia (HJ)	0.32 (0.24 to 0.39)	NSAID+PPI 8/8 NSAID+misoprostol 8/8 COX-2 inhibitors 11/11	100	93 (88-99)
Topical NSAIDs and capsaicin can be effective as adjunctives and alternatives to oral analgesic/anti-inflammatory agents in KJ OA.	Ia (NSAID) Ia(capsaicin)	0.41 (0.22 to 0.59)	7/9 8/9	100	85 (75-95)
IA injections of corticosteroids can be used in KJ or HJ OA and should be considered especially when patients have severe pain not responding satisfactorily to oral analgesic/anti-inflammatory agents or in patients with symptomatic KJ OA with effusions or other signs of local inflammation.	Ib (HJ) Ia (KJ)	0.72 (0.42 to 1.02)	11|13	69	78 (61-95)

Proposition	Level of evidence (LoE)	ES for pain	Frequency recommended in existing guidelines	Level of consensus, %	Strength of Recommendation SOR, %
Injections of IA hyaluronate may be useful in patients with KJ or HJ OA. They are characterized by delayed onset but prolonged duration of symptomatic benefit when compared to IA corticosteroids.	Ia (KJ) Ia (HJ)	0.32 (0.17 to 0.47)	8/9	85	64 (43-85)
Treatment with glucosamine sulphate and/or chondroitin sulphate may provide symptomatic benefit in patients with KJ OA. If no response is apparent within 6 months treatment should be discontinued.	Ia (glucosamine) Ia (chondroitin)	0.45 (0.04 to 0.86) 0.30 (-0.1 to 0.70)	6/10 2/7	92	63 (44-82)
In patients with symptomatic KJ OA glucosamine sulphate and chondroitin sulphate may have structure-modifying effects while diacerein may have structure-modifying effects in symptomatic HJ OA.	Ib (KJ) Ib (HJ)			69	41 (20-62)
The use of weak opioids and narcotic analgesics can be considered for the treatment of refractory pain in patients with KJ and HJ OA when other pharmacologic agents have been ineffective or are contradicted. Stronger opioids should only be used for the management of severe pains in exceptional circumstances. Non-pharmacologic therapies should be continued in such patients and surgical treatments should be considered.	Ia (weak opioids) IV (stronger opioids) IV (other)		9/9	92	82 (74-90)

Notes. Ia – meta-analysis of randomized controllable trials; Ib – randomized controllable tirals; IV – experts' opinion; ES – effect size - is a measure of standard mean difference in treatments (treatment vs. placebo) in units of standard mean deviation of the difference; ES=0.2 – small, ES=0.5 – moderate, ES>0.8 – large; OA – osteoarthritis, KJ – knee joints, HJ - hip joints, NSAIDs – non-steroidal anti-inflammatory drugs, COX – cyclooxygenase.

5.3.2. Substitutes of SF

Joint diseases are accompanied by SF deficit and modification of its properties. First, the SF viscosity decreases owing to depolymerization of hyaluronates with synoviocytes. The lubricant interlayer of the pathologically changed SF in the joint has a low carrying capacity, weakly absorbs impact loads, and “flows out” from the loaded cartilage micropores thus depleting the cartilaginous tissue feeding. In OA, SF inflammatory immune complexes and destructive enzymes are accumulated. This leads to development of degenerative processes in the synovial medium, restricted functional resources of joint and cartilage destruction.

The deficit of the lubricating fluid is compensated, and rheological SF parameters are corrected with use of the preparations called “artificial SF”, “SF substitute” and “SF endoprosthesis”. The last term also assumes that such preparation injected in the joint provides its long-term (for years) fail-free operation similarly to joint endoprostheses. The best representatives of these preparations relieve pain, recover the mobility of “dry” joints, recover the feeding of the cartilaginous tissue and serve chondroprotectors, i.e., protect the cartilage from wear and slow down the development of osteoarthritis.

The first-generation SF substitutes based on aqueous solutions of active polymers or their complexes with biopolymers have appeared in the 1970s.

One of the typical preparations of this kind is 15% solution of polyvinylpyrrolidone (PVP) intended to correct the synovial medium of joints in arthrosis deformans [69]. Hemodez, a 6% solution of PVP is known in medicine as the blood plasma substitute and prolongator of the action of co-administered antibacterial and hormonal drugs. An intra-articular PVP influences inflammation via decreasing permeability of SM, excreting mediators (biologically active agents) from the inflammation focus, inhibiting the activity of enzymes of cellular destruction, desintoxicating tissues, and exerting antihypoxic (aimed to prevent oxygenic starvation) and anti-adhesive effects. Rheological parameters of SF can be simulated to a certain degree by applying PVP together with HA solutions. However, soon, the shortcomings of this substitute have been revealed, such as a low biocompatibility and lubricity (the coefficient of friction in joints after PVP injections was by an order higher than in healthy joints [70]); lower than in SF pH (5.2−7.0 in PVP and 7.4−8.2 in SF); and a weak dependence of viscosity on the rate of shear load application.

PVP is injected in major joints 5 ml once a week together with 25−50 mg of hydrocortisone acetate. This is beneficial because PVP injections may lead to severe pains and exudative phenomena. The treatment effect was maintained during 6 months. The treatment course consisted of 4 to 6 injections with two courses per year. The combination of the preparations has the anti-inflammatory effect, improves the metabolism in the synovial medium, and regulates the functioning of immune cells of SM and SF.

In order to enhance the chondroprotective effect, 15% aqueous solution of PVP was co-administered with PVP hyaluronate or artheparon. The former combination is indicated in treatment of primary and secondary osteoarthritis with functional insufficiency degree I−II without signs of secondary synovitis. The latter combination was used in osteoarthritis with marked cartilage degeneration and osteoarthritis induced by crystal deposition.

The results of clinical approbations have shown PVP injections to improve temporarily the functioning of the joint in 70−80% OA patients; however, the drug is less efficient in rheumatoid arthritis [71].

Hydrogel-based SF substitutes, e.g., dextran- and phospholipids-containing ones are also found in this group [72]. They demonstrate a higher lubricity than PVP but have the same shortcomings at a higher price.

In the early 1990s, pseudosynovia based on sodium salt of carboxymethylcellulose (Na-CMC) with salt components typical of blood plasma [73] was produced. It was not spread in clinical medicine because of low lubricity. The next generation of such preparations [74–76] differed from the prototype in liquid-crystalline compounds of cholesterol with the mesophase within the range of physiological temperatures. The tests with animals proved those SF substitutes to demonstrate an enhanced protective effect towards the cartilage collagen [77]. A lower degree of dystrophic changes and fermentative destruction of the cartilaginous tissue can be attributed to chondroprotective effect.

The second-generation SF substitutes have appeared thanks to the hypothesis of joint homeostatic via recovering the viscosity of pathologically changed SF with use of HA-based preparations [78]. The beneficial effect of the procedure was called viscosupplementation [79]. First, this therapy was used only in Japan, Italy, and Canada. At the turn of the 20th century, it was approved in the USA, European countries, South America, and Australia. Rheumatologists and traumatologists' opinions range from disbelief and cautious optimism [56] to admitting it the main trend in OA treatment [80].

These preparations contain natural HA made from chicken comb or hylan – HA sodium salt. Table 5.6 gives brief information about the basic drugs of this class. We can comment it as follows.

Hyalgan is the first hyaluronic SF substitute. The size and molecular weight (MW) of constituent HA molecules is essentially smaller than those in SF. Hyalgan decreases friction, inhibits inflammation in the joint, influences positively the factors responsible for cartilage regeneration, and helps renew HA in the joint [81].

Synvisc (hylan G–F20) is a compound of two biopolymers whose molecules are linked with cross bonds. Synvisc surpasses healthy SF in viscoelastic parameters. The efficacy of knee joint osteoarthritis treatment with Synvisc is higher than when using NSAIDs [82].

Orthovisc is one of the most recent preparations among SF substitutes. It has the highest HA concentration, a low protein concentration and is characterized by minimal risks of inflammations. Orthovisc co-administered with other drugs reduces the needs in NSAIDs and makes it possible to avoid or postpone surgical intervention [83, 84].

The lubricity of hyaluronic SF substitutes varies under the exposure to the electromagnetic field (see 4.6.4).

The experience of hyaluronate applications in orthopedics has shown that their rheological influence on the synovial medium of OA joints is pathogenetically substantiated and the physiological simulation of joint lubrication with substitutes to replenish the SF secretion and temporarily substitute a pathologically changed synovia is a target biomechanical component in the joint treatment [70, 80, 85]. Topical preparations have been produced to transfer HA through the basal skin membrane in its deep layers.

Nevertheless, the SF substitutes cannot be considered as drugs since thy are only biological analogs to the substances involved in joint metabolism. After injection, HA derivatives cannot remain for a long time in the joint cavity and are incapable of maintaining independently optimal rheological parameters of SF. In osteoarthritis, they undergo enzymatic and free-radical destruction in the joint cavity [86].

Table 5.6. Preparations for Hyaluronic Therapy of Joints

Name and producer	Composition	Administration	MW	Effects
Hyalgan, «Fidia Pharmaceuticals», Padua, Italy; «Artz», Tokyo, Japan	Viscous solution of natural HA	A treatment course consists of 5 intra-articular injections during 4 weeks	0.5–0.73 mln	It relieves pain in knee joints during 6 months and more in most patients owing to increasing SF viscosity, reduces loads to the joint, and prevents side effects of NSAID-therapy.
Neovisc, «Stellar», London, Great Britain; Ontario, Canada	HA solution in physiological solution, 10–15 mg/ml; kinematic viscosity (2÷3)10^{-2} m^2/s	2–3 injections (2 ml) every other week, the repeated course at least after 6 months.	0.5–2.0 mln	They lubricate cartilage, reduce load to OA joints. Low probability of inflammations after injections.
Suplasin, «Bionishe», Montreal and Quebeck, Canada				
Hya–ject, «ORMED GmbH & Co», Freiburg, Germany				
Synvisc, hyalan G–F20, «Biomatrix Inc.», Ridgefield, NJ, USA	Compound of liquid hylan A (9 weight parts) and gel hylan B (1 weigth part) in physiological solution	3 intra-articular injections 7 days apart	6–8 mln	Medicinal effect is due to viscoelasticity and not associated with pharmacological, immunological, and metabolic effects. Synvisc is believed [78] to perform the functions of SF endoprostethis. They relieve pain in OA knee joints for more than 6 months.
Orthovisc, «Anika Therapeutics, Inc.», Woburn, USA	Solution of hylan in physiological solution, 15 mg/ml, viscosity within $5\cdot10^{-2}$ m^2/s	2 or 3 injections 7 days apart		

The pharmacological activity of hyaluronic SF substitutes refers to synoviocytes reaction, which after injection start producing autologous, more competent hyaluronates [87]. In addition, the cartilaginous tissue cells (chondroblasts and chondrocytes) have receptors to hyaluronates making it possible to protect cell membranes from inflammation mediators and free radicals [86]. In *in vitro* experiments, HA inhibits hemotaxis (directed motion of chemical substances), leucocyte migration, phagocytosis reactions, proliferation of lymphocytes, and adhesion of Monocytes; reduces the synthesis of PG-E_2 (hormone-like substance produced by cartilage cells) and bradykinin (biologically active peptide); and modulates the secretion of cytokines (protein or polypeptide molecules that are mediators of intercellular interactions) and inflammation mediators [87].

The therapeutic effect of HA-based preparations is the result of the improvement of rheological characteristics of the lubricating layer in the joint as well as increasing protection of the cartilage from wear and destruction of the cartilage tissue under enzymatic reactions. The pain is relieved and the functional state of joints improves in 75–77% of patients [84].

The best results were achieved when the preparations were injected at early osteoarthrosis stages. SF substitutes are not introduced intra-articularly in osteoarthrosis exacerbations accompanied by effusions and in infectious arthritis. The producers warn against injections of hyaluronic preparations in para-articular tissues as well as intra-articularly to patients having allergy to proteins, pregnant women, and children. After injections of SF substitutes, discomfort, shirt-term pains and exudates occurrence are possible [88].

At the turn of 21st century, a demand of creating high-efficient drugs with minimum side effects, so-called super-agents arose in orthopedics [89]. One may assume that their components demonstrate a perfect biocompatibility and actively affect the biological mechanisms of friction reduction in joints as well as inhibition of mechanical and enzymatic destruction of cartilage.

5.3.3. Autologous Blood Serum

The ideology of creation of super-agents for intra-articular injections presumes them to possess a high lubricity. In pathologically changed joints they should ensure the lubrication comparable to the friction of healthy joints with the coefficient of friction $f = 0.002–0.005$ under load $p \sim 3$ kPA [90]. The present-day views on biotribology are based on experimental findings obtained by atomic force microscopy and biochemical and tissue engineering methods [91, 92].

A hypothesis on the role of phospholipids in the synovial medium functioning explains the boundary lubrication in joints and hydrophobia of the cartilage surface [91]. As noted in 1.3.1, lipids are found in all living cells where they perform numerous functions, e.g., make an energy reserve, take part in the development of waterproof films and transfer of nervous impulses, etc. In a normal joint, phospholipids are major constituents (up to 61%) of lipids [93]. The ground substance of phospholipids – phosphatidylcholines (PC) – demonstrates high surface activity. PC (or lecitines and cholin phosphoglycerides) belong to the group of complex lipids whose molecules consist of alcohol, high-molecular weight fatty acids, and other components.

In a healthy joint, PC molecules are adsorbed on the rubbing cartilage surface that carries negative charge [94]. A diagram of the adsorbed layer is shown in Fig. 1.9. A specific structure of the adsorption layer provides a high load capacity and boundary lubrication of the cartilage-cartilage friction pair [91]. Neutral hydrocarbon chains of fatty acids make densely packed "tails" of PC molecules. Such arrangement transforms the hydrophilic phase of proteoglycans in the cartilage surface layer to a hydrophobic surface. The layer of adsorbed phospholipids ensures lubrication of joint endoprostheses after they have been implanted [96].

At the same time, another lubrication theory implies formation – on the cartilage surface – of specific lubricating structures secreted by fibroblasts and chondrocytes. Their emergence can be attributed to the fact that boundary lubrication takes place even in arthrosis-afflicted joints where SF has lost its natural viscosity maintained by HA. English tribologist D. Swann has extracted, from SF, glycoproteid of MW = 227 and proposed the term "lubricin" to denote the boundary lubricating layer containing it on the cartilage surface [97]. Blood plasma proteins are constituents of glycoproteids. Lubricin has attracted the attention of biotribologists as the nanosized lubricating layer that ensures boundary lubrication of cartilages. Later, the biochemical extraction was used to extract the protein of MW = 345 as the major lubricin component from the nanosized layer on the cartilage surface [98]. After that, the secretion of lubricin by chondrocytes was discovered [99] and it was set that the lubricin level was reduced in the joints with traumatic synovitis [100]. In the experiments with making use of atomic force microscopy, it has been found that HA molecules adsorbed on the rubbing surface synergetically improve the lubricity of lubricin [101].

These theories summarize the development of concepts on boundary lubrication in joints. First, it may be conceived that a natural lubricant of joints always ensures boundary lubrication of cartilages. Second, the adsorption lubricating film is formed from the substances found in blood serum and/or chondrocytes secreted by fibroblasts and chondrocytes. Third, the latter need a raw material in the form of blood serum proteins to secrete lubricin. Therefore, failures in the functioning of an "intelligent" joint that occur most often because of lacking provision of SM with serum (in Fig. 1.4 it is designated by the red line "bloodstream – SM") are compensated by blood serum-based intra-articular injections.

It can be conceived that injectable blood serum provides a better nourishment and lubrication of cartilages than the pathologically changed SF found in the joint. Immune damages are localized in the synovial medium of the joint and involved other organism's systems, in particular, the bloodstream, to a lesser extent. The idea of creating a medicinal BS + PC (pharmaceutical composition) complex looks promising. Such an agent would temporality perform all SF functions normalizing the structure and interrelation of the components of the synovial medium of the joint. Consequently, the medicinal effect aims at chondroprotection rather than just the replacement of SF with its endoprostheses.

Serum-based SF substitutes have the following advantages:

1) high biocompatibility of a substitute when the donor's serum matches the patient's blood group and absolute biocompatibility when using the autologous patient's blood serum (autologous serum) as a susbstitute base;

2) biochemical composition of the serum is closer to natural SF compared to other biological fluids of human organism and differs from SF only by the absence of hyaluronates;

3) availability of liquid-crystalline derivatives of cholesterol in both serum and SF;

4) improvement of lubricity under the effect of the joint biofield (shown below);

5) individual autologous serum-based substitutes for each patient and the absence of deficit and expensive components.

These arguments have formed the basis for a principally novel approach, advanced in [102], to the creation of third-generation SF substitutes based on blood serum [103, 104]. A prerequisite to their creation was a record-low lubricating ability of blood serum of groups I–IV compared to other liquids. The following experimental findings are helpful to understand what this fluid is like.

The coefficient of friction was registered by a pendulum tribometer described in 4.6.3 whose support (UHMWPE – Co-Cr-Mo alloy) is provided with an electromagnet coil. In addition, its variation was recorded under the effect of the electromagnetic field when the unit was lubricated with artificial SF components and their compositions (Table 5.7). In the experiments, the following fluids were used: blood serum (BS), group IV, SF taken from conventionally healthy knee joint (with patient's consent) with blood group IV; and HA according to Technical Specifications 42.KBC 146-78. The viscosity of the fluids was evaluated by a Guess viscosimeter relative to the viscosity of distilled water. The friction conditions were: pressure in the tribometer support $p = 0.3$ MPa, sliding velocity $v = 0.1$ m/s, and magnetic field stress on the friction surface $H = 1{,}2$ KA/m. The measurement results are shown in Fig. 5.5. Their analysis allows the following conclusions to be drawn:

1) all studied fluids, like natural SF (curve *5*), are susceptible to the magnetic field and respond to it by reducing coefficient of friction;

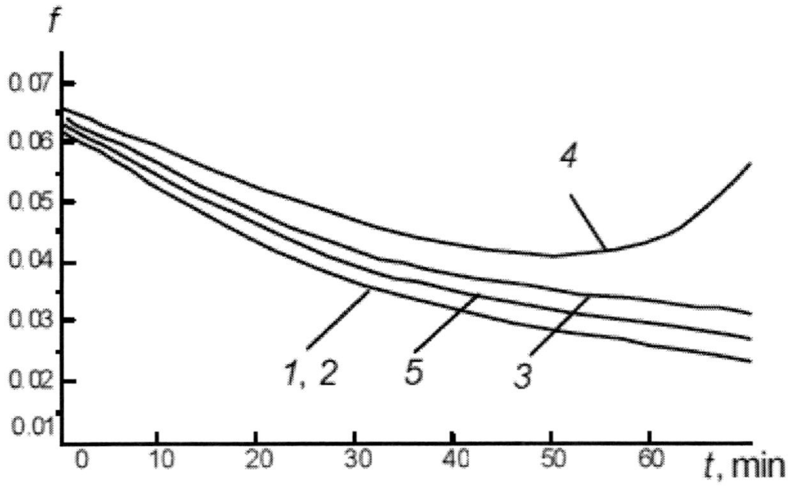

Figure 5.5. Coefficient of friction in tribometer support vs. duration of application of magnetic field and lubricating fluid composition. Curve numbers correspond to composition numbers in Table 5.7.

Table 5.7. Lubricating fluids

N	Composition	Viscosity, relative units.
1	BS	2.0
2	BS+ HA (2.0 g/l)	2.1
3	BS+ HA (3.5 g/l)	3.1
4	BS+ HA (4.5 g/l)	4.5
5	SF	3.1

2) the lowest f corresponds to BS and artificial SF with minimal addition of HA (*1*, *2*) having minimal viscosity;

3) excessive HA amounts (*4*) essentially increase the viscosity of the lubricating fluid and decrease the efficiency of field exposure on the lubricating film.

The similar dependences are typical of the compounds of BS with hyaluronic substitutes such as BS – Hyalgan, Hya-ject, and Synvisc [105]. Figure 5.6 shows the concentration dependences of f in the pendulum tribometer support when the support is lubricated with these compounds and long-term (50 min) exposure of constant magnetic field ($H = 1.2$ kA/m) on the lubricating film.

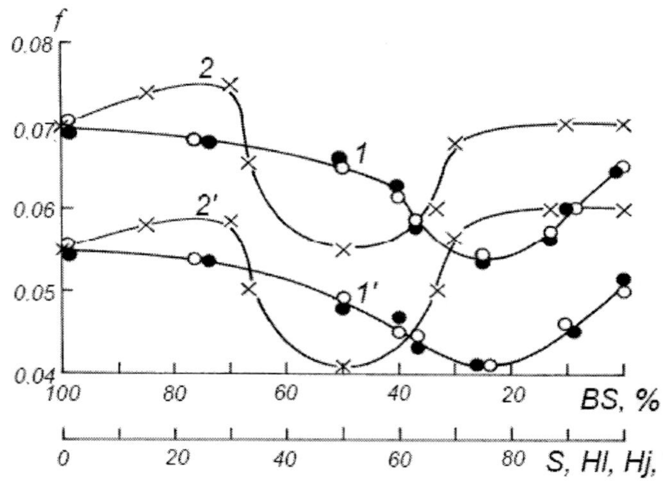

Figure 5.6. Coefficient of friction vs. composition of lubricating fluids exposed to magnetic field in the moving joint. Drug compositions: *1* and *1'* – BS + Hyalgan (Hl, light dots) and BS + Hya–ject (Hj, dark dots); *2, 2'* – serum + Synvisc (S). *1, 2* – the field is off; *1', 2'* – the field is turned on.

It is seen that the addition of Hyalgan and Hya-ject in BS leads to similar results. Minimum on curves *1* и *1'* is due to competitive influence of counteracting factors. The HA addititve increases the BS viscosity that in its initial state leaks out under load from the supports. With increasing viscosity, the lubricating film in the support is stabilized and its thickness increases. Therefore, an increase of additive within 50% results in friction transition to the boundary lubrication regime and monotonous decrease of *f*. Minimum in the region of additive concentration C = 45–85% evidently corresponds to the formation of a stable lubricating film consisting of complex compounds based on protein and liquid-crystal components of BS with addition of HA molecules. Excess of the latter at C > 85% essentially increases the viscosity of the lubricating layer, which causes the growth of coefficient of friction.

The BS + Synvisc mixtures show more complex concentration dependence. The initial growth of *f* with increasing concentration of the additive within 25% is related to a large viscosity of Synvisc ($\eta \sim 0.05$ Pa·s). Minimum at C ~ 50%, like in the previous case, evidently corresponds to the formation of complex structures (similar to those existing in healthy SF) with involvement of macromolecules of protein, hyalan, and liquid-crystal derivatives of cholesterol. An increase in hyalan concentration above limits corresponding to its complete binding in the complex compounds results in increasing friction within a certain constant value.

Therefore, minimum friction should be chosen as a criterion for optimization of hyaluronate content of BS-based synovia substitutes. A hypothesis has been advanced [105] that once SF substitutes are injected, under the effect of the biofield and friction, the compounds arise in the lubricating layer of the joint based on proteins, hyaluronates, and liquid-crystal derivatives of cholesterol that are similar to the structures existing in a healthy SF.

Autologous serum as a SF substitute was approbated with involvement of volunteers with degenerative-dystrophic changes of hip joints stages 1–3 by Kellgren-Lawrence (J. Kellgren и J. Lawrence, British rentgenologists) [106].

Experiments with synovia and serum were carried out under compliance with the ethical norms established at the 18th (Helsinki, 1964) and 41st (Hong Kong, 1989) World Medical Assemblies.

The patients were chosen according to the following criteria:

1) the patients aged between 40 and 65 years old,
2) OA stages 1–3 by Kellgren-Lawrence,
3) exception of intra-articular application of chondroprotectors during 6 months before trial,
4) exception of intra-articular injections of glucocorticoids during 2 months before trial,
5) informed patient's consent.

Exception criteria:

1) uncontrollable somatic diseases,
2) contradictions for joint aspiration,
3) psychic disorders in the history.

The scale (Table 5.8) [107] was used to evaluate the changes in knee joint functioning in the course of treatment based on the HSS (Hospital for Special Surgery, New York) rating system [108] and Knee Society [109] aimed to compare the results of knee arthroplasty. According to this scale, the healthy joint function corresponds to 100 points. By scoring the state of the damaged joint, one can conceive the degree of function losses and level of its recovery in treatment.

The treatment with autologous blood serum not containing any pharmaceutical preparations was performed in the following manner. The serum was prepared and conserved following the standard technique [11] in sterile conditions. At the blood transfusion station, 300–400 ml of patient's blood was taken in a flask without stabilizer. In 48 hours after the blood had been taken, the serum was aspirated and filtered, and simultaneously bacteriological control was performed. The serum sealed in ampoules 5 ml in volume was kept at T = +2 °C. The preparation was introduced in the cavity of degenerated joints threefold 7 to 10 days apart. The volume of the serum per injection varied from 5 to 10 ml depending on individual sensations. The injections stopped if a slight arching occurred in the joint. It was reported that in each next injection the volume of injected autologous serum increased by 3–5 ml. In patients with two-sided joint disorder, the preparation was injected in both joints during one procedure. Other drugs were withdrawn during treatment with autologous serum. The function of joints was assessed before treatment and after 2–3 days. The control evaluation of joint functioning was performed at least after a month after the third injection [107].

Table 5.8. The Scale for Evaluation of Knee Joint Functioning in Local Therapy

Attribute	Points
I. Pain	Total 40 points
None	40
At rest none	20
mild	15
moderate	10
severe	0
In walking no pain	20
initial	15
mild	10
moderate	5
severe	0
II. Walking	Total 20 points
Is possible during 2 to 3 hours	20
within an hour	15
within 30 minutes	10
impossible	0
III. Range of motion	Total 20 points
Full	20
Moderately limited (motion deficit within 45%)	15
Strongly limited (motion deficit within 90 %)	10
Joint rigidity	0
IV. Strength of extensors of knee joint in sitting position	Total 10 points
Patient raises and holds his ankle in horizontal position	10
Patient raises his ankle but cannot hold it	5
Patient cannot raise his ankle	0
V. Therapy efficacy	Total 10 points
Drugs are not used	10
Analgesics: not used	
reduced dose	1
the same dose	0
NSAID: not used	2
reduced dose	1
the same dose	0
Joint aspiration: yes	0
no	2
Intra-articular CS: yes	0
no	2
Attitude to surgical treatment: agree	0
not agree	2
VI. Subtraction	The points are subtracted from the total sum
Claudication	1
A stick	1
One crutch	2
Two crutches	3
Stiffness in joint after being in constrained position	1
Crepitation in motion	1
Joint swelling	1

The recent results of clinical investigations performed on 19 joints are as follows. The initial mean value of knee joint function in patients who agreed to take autologous serum injections was 55 points. After three injections, the function increased sequentially up to 72, 80, and 85 points. The control evaluation of the state of the treated joints was 80 points. A difference in efficacy of treating men and women was not reported. The patients reported pain relief, slippery joint sensation, disappearance of crepitation and stiffness, and ability to stay longer in constrained position without pain in the leg. This is because the autologous serum filling the cavity of the pathologically altered joint first, temporarily normalizes protein, aqueous, and saline metabolism, trophism of joint tissues, and synthesis of HA with synoviocytes and chondrocytes. Second, autologous serum has a better lubricity than the pathologically changed SF. Third, the autologous serum dissolves HA inclusions found in SM cells and cartilaginous tissue thus forming complex compounds analogous in chemical composition to healthy SF.

In the course of investigation, no negative results were reported. Statistical processing of the results confirmed a high efficacy of autologous serum injections both during treatment and after 1 to 7 months. Autologous serum makes it possible to get around the problem of biological incompatibility and expensiveness of hyaluronic SF substitutes as well as avoid hematogeneous infections in patients during treatment.

Modification of Serum with Medicinal Preparations

The findings of autologous serum treatment have shown the advisability of its modification with drugs of directed action. The modification can be performed most safely in the patient's organism. A drug is chosen with regard to etiopathogenesis of osteoarthritis based on the history and analysis of the most expedient and efficient drugs for a given patient. Depending on its pharmaceutical form, the drug is introduced in the patient's organism orally, intramuscularly, or intravenously. Once the blood is saturated with active drug components, the biosynthesis of a new transport medicinal complex occurs in the blood serum. Its composition is individual since the patient's blood serum has a certain individual number of protein molecules binding the active substance of the drug. The patient's organism sets the medicinal concentration of the drug that forms a medicinal complex with the serum in a natural manner

The groups of the patients with osteoarthritis of the knee joint – trial (36 patients and 41 joints) and control (29 patients) ones were formed as the need arose to treat the joints. The etiopathogenetic correlation between osteoarthritis and its cause leading to the disease or aggravation of its clinical course was set based on the history, and SF and blood test results.

Most patients of the trial group have been said that arthroplasty of the affected joint is unavoidable and their consent was obtained. The treatment went in line with the technique approved by the Ministry of Health of the Republic of Belarus [111] in the following manner. A target medicinal preparation (MP) was administered to the patient orally or intramuscularly. As soon as MP at its maximal concentration in blood had been introduced, (within the half-life period) 30 ml of blood was taken from the elbow vein. The syringe was incubed at 18–20 °C under aseptic conditions in the vertical position. Upon fractioning, 5-7 ml of serum was obtained containing the complex of MP with protein, fibrin clot, and sediment of blood cells. The serum obtained was taken with the second sterile syringe whose needle was replaced with a sterile one before an intra-articular injection. Intra-articular modified autologous serum was injected threefold 5 to 7 days apart. The volume of the first injection was 4-5 ml, the second and third – 5–7 ml. The patients of the trial group did not receive any other drugs.

The patients of the control group suffer from either traumatic or rheumatoid monoosteoarthritis. The traumatic osteorathritic patients received NSAIDs and physiotherapy and were injected intra-articularly with diprospane or kenalog. In the patients with rheumatoid arthritis the standard medication was accompanied by three (7 days apart) kenalog or diprospane (7 days apart) injections.

According to the scale shown in Table 5.8 the joint functioning was evaluated before treatment, after each injection, and in 5-6 months after treatment. The significance of the therapeutic effect was determined by meta-analysis described in the Cochrane Database Systematic Review [112] devoted to critical discussion of evidence of the efficacy of viscosupplementation of OA knee joint (*viscosupplementation* is a treatment intended to improve the viscoelasticity of SF).

The safety of new drug application was evaluated by clinical manifestations and dynamics of laboratory tests (cytological and biochemical blood test and urine test) during treatment.

Clinical examination of the patients of both groups has shown the following.

The patients with posttraumatic osteoarthritis reported bone fractures, meniscectomy, and/or plasty of cruciate ligament in their anamnesis. The cellular and biochemical compositions of SF were within normal limits. In microscopy of SF smears, singular multinuclear cells were detected. General and biochemical blood tests were within normal limits or pointed to positive C-reactive protein.

The duration of rheumatoid arthritis exceeded 7 years with a beneficial effect of corticosteroid therapy. The neutrophil leucocyte content of the SF smears set by microscopy varied within 55–87 %; also, rhagocytes were detected. The whole protein was increased up to 53 g/l, mainly because of γ-globulins, fibrin, and C-reactive protein. Blood tests pointed to an increasing leucocyte and lymphocyte amount and growing ESR. The diagnosis was confirmed by positive C-reactive protein and rheumatoid factor, dysproteinemia in the form of increasing fractions of α_2- and γ-globulins in the biochemical analysis as well as antigens of histocompatibility HLA DR4, Dw4, and DQ7.

More than 5 years ago, nine patients suffered from bacterial arthritis with primary OA of knee joints as the result of intra-articular kenalog injections. Afterwards, these patients experienced exacerbations of pain and synovitis 3-4 times a year. In exacerbations, the SF volume reached 80 ml, viscosity decreased sharply, and cytosis exceeded 5×10^{10}/l because of neutrophils. In one patient, *St. epidermidis* was detected in SF in exacerbation. Inflammatory SF alterations manifest in lowering viscosity, turbidity, fibrin thread availability, increasing neutrophils leucocytes up to 71%, decreasing glucose concentration, and increasing lactic acid concentration. In exacerbations, the growth of neutrophil leucocytes, increasing ESR, and sharply positive C-reactive protein were detected in the blood tests.

Viral synovitis was diagnosed based on epidemiological anamnesis: a pain syndrome and synovitis in osteoarthritic knee joints occurred in 1.5 weeks after exacerbation of herpetic infection in three patients and in 5-7 days after flu in three others. A week after disappearance of skin manifestations of herpetic infection and 2 weeks after respiratory infection was cured, nonspecific moderately pronounced inflammatory changes were detected in the patients' blood.

For target modification of serum, single doses of drugs conventionally used for above-listed disease were taken. Doxycycline, Arbidol, Cycloferone, Polcortololone, and Diclofenac were administered orally or intramuscularly. Maximum drug concentration in the blood was determined based in instructions for their application. Thus, 93% of an oral Doxycycline dose of 200 mg binds to blood proteins in 2 hours and its maximum therapeutically efficient concentration 2.6 μkg/l is set [113]. Doxycycline has both antibacterial and chondroprotective effects owing to inhibition of matrix metalloproteinases and nitrogen oxide synthase.

Maximum concentration of Arbidol in blood plasma is set 1.5 hours after 100 mg of the drug is received. Arbidol makes complex compounds with albumin in the blood that prevent from the contact and invasion of viruses in the cells of joint tissues and inhibit the confluence of lipid membrane of the virus with cellular membranes [114].

Cycloferone is a low-molecular inductor of interferone having a wide spectrum of biological activity (immune modulating, antiviral, anti-inflammatory, etc.) [115]. The blood enriched with cycloferone was taken 1-2 hours after intramuscular and intravenous injection of 0.25 g.

After taking a minimal single dose of Polcortlone (4 mg), its active substance triamcinolone is absorbed from the gastrointestinal tract (20–30% bioavailability). After 1-2 h, its maximum concentration in patient's blood is set. Triamcinolone binding to serum proteins (mainly to globulins) is 40% [116].

Diclofenac is totally absorbed from the intestine once taken orally. In first passage it is metabolized in the liver after which about a half of the drug enters the blood. Binding of Diclofenac to serum proteins is 99%. After 2 to 4 h, its maximum concentration in blood is registered [117].

In the trial group, the Doxyxycline-saturated serum was injected in the knee joints in 8 patients suffered with posttraumatic osteoarthritis and one patient with bacterial synovitis (based on revealed susceptibility *St. epidermidis* detected earlier to Doxycycline). The rheumatoid arthritis patients were injected intra-artucularly with the composition of autologous serum and Polcortolone. Ardibol-modified serum was injected to the patients with flu and Cycloferone-modified serum was used in exacerbations of herpetic infection. Diclofenac was bound to serum to stop articular syndrome in exacerbations of posttraumatic osteoarthritis in four patients and in eight patients with old bacterial arthritis.

The treatment results are given in Table 5.9.

The above results correspond to the category of randomized controlled trials: the trial period exceeded 2 months and all patients were maintained throughout the study (allowed within 50%) [112]. Meta-analysis shows that in all patients 95% confidence intervals for the difference of mean values of therapeutic effect in the trial and control groups does not intersect zero, which indicates the efficacy of trament in the trial group. The heterogeneity of the results was statistically significant. A value of therapeutic effect of the new method for osteoarthritis treatment shown as a weighted difference of mean with 95% confidence intervals was 5.01. This is the evidence of the advantage of the new method over the conventional one.

All the patients from the trial group reported pain relief in joints under loads and its significant reduction or even disappearance at rest. During treatment, complications and allergic reaction were not registered. The dynamics of the laboratory analysis results has revealed a stable tendency to reducing pathological deviations and normalization of organism's functions. 5–6 moths after the last injection the function of joints in all the patients of the trial group maintained at the achieved level. At the same time, the doses of anti-inflammatory and analgesic drugs were tapered and a necessity of endoprosthetics denied. In the patients of the control group the therapeutic effect maintained within 6 months after treatment at the same doses of maintaining drugs.

Table 5.9. The Results of Knee Joint Treatment with Autologous Serum Modified with MP in Patient's Organism

OA Etiology	Number of treated joints	Average patient's age	Evaluation of joint function (mean score)		
			Before treatment	After 1, 2, and 3 injections	After treatment course (months)
Trial group					
Posttraumatic	14	54	57	76/79/89	88 (6)
Rheumatoid	11	59	48	66/76/78	76 (6)
Bacterial	9	48	51	62/81/87	86 (6)
Viral	7	45	56	63/75/78	77 (5)
Control group					
Posttraumatic	16	52	56	61/68/79	77 (6)
Rheumatoid	13	54	47	49/58/68	67 (6)

It may be conceived that the clinical effect of the treatment of the trial group patients has been achieved thanks to the fact that the drug bound to serum proteins enters directly the affected joint passing metabolically active organs and the fibrously affected joint capsule. In the joint cavity, the drug dissociates from the protein transport complex and has a medicinal effect on the synovial medium of the joint. This allows minimization of the drug dose and reduction of adverse reactions. Instead of pathologically altered SF containing tissue decay products, anti-inflammatory cytokines, matrix metalloproteinases, etc., an injected preparation rich in proteins, carriers of biologically active substances, enters the joint cavity thanks to which the trophism of the joint as well as protein, aqueous, and saline metabolism are normalized. The lubricity of such drug is considerably higher than that of the pathologically altered SF [118]. Pain is relieved owing to better sliding of the degenerated bone surface. Surely, the mechanisms of beneficial effects of drug-modified blood serum in osteoarthritis patients need further understanding. It is required to conceive whether maximum concentration of the drug naturally bound to autologous serum proteins is optimal for joint treatment. Nevertheless, a marked positive effect of such preparations in knee joint osteoarthritis treatment has been established. A course therapy with serum-based preparations is advisable to include in the recommendations on osteoarthritis management in the cases of inefficiency of and/or contradictions to long-term administration of analgesic and anti-inflammatory drugs.

Treatment of osteoarthritis with autologous blood serum can be implemented in hospitals and polyclinics following the standard technique of intra-articular injections. Preliminary saturation of serum with a target drug in the patient's organism occurring in a sealed volume and under sterile conditions allows minimization of probability of septic complications and making the procedure time- and cost-efficient. Primary results of laboratory and clinical studies indicate the advisability of further research into metabolic effects of medicinal compositions based on blood serum.

The findings cited above indicate that a new trend in transfusion-infusion therapy has been fumed called transfusion chondroprotection intended for treatment of osteoarthritis with autologous blood serum affiliating to the patient's or donor's blood of the same group. The above-discussed results indicate that a new trend in transfusion-infusion therapy has developed, namely, transfusion chondroprotection, which aims to treat osteoarthritis with autologous patient's blood or donor blood of the same group. Necessity to develop works in this direction by immunologists, virologists, and microbiologists is evident. Development of immune-modulating drugs for OA treatment that inhibit catabolic processes in joints by regulating intercellular and intermolecular anti-inflammatory interactions allows improvement of the patients' quality of life, widening of their functional possibilities, and weakening of the urgency of the global problem of joint pathology.

Acknowledgments

The following main trends of affecting the synovial medium of joints have taken shape in the methodology of arthrological treatment:

1) chondroprotection conducted both pharmacologically and through local therapy using intra-articular injections of blood serum-based drugs;

2) development of new-generation medicinal preparations actively affecting immune reactions in joint, primarily, immunosuppressive drugs inhibiting the development of pathological states of the joint wherein the immune response to an antigen invaded by infectious agents is enhanced with maintained normal immune response to other antigens;

3) orientation of physiotherapy to compensation of weaker biophysical fields in pathologically altered joints and activization of processes that occur in the synovial medium of joints at the biochemical, biophysical, and biomechanical levels.

These trends define the medicinal effects on SF as a multifunctional substance responsible for metabolism in joints and immunization of the synovial medium of joints.

References

[1] *Diagnostics and treatment of internal diseases. Handbook for physicians in 3 Vol.* Ed. Komarov, FI. Vol 1. Diseases of cardio-vascular system, rheumatic diseases. Moscow: Medicine, 1991.

[2] Soroka, NF; Yagur, BE. *Rheuamtoid arthritis: problems of diagnostics and treatment: a reference book.* Minsk: Belarus, 2000.

[3] Champion, GD; Feng, PH; Azuma, T; et al. NSAID-induced gastrointestinal damage. *Drugs,* 1997, Vol 53, 6–19.

[4] Sigidin, YaA; Shvartz, TYa; Arzamastsev, AP; Liberman, SS. *Drug therapy of inflammations*. Moscow: Medicine, 1988.

[5] Grosser, T; Fries, S; FitzGerald, GA. Biological basis for the cardiovascular consequences of COX-2 inhibition: therapeutic challenges and opportunites. *J. Clin. Invest.* 2006, Vol 116, 4–15.

[6] Belousov, YuB; Moiseev, VS; Lepakhin, VK. *Clinical pharmacology and pharmacotherapy: a handbook for physicians*. Moscow; Unversum, 1993.

[7] Non-sterioidal anti-inflammatroy drugs (Editor's article). *Klin. Pharm. Pharmakoter.* 1994, N 3, 6–7.

[8] Loeb, DS; Ahlquist, DA; Talley, NJ. Management of gastroduodenopathy associated with use of nonsteroidal anti-inflammatory drugs. *Mayo Clin. Proc.* 1992, Vol 67, 354–364.

[9] Espinosa, L; Lipani, J; Poland, M; Wallin, B. Perforations, ulcers and bleeds in a large, randomized, multicenter trial of namubetone compared with diclofenac, ibuprofen, naproxen and piroxicam. *Rev. Exp. Rheumatol.* 1993, Vol 20, Suppl I, 324.

[10] Marcus, AL. Aspirin as prophylaxis against colorectal cancer. *N. Engl. J. Med.* 1995, Vol 333, 656–658.

[11] Lieber, CS. Medical disorders of alcoholism. *N. Engl. J. Med.* 1995, Vol 333, 1058–1065.

[12] Guslandi, M. Gastric toxicity of antiplatelet therapy with low-dose aspirin. *Drugs.* 1997, Vol 53, 1–5.

[13] Insel, PA. *Analgesic-antipyretic and anti-inflammatory agents and drugs employed in the treatment of gout.* In: Goodman & Gilman's. The pharmacological basis of therapeutics. 9th Ed. McGraw-Hill, 1996, 617–657.

[14] Noble, S; Balfour, J. Meloxicam. *Drugs.* 1996, Vol 51, 424–430.

[15] Perneger, TV; Whelton, PK; Klag, MJ. Risk of kidney failure associated with the use of acetaminophen, aspirin, and nonsteroidal anti-inflammatory drugs. *N. Engl. J. Med.* 1994, Vol 331, 1675–1712.

[16] Lieber, CS. Medical disorders of alcoholism. *N. Engl. J. Med.* 1995, Vol 333, 1058–1065.

[17] Gillis, JC; Brogden, RN. Ketorolak. A reappraisal of its pharmacodinamic and pharmacokinetic properties and therapeutic use in pain management. *Drugs.* 1997, Vol 53, 139–188.

[18] Mashkovskii, MD. *Medical Drugs. In 2 Vol.* Moscow: Medicine, 1998.

[19] Schumacher, HR; Chen, LX. Injectable corticosteroids in treatment of arthritis of the knee. *Amer. J. of Medicine*. 2005, Vol 118, 1208–1214.

[20] Beresten', TI; Trofimova, TM. Treatment of Rheumatoid Arthritis with Gold Preparations under its concentration control in plasma serum. *Ther. Archive.* 1980, N 2, 102–106.

[21] Langford, CA; Klippel, JH; Balow, JE; James, SP; Sneller, MC. Use of cytotoxic agents and cyclosporine in the treatment of autoimmune disease. Part I: Rheumatologic and renal diseases. *Ann. Intern. Med.* 1998, Vol 128, 1021–1028.

[22] Korzh, AA; Chernykh, VP; Filippenko, VA; et al. *Diagnostics and conservative treatment of diseases and injures of locomotor system.* Ref. book in 8 books. Book 2: Osteoarthrosis. Kharkov: Basis, 1997.

[23] Nasonova, VA; Nasonov, EL; Alekperov, RT; Alekseeva, LI; et al. *Rational pharmacotherapy of rheumatic diseases.* Moscow: Littera, 2003.

[24] *Clinical rheumatology.* Ed. Mazurov, VI. Moscow: Medicine, 2004.

[25] Sigidin, YaA; Guseva, NG; Ivanova, MM. *Diffusive diseases of connective tissue.* Moscow: Medicine, 2004.

[26] Nasonov, EL. *Rheumatology. Clinical recommendations.* Moscow: GEOTAR-MED, 2007.

[27] Yasnogorodskii, VG. *Electrotherapy.* Moscow: Medicine, 1987.

[28] Ulashchik, VS; Lukomskii, IV. *General physiotherapy.* Minsk: InterPressSerice, 2004.

[29] Vyalko, VV; Berglezov, MA; Ugnivenko, VI. *Low-frequency lasers in traumatology and orthopedics.* Moscow: CITO, 1998.

[30] Cherniakova, YuM; Pinchuk, LS; Lobanovskii, LS; Drozd, ES; Chizhik, SA. Structure and magnetic susceptibility of lubricating fluids of the synovial joint. *J. Friction and Wear.* 2011, Vol 32, N 1, 54–60.

[31] Shipulina, IA; Averyanova, NI. *Foundations of physiotherapy: A handbook for medical universities.* Rostov-on-Don: Fenix, 2007.

[32] Kuskov, AS; Lysikova, OV. Balneology and recreational tourism. Rostov-on-Don: Fenix, 2004.

[33] Zeman, MA. *Technique of dressing.* St Petersbusr: Piter, 1994.

[34] Movshovich, IA. *Surgical orthopedics. Manual for physicians.* Moscow: Medicine, 1994.

[35] Brittberg, M; Lindahl, A; Nilsson, A; et al. Treatment of deep cartilage defects in the knee with autologous chondrocyte transplantation. *N. Eng. J. Med.* 1994, Vol 331, 889–895.

[36] Mandelbaum, B; Browne, J; Fu, F; et al. Articular cartilage lesions of the knee. *J. Sport Med.* 1998, Vol 26, N 6, 853–860.

[37] *International Cartilage Repair Society Documentation and Classification System.* Freiburg, Switzerland, Newsletter 1, March, 1998, 5–8.

[38] Luano-Ravina, A; Jato Dias, M. Autologous chondrocyte implantation: a systematic review. *Osteoarthritis Cartilage.* Vol 14, 47–51.

[39] Methodical instructions N 2001/25 of the Ministry of Health RF. *Consilium Medicum,* 2003, Vol 5, N 2, 109–110.

[40] Rutskii, AV; Rylyuk, AF. *Surgery and topographic anatomy of low extremity and spine.* Minsk: BelGIUV, 1993, Part 1.

[41] Astapenko, MG; Pavlov, VP. *Aspiration of joints and intra-articular introduction of steroid hormones in therapeutic practice.* Moscow: Medicine, 1973.

[42] Soroka, NF. *On rheumatoid arthritis (questions and answers).* Minsk: Belarus, 1992.

[43] Golikova, NM; Vyal'ko, VV. *Intra-articular injection therapy in complex treatment of arthrosis deformans of the knee joint.* In: Diagnostics and treatment of injuries and diseases of locomotor system. Collection of papers CITO, 1987, 33–37.

[44] Emkey, RD; Lindsay, R; Lissy, J; et al. The systemic effect of intra-articular administration of corticosteroid on markers of bone formation and bone resorbtion in patients with rheumatoid arthritis. *Arthritis Rheum.* 1996, Vol 39, 277–282.

[45] Walsh, U; Wong, CA; Pringle, M; Taffersfield, AE. Use of oral corticosteroids in the community and the prevention of secondary osteoporosis: across sectional study. *BMJ.* 1996, Vol 313, 344–346.

[46] Cherniakova, YuM; Pinchuk, LS; Kravtsov, AG; Kadolich, ZhV; Nikolaev, VI. Tribological and electret-thernal analysis of drugs for local joint therapy. *Zh. Tech. Phys.* 2005, Vol 75, Issue 5, 119–123.

[47] Alekseeva, LI. Promises of chondroprotective therapy of osteoarthrosis. *Nauch. Pract. Rheumat.* 2003, N 4, 83–86.

[48] Zaitseva, EM; Alekseeva, LI; Smirnov, AV; Nasonov, AL. Magentoresonance imaging in osteoarthrosis. *Nauch. Pract. Rheumat.* 2006, N 5, 59–75.

[49] Crues, JV; Rye, RK. *MRI of the knee*. In: Magnetic Resonance Imaging. Vol II. NY: Raven Press, 1992, 2391–2403.

[50] Lauterbur, PC. Image formation by induced local interactions examples employing nuclear magnetic resonance. *Nature.* 1973, Vol 243, 190–193.

[51] M Pritzker, KP; Gay, S; Jimenez, SA; et al. Osteoarthritis cartilage histopathology: grading and staging. *Osteoarthritis Cartilage.* 2006, Vol. 14, 13–29.

[52] Brederick, LS; Turner, DA; Renfrew, DL; et al. Severity of articular cartilage abnormality in patients with osteoarthritis: evalution with fast spin-echo MR vs arthroscopy. *Am. J. Röentgenol.* 1994, Vol 162, N 1, 99–103.

[53] Karvonen, RL; Negendank, WG; Fraser, SM; et al. Articular cartilage defects of the knee: correlation between MRI and gross pathology. *Ann. Rheum. Dis.* 1990, Vol 49, 672–675.

[54] Yasui, T; Akatsuka, M; Tobetto, K; et al. The effect of hyaluronan on interleukin 2 induced prostaglandin E2 production in human osteoarthritis synovial cells. *Agents Action.* 1992, Vol 37, 1556.

[55] Ghosh, P. The role of hyaluronic acid (hyaluronan) in health and disease: interactions with cells, cartilage and components of the synovial fluid. *Clin. Exp. Rheumatol.* 1994, Vol 12, 75–82.

[56] Sushchuk, EA. *Evaluation of efficacy of hyaluronic acid preparation in posteoarthritis management in terms of evidence medicine*. Moscow: LiniaPRINT, 2007.

[57] Patent 6486307 US. *Preparation of glucosamine hydrochloride*. Gandhi, DR; Laidler, JK. ICI A 61K. 2002.

[58] Patent 5847107 US. *Method of preparing mixed glucosamine salts*. De Wan, M; Volpi, G. ICI A 61K. 1998.

[59] Pavelka, K; Gatterova, J; Giacovelli, G; et al. Glucosamine sulfate prevents total joints replacement in the long-term follow-up of knee osteoarthritis patients. *Arthritis Rheum.* 2004, Vol 49, Suppl, A 251.

[60] Krigstein, OS; Golubev GSh. Evaluation of evidences of efficacy of drugs pretending to be structure-modifying ones (2-004-2007). Part 1. *Zdravookhranenie.* 2009, N 11, 39–52.

[61] Nasonov, EL; Alekseeva, LI. Chondrotin sulphate (structum) in osteoarthrosis treatment: pathogenetic justification and clinical activity. *Ter. Arkhiv.* 2001, Vol 73, N 11, 87–89.

[62] Uebelhart, D; Thonar, E; Zhang, J; Williams, J. Protective effect of exogenous 4.6sulfate in the acute degradation of articular cartilage in the rabbits. *Osteoarthritis Cartilage.* 1998, Vol. 6, Ssuppl A, 613.

[63] Alekseeva, LI; Benevolenskaya, LI; Nasonov, EL; Chichasova, NV; Karyakin, AN. Structum (chondroitin sulfate) a new remedy for osteoarthrosis treatmen. *Ter. Arkhiv.* 1999, N 5, 51–53.

[64] Uebelhart, D; Thonar, E; Delmas, P; et al. Effects of oral chondroitin sulfate on the progression of knee osteoarthritis: a pilot study. *Osteoarthritis Cartilage.* 1998, Vol 6, Suppl A, 39–46.

[65] Brandt, KD. *Management of osteoarthritis*. In: Kelleys textbook of rheumatology. 6th Ed. 2001, 1419–1432.

[66] Golubev, GSh; Krigstein, OS. Estimation of evidence of drug efficacy pretending to be called structure-modifying preparations. *Int. J. Med. Practice*. 2005, N 2, 38–52.

[67] Burmakova, GM; Natsvlishvili, ZG. Application of Repisan in treatment of osteoarthrosis of knee joints. *NN Priorov Vestnik traumatol. and orthop.* 2005, N 3, 52–57.

[68] Krigstein, OS; Golubev, GSh. Estimation of evidence of drug efficacy pretending to be called structure-modifying preparations (2004–2007). Part 1. *Zdravookhranenie*. 2009, N 12, 26–39.

[69] Vasilenkaitis, VV. *Clinical biomechanical principles of intra-articular application of artificial synovial fluid in osteoarthrosis deformans*. In: Proc of Research Institute of Exp and Clin Medicine, Ministry of Health of Lithuania, Vilnius: Mokslas, 1983, Issue 18, 81–84.

[70] Vyrva, OE. Artificial synovial fluid in treatment of knee joint pathology. *Orthop. Traumatol. Prosth*. 2000, N 2, 146–150.

[71] Khasan, R; Shibalkin, VD. Experience of treatment with polyvinylpyrrolidone of osteoarthrosis deformans of the knee joints. *Rheumatologia*. 1985, N 3, 40–43.

[72] Patent 0185179 WO. *Biological lubricant composition and method of applying lubricant composition*. Laberge, M; Lickfield, G; Budrick, J-AM. IPC A 61K 31/721, 31/685; A 61L 27/20, 27/52; A 61P 41/00. 2001.

[73] Patent 1391577 US. *Pseudo-synovial plastic body fluids and method of preparing some*. Homsy, CA. IPC C 08L 1/28, A 61K 317/15. 1975.

[74] Patent 5238929 US. *Correction of tribology of arthritis-affected joints and medicine for its implementation*. Koupchinov, BI; Ermakov, SF; Beloenko, ED; et al. IPC A 61K 31/56. 1993.

[75] Patent 2033162 RF. *Artificial synovial fluid*. Kupchinov, BI; Beloenko, ED; Ermakov, SF; et al. IPC A 61K 31/79. 1995.

[76] Patent 898 BY. *Artificial synovial fluid*. Kupchinov, BI; Beloenko, ED; Ermakov, SF; et al. IPC A 61K 31/79. 1995.

[77] Beloenko, ED; Kupchinov, BI; Ermakov, SF; et al. Experimental substantiation of liquid-crystal state of joint synovial lubricating medium. *Vesti NAN Belarus Medical Ser*. 2001, N 1, 79–85.

[78] Swann, DA; Radin, EL; Nazimiec, M; Wessler, PA; Curran, N; Levinner, G. Role of hyaluronic acid in joint lubrication. *Ann. Rheum. Dis*. 1974, Vol 33, 318–330.

[79] Balazs, EA; Denlinger, JZ. Viscosupplementation a new concept in the treatment of osteoarthritis. *J. of Rheum*. 1993, Vol 20, Suppl 39, 3–9.

[80] Marshall, KW. Intra-articular hyaluronan therapy. *Current Opinion in Rheumatology*. 2000, N 12, 467–474.

[81] Makeu, E; Aural, X; Dougados, M. A hyaluronan preparation (500–730 kDA) in treatment of osteoarthritis: a review of clinical trials with Hyalgan. *Int. J. Clin. Pract*. 2002, Vol 56, N 10, 804–813.

[82] Vad, VB; Sakalkale, D; Sculco, TP; et al. Role of hylan G–F20 in treatment of osteoarthritis of the hip joint. *Arch. Phys. Med. Rehabil.* 2003, Vol 84, 1224–1226.

[83] Tanaka, N; Sakanashi, H; Sato, E; et al. Intra-articular injection of high molecular weight hyaluronan after arthrocentesis as treatment for rheumatoid knees with joint effusion. *Rheumatol. Int*. 2002, Vol 22, N 4, 151–154.

[84] Axe, MJ; Shields, CL. Potential application of hyaluronans in orthopaedics. Degenerative joint disease, surgical recovery, trauma and sports injuries. *Sports Med.* 2005, Vol 35, N 10, 853−864.

[85] Kelly, MA; Goldberg, VM; Healy, WZ; et al. Osteoartritis and beyond: a consensus on the past, present and future of hyaluronans in orthopaedics. *Orthopaedics.* 2003, Vol 26, 1064−1079.

[86] Scott, JE. Hyaluronan, multum in parvo. *Europ. J. of Rheumatology and Inflammation.* 1995, Vol 15, N 1, 3−8.

[87] Abatangelo, G; O'Regan, M. Hyaluronan: biological role and function in articular joints. *Europ. J. of Rheumatology and Inflammation.* 1995, Vol 15, N 1, 9−16.

[88] Goldberg, VM; Buckwalter, JA. Hyaluronans in the treatment of osteoarthritis of the knee: evidence for disease-modifying activity. *Osteoarthritis Cartilage.* 2005, Vol 3, N 3, 216−224.

[89] Soroka, NF. Clinical rheumatology at the turn of the century. *Zdravookhranenie.* 2001, N 5, 2−7.

[90] Charnley, J. *Low friction arthroplasty of the hip − theory and practice.* Berlin: Springer-Verlag, 1979.

[91] Hills, BA; Crawford, RW. Normal and prosthetic synovial joints are lubricated by surface-active phospholipid. A hypothesis. *J. of Arthroplasty.* 2003, Vol 18, N 4, 499−505.

[92] Jay, GD. Lubricin and surfacing of artificial joints. *Current Opinion in Orthopaedics.* 2004, Vol 15, 355−359.

[93] Rabinowitz, JL; Gregg, JR; Nixon, JE. Lipid composition of the tissues of human knee joints. II. Synovial fluid in trauma. *Clin Orthop Rel Res*, 1984, Vol 190, 292−300.

[94] Glosh, P. *Anti rheumatic drugs and cartilage.* In: *Bailliere's clinical rheumatology.* Ed. Brooks, P. London: Bailliere, 1988, 310−333.

[95] Hills, BA. *The biology of surfactant.* Cambridge: Cambridge University Press, 1988.

[96] Bell, J; Tipper, JL; Ingham, E;, et al. The influence of phospholipid concentration in protein-containing lubricants on the wear of ultra-high molecular weight polyethylene in articular hip joints. *Proc. Inst. Mech. Eng.* 2001, H, 215−259.

[97] Swann, DA; Silver, FH; Slayter, HS; et al. The molecular structure and lubricating ability of lubricin isolated from bovine and human synovial fluids. *Biochem. J.* 1985, Vol 225, 195−201.

[98] Schumacher, BL, Block, JA; Schmid, TM; et al. A novel proteoglican synthesized and secreted by chondrocytes of the superficial zone of articular cartilage. *Arch. Biochem. Biophys.* 1994, Vol 311, 144−152.

[99] Flannery, CR; Hughes, CR; Schumacher, BC; et al. Articular cartilage superficial zone protein (SZP) is gomologous to megakaryocyte stimulating factor precursor and a multifunctional proteoglycan with potential glowth − promoting, cytoprotective and lubricating properties in cartilage metabolism. *Biochem. Biophys. Res. Comun.* 1999, Vol 234, 535−541.

[100] Jay, GD; Khaled, EA; Zack, J; et al. Lack of chondroprotection occurs amond emergency department patients with knee joint synovitis. *J. of Rheum.* 2004, Vol 31, 557−564.

[101] Tadmor, R; Chen, N; Israelishvili, J. Normal and chear forces between mica and model membrane surfaces with absorbed hyaluronan. *Macromolecules.* 2003, Vol 36, 9516–9526.

[102] Cherniakova, YuM. *Optimization of diagnostics and treatment of synovitis by controlling the biophysical properties of the synovial fluid.* Cand Sci Med Dissertation, Minsk, 2006.

[103] Patent 9146 BY. *Artificial Synovial Fluid.* Cherniakova, YuM; Pinchuk, LS; Beloenko, ED; et al. IPC A 61K 35/16, 47/36. 2007.

[104] Patent 10230 BY. *Methods for treatment of osteoarthritis deformans.* Pinchuk, LS; Chernyakova, YuM; Kadolich, ZhV; et al. IPC A 61K 35/16. 2008.

[105] Beloenko, ED; Cherniakova, YuM; Pinchuk, LS. Tribological substantiation of chondroprotection with autologous blood serum and hyaluronates, *Dokl. NAN of Belarus.* 2007, Vol 51, N 2, 72–75.

[106] Kovalenko, VN; Shuba, NM. *Reumatic diseases: nomenclature, classification, standards of diagnostic and treatment.* Kiev: OOO Katran Group, 2002.

[107] Nikolaev, VI; Chernyakova, YuM; Pinchuk, LS; Linkevich, ER; Beloenko, ED. Local therapy of gonarthrosis with patient's autologous blood serum. *Vesti NAN of Belarus Medical Ser.* 2006, N 4, 50–53.

[108] Insall, JN, Ravanat, CS; Aglietti, P; et al. A comparison of four models of total knee-replacement prostheses. *J. Bone Joint Surg.* 1976, Vol 58A, 754–765.

[109] Insall, JN; Dorr, LD; Scott, RD; et al., Rationale of the knee society clinical rating system . *Clin. Orthop.* 1989, Vol 248, 13–14.

[110] Filatov, AN; Bomolova, LG; Andrianova, LG. *Dry blood plasma.* Leningrad: Medicine, 1964.

[111] Instruction N 058-0609 on application *Method of intra-articular chodrorpotection of joints with autologous blood serum modified with doxycycline.* Appr By Ministry of Health, BY. Minsk, 2010.

[112] Bellami, N; Campbell, J; Robinson, V; et al. Viscosupplementation for the treatment of osteoarthritis of the knee. *Cochrane Database Syst. Rev.* 2006, N 2, CD005321.

[113] *Instruction on medical use of doxycycline hydrochloride capsules 0.1 g.* Appr by Ministry of Health BY, Reg N 05/07/122. 2005.

[114] *Instruction on medical application of Arbidol®.* Appr by the Directive of Federal Service, RF on control in health care, 2008.

[115] *Instruction on medical application of Cycloferon.* Reg N PN 0010149/03, Reg Date Dec 23, 2005.

[116] *Instruction on the application of Polcortolon.* Reg N P 013540/01-2001, Reg date Dec 07, 2001.

[117] *Instruction on medical application of Diclofenac-sodium.* Reg N 05/01/36. Appr by Ministry of Health, BY Nov 27, 2003.

[118] Cherniakova, Yu. *Chondroprotection by means of tribological adaptation of joint pharmacotherapy.* In: Book of Abstr of SICOT/SIROT XXIVth TWC, 2008, 1481.

Conclusions

In 2000, Director-General of the World Health Organization G. Brundtland announced the Bone and Joint Decade 2000–2010. This decennial campaign aimed to solve arthrological problems of top priority:

- weaken the burden that musculoskeletal diseases exert on the society worldwide;
- empower people to participate in their own care;
- promote cost-effective prevention and treatment;
- focus the orthopedists' interest on the mechanisms of development of joint disorders and new technologies of treatment of musculoskeletal conditions.

Koffi Annan, Secretary-General of UN, said in 2001: "Musculoskeletal diseases have become the most often cause of the suffering and lost capacity for work of millions of people. UN, WHO, nation-wide and international associations of medical professionals and patients should jointly promote the ideas of the Bone and Joint Decade" thus accentuating a global nature of the problem. Tremendous progress achieved during recent years in many orthopedic fields allows us to critically evaluate the opinion expressed by Russian physician A. S. Zalmanov in the 1920s: "There is no sadder story than the science about arthritis and rheumatic diseases. This is a story about total helplessness of the medical science and total blindness of human intellect". Advances in arthrology achieved in the 21st century were possible in part owing to research into synovial fluid as a multifunctional immune-competent environment. The advances can be summarized as follows.

A. Research in orthopedics has been developed at the interface of medical science and physics and chemistry. As a result, the researchers have disclosed a liquid-crystal state of the SF lubricating film, synovia quasi-electret effect, and susceptibility to the electromagnetic field shown in changes in synovia physicochemical structures and biophysical properties.

B. Methods and tools of up-to-date tribological studies of synovial joints allow experiments to be carried out at nano-sized scales. Weak electromagnetic fields that simulate the biophysical field of joint are helpful to study the lubricity of synovia boundary layers. A new trend has emerged in orthopedics that is associated with tribological monitoring of drugs intended for intra-articular injections. By making use of atomic force microscopy, *in vitro* studies of the structure of lubricating layers in a joint enable specialists to establish mechanisms of cartilage boundary lubrication and super lubrication with involvement of phospholipids and glycoproteids.

C. An approach to the investigation of the etiology of acute rheumatic conditions as systemic diseases of connective tissue and SF has been developed. Evidence of persistence of infectious agents (DNA of chlamydiae and spirochetes) that invade into SF and joint tissues has been obtained. Specialists are making efforts to determine the contribution of the etiology of retroviral and other latent infections in the development of rheumatoid diseases, systemic lupus erythematosus and some other systemic diseases of connective tissue.

D. A predisposing role of genetic types of human organism (histocompatibility antigens and their subtypes) in the onset of rheumatic diseases – rheumatoid arthritis, Bekhterev's disease, psoriatic arthritis, and postenterocolitic arthritis – has been established. Views have been developed about rheumatoid arthritis as a genetically predisposed disease that is governed by a set of polygenic systems and their interaction with the factors of synovial medium. A dependence of rheumatic diseases on the antigenic structure of SF and joint tissues has been set. One of the mechanisms of development of systemic diseases of synovial joints proved to occur with participation of molecular mimicry defined as a similarity between the structure of antigenic determinants (so-called epitopes) of an infectious agent and that of the synovial membrane and synovia.

E. Capabilities of diagnostics of systemic diseases of joint tissues have been enhanced thanks to identification of antibodies that react with autologous antigens of the cells of synovial medium including cell nucleus, cytoplasm, and other structural elements. Now we can follow up the activity of systemic lupus erythematosus and predict its current by the number of antibodies to DNA in SF and blood serum. A significant interest is focused on the study of antiphospholipid syndrome. It can be diagnosed through detection of autologous antibodies to phospholipids in blood serum and synovial effusions.

F. Up-to-date strategy of treatment of arthritis involves an active therapy immediately after the diagnosis has been set. It includes a concurrent therapy of joints with application of slowly acting drugs, new NSAIDs (selective COX-2 inhibitors) and SF substitutes, primarily, based on blood serum. A methodology of modification of donor's blood serum with active components (antigens, antibodies, cytokines, etc.) intended to obtain an individual drug for each particular case is now progressing.

G. Advances in fundamental sciences such as molecular biology, virology, genetics, immunology, and pharmacology could be of great help in making progress in the treatment of musculoskeletal disorders. Decoding of the etiology of basic rheumatic diseases can contribute to the development of beneficial technologies based on genetic-level intervention into metabolic processes. Modern computerized development and controllable synthesis of pharmacological preparations for joint treatment are intended to create super-drugs or new-generation drugs that are extremely effective and induce minimum adverse reactions.

The conception of synovial joint as an intelligent friction assembly implies that biophysical mechanisms of joint operation comprise a stage of interaction of joint tissues and synovial fluid. The latter is perfectly biocompatible with the surrounding tissues, performs vital functions, and carries immunological information. Synovial fluid being the main element of the intelligent friction assembly is the most readily accessible and extremely valuable, especially at early stages of diseases, as the source of information necessary to diagnose a joint state. Complex controllable application of drugs of different pharmacological groups as well as substantiated schemes and techniques of their introduction into synovial medium, concurrently with healing physical factors, ensure chondroprotection and improved joint functioning.

INDEX

A

B

C

D

G

H

I

J

K

L

M

N

O

P

Q

R

S

T

U

V

W

X

Y

Z